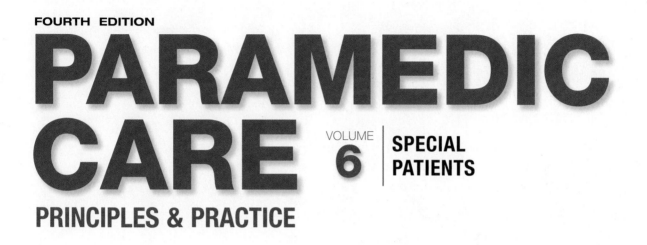

FOURTH EDITION

PARAMEDIC CARE

PRINCIPLES & PRACTICE

VOLUME **6** | **SPECIAL PATIENTS**

FOURTH EDITION

PARAMEDIC CARE

CARE

VOLUME **6** | **SPECIAL PATIENTS**

PRINCIPLES & PRACTICE

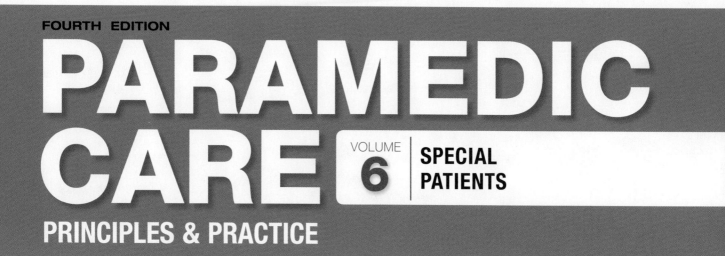

BRYAN E. BLEDSOE, DO, FACEP, FAAEM, EMT-P

Professor of Emergency Medicine
Director, Prehospital and Disaster Medicine Fellowship
University of Nevada School of Medicine
Attending Emergency Physician
University Medical Center of Southern Nevada
Medical Director, MedicWest Ambulance
Las Vegas, Nevada

ROBERT S. PORTER, MA, EMT-P

Senior Advanced Life Support Educator
Madison County Emergency Medical Services
Canastota, New York

RICHARD A. CHERRY, MS, EMT-P

Director of Training
Northern Onondaga Volunteer Ambulance
Liverpool, New York

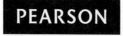

PEARSON

Boston   Columbus   Indianapolis   New York   San Francisco   Upper Saddle River
Amsterdam   Cape Town   Dubai   London   Madrid   Milan   Munich   Paris   Montreal   Toronto
Delhi   Mexico City   São Paulo   Sydney   Hong Kong   Seoul   Singapore   Taipei   Tokyo

Library of Congress Cataloging-in-Publication Data

Bledsoe, Bryan E., (Date)
  Paramedic care: principles & practice / Bryan E. Bledsoe,
    Robert S. Porter, Richard A. Cherry. — 4th ed. p. ; cm.
  Includes bibliographical references and index.
  ISBN-13: 978-0-13-211231-4 (v. 6 : alk. paper)
  ISBN-10: 0-13-211231-0 (v. 6 : alk. paper)
  I. Porter, Robert S., (Date) II. Cherry, Richard A. III. Title.
  [DNLM: 1. Emergencies. 2. Emergency Medical Services.
    3. Emergency Medical Technicians. 4. Emergency Treatment. WB 105]
  616.02'5—dc23
                                        2011034904

Publisher: Julie Levin Alexander
Publisher's Assistant: Regina Bruno
Editor-in-Chief: Marlene McHugh Pratt
Senior Managing Editor for Development: Lois Berlowitz
Editorial Project Manager: Deborah Wenger
Assistant Editor: Jonathan Cheung
Director of Marketing: David Gesell
Marketing Manager: Brian Hoehl
Marketing Specialist: Michael Sirinides
Managing Editor for Production: Patrick Walsh
Production Liaison: Faye Gemmellaro
Production Editor: Mary Tindle, S4Carlisle Publishing Services
Manufacturing Manager: Ilene Sanford

Creative Director: Blair Brown
Cover and Interior Design: Kathryn Foot
Interior Photographers: Nathan Eldridge, Michael Gallitelli, Michal Heron, Ray Kemp/Triple Zilch Productions, Carl Leet, Kevin Link, Richard Logan, Scott Metcalfe
Cover Image: © corepics/Shutterstock
Managing Photography Editor: Michal Heron
Editorial Media Manager: Amy Peltier
Media Project Manager: Lorena Cerisano
Composition: S4Carlisle Publishing Services
Printer/Binder: Courier/Kendallville
Cover Printer: Lehigh-Phoenix Color/Hagerstown

Notice

The author and the publisher of this book have taken care to make certain that the information given is correct and compatible with the standards generally accepted at the time of publication. Nevertheless, as new information becomes available, changes in treatment and in the use of equipment and procedures become necessary. The reader is advised to carefully consult the instruction and information material included in each piece of equipment or device before administration. Students are warned that the use of any techniques must be authorized by their medical advisor, where appropriate, in accordance with local laws and regulations. The publisher disclaims any liability, loss, injury, or damage incurred as a consequence, directly or indirectly, of the use and application of any of the contents of this book.

Brady
is an imprint of

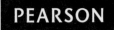

www.bradybooks.com

10 9 8 7 6 5 4 3 2 1
ISBN 10:   0-13-211231-0
ISBN 13: 978-0-13-211231-4

DEDICATION

This text is respectfully dedicated to all EMS personnel who have made the ultimate sacrifice. Their memory and good deeds will forever be in our thoughts and prayers.

BEB, RSP, RAC

DETAILED CONTENTS

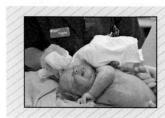

CHAPTER 5 ● Geriatrics 137

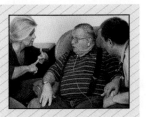

CHAPTER 6 ● Abuse, Neglect, and Assault 182

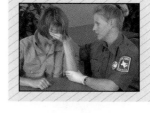

CHAPTER 7 ● The Challenged Patient 195

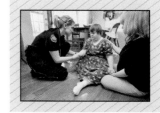

CHAPTER 8 ● Acute Interventions for the Chronic Care Patient 211

Today's paramedics are professional health care clinicians and practitioners of emergency field medicine. The present paramedic curriculum provides both a broad-based medical education and a specific intensive training program designed to prepare paramedics to perform their traditional role as providers of emergency field medicine. The curriculum also provides a broad foundation in anatomy and physiology, patient assessment, pathophysiology of disease, and pharmacology that allows paramedics to expand their roles in the health care industry. The seven-volume *Paramedic Care: Principles & Practice* and, in particular, *Volume 6, Special Patients,* reflect these broad and specific purposes.

This volume provides paramedic students with information they need about special populations. The first five chapters discuss medical emergencies involving special patient populations: gynecology, obstetrics, neonatology, pediatrics, and geriatrics. The sixth chapter looks at abuse, neglect, and assault of all patient populations. The final two chapters discuss patients with special challenges and issues dealing with chronic care.

OVERVIEW OF THE CHAPTERS

CHAPTER 1   Gynecology is devoted to the recognition and treatment of emergencies arising from the female reproductive system. The chapter provides an overview of female reproductive anatomy and physiology. This is followed by a discussion of common gynecologic emergencies.

CHAPTER 2   Obstetrics pertains to both normal delivery of a baby in the prehospital setting and various abnormal conditions and emergencies that may occur in association with childbearing. Following a review of the anatomic and physiologic changes that occur with pregnancy, the chapter addresses emergencies that may arise before, during, or after childbirth.

CHAPTER 3   Neonatology introduces the paramedic student to the specialized world of neonates. The neonate is a child less than one month of age. These patients have very different problems, and their treatment must be modified to accommodate their size, anatomy, and physiology. This chapter presents a detailed discussion of neonatology with a special emphasis on neonatal resuscitation in the field setting.

CHAPTER 4   Pediatrics presents a detailed discussion of pediatric emergencies. Children are not "small adults." They have special needs and must be approached and treated differently from adults. This chapter provides an overview of the common and uncommon pediatric emergencies encountered in prehospital care, with special emphasis on recognition and treatment. Specialized pediatric assessment techniques and emergency procedures are presented in detail.

CHAPTER 5   Geriatrics is a detailed presentation of emergencies involving elderly patients. The elderly are the fastest-growing group in our society. A significant number of EMS calls involve elderly patients. This chapter reviews the anatomy and physiology of aging. It then presents a detailed discussion of the assessment and treatment of emergencies commonly seen in the elderly.

CHAPTER 6   Abuse, Neglect, and Assault presents a timely discussion of the needs of victims of abuse, neglect, or assault. This chapter provides important information that will aid the paramedic in detecting abusive or otherwise dangerous situations. EMS personnel are often the first, and occasionally the only, health care personnel to encounter the victim of abuse, neglect, or assault. Therefore, it is essential that abusive situations be recognized early and the appropriate personnel and authorities notified.

CHAPTER 7   The Challenged Patient addresses patients with special physical, mental, or cultural needs. Paramedics must be familiar with techniques for successful assessment and treatment of these patients. Because a medical emergency can be an extremely frightening event for the challenged patient, the paramedic must be skilled in strategies that reduce stress for these special patients.

CHAPTER 8 Acute Interventions for the Chronic Care Patient offers an important discussion of the role of EMS personnel in treating home care patients and patients with chronic medical conditions. With declining hospital revenues, more and more patients are being cared for at home—either by family members or by home care personnel. Paramedics are often summoned when a home care patient deteriorates or otherwise suffers a medical or trauma emergency. It is essential that prehospital personnel have a fundamental understanding of home health care as well as a basic knowledge of the medical devices and technology routinely used in home care. This chapter details the paramedic's role in assessing, treating, and managing home care patients.

ACKNOWLEDGMENTS

INSTRUCTOR REVIEWERS

The reviewers of *Paramedic Care: Principles & Practice, Fourth Edition, Volume 6* have provided many excellent suggestions and ideas for improving the text. The quality of the reviews has been outstanding, and the reviews have been a major aid in the preparation and revision of the manuscript. The assistance provided by these EMS experts is deeply appreciated.

G. Paul Cooper, MS, CCEMT-P
Emory University
Atlanta, GA

William A. Johnson, EMT-P
Adjunct Faculty EMT/Paramedic
Program
MassBay Community College
Framingham, MA

Jason Kodat, MD, EMT-P
Resident Physician
Allegheny General Hospital
Pittsburgh, PA

Lawrence "Boogie" Molina, BS, NREMT-P, CCEMTP, MPH
Flight Paramedic
East Bay Regional Park Police
Air Support Unit
Hayward, CA

Dennis Di Sarro, M.Ed/ITS
Program Director
Emergency Services Programs
Edison State College

Jason O. Wilson, AAS EMS
Paramedic
Spartanburg EMS
Spartanburg, SC

We also wish to express appreciation to the following EMS professionals who reviewed the corresponding third edition of Paramedic Care: Principles & Practice. *Their suggestions and perspectives helped to make this program a successful teaching tool.*

Mike Dymes, NREMT-P
EMS Program Director
Durham Technical Community College
Durham, NC

Joyce Foresman-Capuzzi, RN, BSN, CEN, CPN, CTRN, EMT-P
Temple Health System Transport Team
Philadelphia, PA

Darren P. Lacroix
Del Mar College
Emergency Medical Service Professions
Corpus Christi, TX

Greg Mullen, MS, NREMT-P
National EMS Academy
Lafayette, LA

Deborah L. Petty, BS, EMT-P I/C
Training Officer
St. Charles County Ambulance District
St. Peters, MO

B. Jeanine Riner, MHSA, BS, RRT, NREMT-P
GA Office of EMS and Trauma
Atlanta, GA

Mark A. Simpson, AS, BS, MSN, RN, NREMT-P
Program Director
Northwest-Shoals Community College
Muscle Shoals, AL

Allen Walls
Department of Fire & EMS
Colerain Township, OH

Brian J. Wilson, BA, NREMT-P
Education Director
Texas Tech School of Medicine
El Paso, TX

PHOTO ACKNOWLEDGMENTS

All photographs not credited adjacent to the photograph or in the photo credit section below were photographed on assignment for Brady/Prentice Hall/Pearson Education.

Organizations

We wish to thank the following organizations for their valuable assistance in creating the photo program:

Bound Tree University
Dublin, OH. www.boundtreeuniversity.com

Canandaigua Emergency Squad
Canandaigua, NY

Flower Mound Fire Department
Flower Mound, TX

Children's Hospital St. Louis/BJC Health Care
St. Louis, MO

Christian Hospital/BJC Health Care
St. Charles, MO

Tyco Health Care/Nellcor Puritan Bennet
Pleasanton, CA

Wolfe Tory Medical
Salt Lake City, UT

Winter Park Fire-Rescue
Winter Park, FL
Chief James E. White
Deputy Chief Patrick McCabe

City of Winter Park, FL
Kenneth W. Bradley, Mayor

Technical Advisors

Thanks to the following people for providing technical support during the photo shoots in Winter Park, Florida:

Andrew Isaacs, EMS Captain
Tod Meadors, EMS Captain
Dr. Tod Husty, Medical Director

Richard Rodriguez, EMS Captain
Jeff Spinelli, Engineer-Paramedic

Models

Thanks to the following people from the Flower Mound Fire Department, Flower Mound, Texas, and from Winter Park Fire-Rescue, Winter Park, Florida, who provided locations and/or portrayed patients and EMS providers in our photographs:

FAO/Paramedic Wade Woody
FF/Paramedic Tim Mackling
FF/Paramedic Matthew Daniel
FF/Paramedic Jon Rea
FF/Paramedic Waylon Palmer
FF/EMT Jesse Palmer
Captain/EMT Billy McWhorter
Linda Kirk, Director, Winter Park Towers,
    Winter Park, FL

Andrew Isaacs
Richard Rodriguez
Tod Meadors
Jeff Spinelli
Mark Vaughn
Victoria Devereaux
Teresa George

BRYAN E. BLEDSOE, DO, FACEP, FAAEM, EMT-P

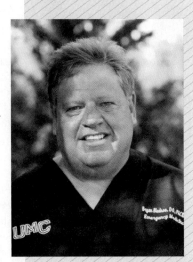

Dr. Bryan Bledsoe is an emergency physician, researcher, and EMS author. Presently he is Professor of Emergency Medicine and Director of the EMS Fellowship program at the University of Nevada School of Medicine and an Attending Emergency Physician at the University Medical Center of Southern Nevada in Las Vegas. He is board-certified in emergency medicine. Prior to attending medical school, Dr. Bledsoe worked as an EMT, a paramedic, and a paramedic instructor. He completed EMT training in 1974 and paramedic training in 1976 and worked for six years as a field paramedic in Fort Worth, Texas. In 1979, he joined the faculty of the University of North Texas Health Sciences Center and served as coordinator of EMT and paramedic education programs at the university.

Dr. Bledsoe is active in emergency medicine and EMS research. He is a popular speaker at state, national, and international seminars and writes regularly for numerous EMS journals. He is active in educational endeavors with the United States Special Operations Command (USSOCOM) and the University of Nevada at Las Vegas. Dr. Bledsoe is the author of numerous EMS textbooks and has in excess of 1 million books in print. Dr. Bledsoe was named a "Hero of Emergency Medicine" in 2008 by the American College of Emergency Physicians as a part of their 40th anniversary celebration and was named a "Hero of Health and Fitness" by *Men's Health* magazine as part of their 20th anniversary edition in November of 2008. He is frequently interviewed in the national media. Dr. Bledsoe is married and divides his time between his residences in Midlothian, TX, and Las Vegas, NV.

ROBERT S. PORTER, MA, EMT-P

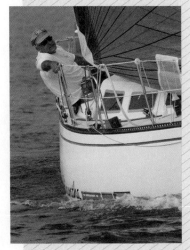

Robert Porter has been teaching in emergency medical services for 38 years and currently serves as the Senior Advanced Life Support Educator for Madison County (New York) Emergency Medical Services. Mr. Porter is a Wisconsin native and received his bachelor's degree in education from the University of Wisconsin. He completed his paramedic training at Northeast Wisconsin Technical Institute in 1978 and earned a master's degree in health education at Central Michigan University in 1990.

Mr. Porter has been an EMT and an EMS educator and administrator since 1973 and obtained his certification and national registration as an EMT-Paramedic in 1978. He has taught both basic and advanced EMS courses in the states of Wisconsin, Michigan, Louisiana, Pennsylvania, and New York. Mr. Porter conducted one of the nation's first rural paramedic programs and developed a university-based, two-year paramedic program. Mr. Porter served for more than ten years as a paramedic program accreditation-site evaluator for the American Medical Association and is a past chair of the National Association of EMTs—Society of EMT Instructor/Coordinators. Mr. Porter also served for 15 years as a flight paramedic with the Onondaga County Sheriff's Department air medical service, AirOne. He has authored Brady's *Paramedic Care: Principles & Practice, Essentials of Paramedic Care, Intermediate Emergency Care: Principles & Practice, Tactical Emergency Care,* and *Weapons of Mass Destruction: Emergency Care,* as well as the workbooks accompanying this text. When not writing or teaching, Mr. Porter enjoys offshore sailboat racing and home restoration.

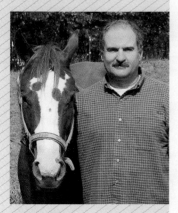

RICHARD A. CHERRY, MS, EMT-P

Richard Cherry is the Director of Training for Northern Onondaga Volunteer Ambulance (NOVA) in Liverpool, New York, a suburb of Syracuse. He recently retired from the Department of Emergency Medicine at Upstate Medical University where he held the positions of Director of Paramedic Training, Assistant Emergency Medicine Residency Director, Clinical Assistant Professor of Emergency Medicine, and Technical Director for Medical Simulation. His experience includes years of classroom teaching and emergency fieldwork. A native of Buffalo, Mr. Cherry earned his bachelor's degree at nearby St. Bonaventure University in 1972. He taught high school for the next ten years while he earned his master's degree in education from Oswego State University in 1977. He holds a permanent teaching license in New York State.

Mr. Cherry entered the emergency medical services field in 1974 with the DeWitt Volunteer Fire Department, where he served his community as a firefighter and EMS provider for more than 15 years. He took his first EMT course in 1977 and became an ALS provider two years later. He earned his paramedic certificate in 1985 as a member of the area's first paramedic class.

Mr. Cherry has authored several books for Brady. Most notable are *Paramedic Care: Principles & Practice, Essentials of Paramedic Care, Intermediate Emergency Care: Principles & Practice,* and *EMT Teaching: A Common Sense Approach.* He has made presentations at many state, national, and international EMS conferences on a variety of teaching topics. He and his wife, Sue, run a summer horse-riding camp for children with special needs on their property in West Monroe, New York. He also plays guitar in a Christian band.

Welcome to

PARAMEDIC CARE PRINCIPLES & PRACTICE

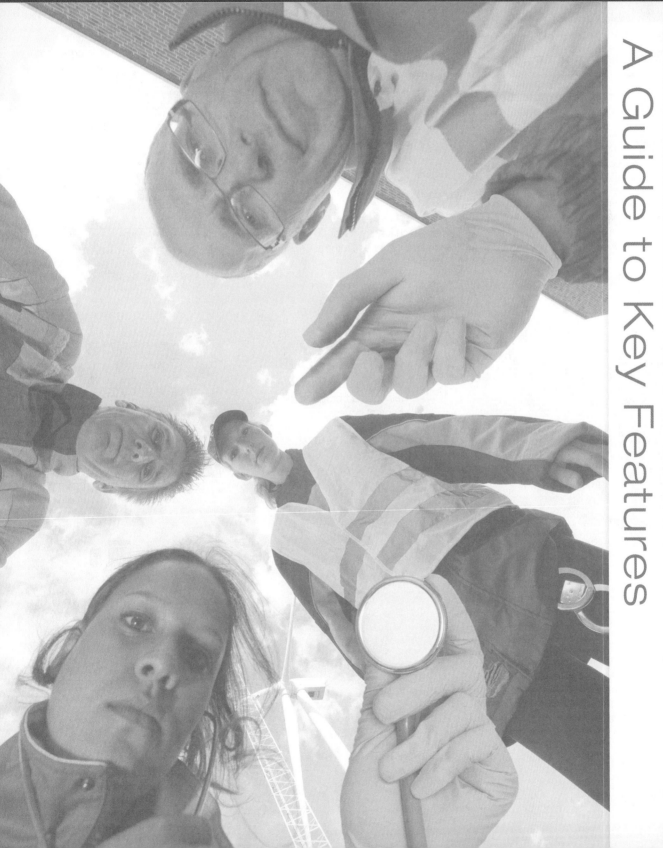

A Guide to Key Features

Emphasizing Principles

CHAPTER OBJECTIVES

Terminal Performance Objectives and a separate set of Enabling Objectives are provided for each chapter.

KEY TERMS

Page numbers identify where each key term first appears, boldfaced, in the chapter.

TABLES

A wealth of tables offers the opportunity to highlight, summarize, and compare information.

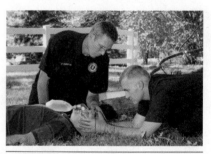

TABLE 4-2	Common Infectious Diseases		
Disease	**Mode of Transmission**	**Incubation Period**
AIDS (acquired immune deficiency syndrome)	AIDS- or HIV-infected blood via intravenous drug use, semen and vaginal fluids, blood transfusions, or (rarely) needlesticks. Mothers also may pass HIV to their unborn children.	Several months or years
Hepatitis B, C	Blood, stool, or other body fluids, or contaminated objects.	Weeks or months
Tuberculosis	Respiratory secretions, airborne or on contaminated objects.	2 to 6 weeks
Meningitis, bacterial	Oral and nasal secretions.	2 to 10 days
Pneumonia, bacterial and viral	Oral and nasal droplets and secretions.	Several days
Influenza	Airborne droplets, or direct contact with body fluids.	1 to 3 days
Staphylococcal skin infections	Contact with open wounds or sores or contaminated objects.	Several days
Chicken pox (varicella)	Airborne droplets, or contact with open sores.	11 to 21 days
German measles (rubella)	Airborne droplets. Mothers may pass it to unborn children.	10 to 12 days
Whooping cough (pertussis)	Respiratory secretions or airborne droplets.	6 to 20 days
SARS (severe acute respiratory syndrome)	Airborne droplets and personal contact.	4 to 6 days

PHOTOS AND ILLUSTRATIONS

Carefully selected photos and a unique art program reinforce content coverage and add to text explanations.

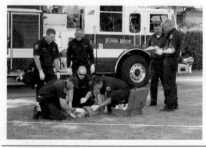

● **Figure 3-3** During the primary assessment of your patient, you will look for and immediately treat any life-threatening conditions.

● **Figure 3-7** As leader of the EMS team, the paramedic must interact with patients, bystanders, and other rescue personnel in a professional and efficient manner.

CONTENT REVIEW

Screened content review boxes set off from the text are interspersed throughout the chapter. They summarize key points and serve as a helpful study guide—in an easy format for quick review.

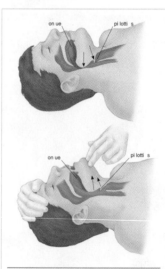

CONTENT REVIEW

► Steps of Primary Assessment

- Form a general impression
- Stabilize cervical spine as needed
- Assess baseline mental status
- Assess and manage airway
- Assess and manage breathing
- Assess and manage circulation
- Determine priorities

● **Figure 2-4** The head-tilt/chin-lift maneuver in an adult.

SUMMARY

This end-of-chapter feature provides a concise review of chapter information.

SUMMARY

The scene size-up is the initial step in the patient care process. Sizing up the scene and situation begins at your initial dispatch and does not end until you are clear of the call. As the call unfolds, you should be making constant observations and adjustments to your plan of action. Remember that your safety and the safety of your partner are paramount—it is hard to effectively treat both yourself and others.

Scene size-up should be practiced so much that it becomes second nature to you. It is like noticing veins on people in public after you begin starting IVs. (You have all done it—looked across the room at the back of someone's hand and noticed what nice veins they had.) Sizing up a scene is no different. After a while you begin to notice mechanisms of injury and other important details almost subconsciously. But be careful and do not get complacent! Always make it a point to pause for just a few seconds and consciously look around the scene before proceeding into any situation.

Scene size-up is not a step-by-step process, but a series of decisions you make when confronted with a variety of circumstances that are often beyond your control. It is a way to make order out of chaos, keep yourself and your crew safe, and ensure that all necessary resources are focused on patient care and outcomes. With time and experience, you will learn to perform a scene size-up quickly and focus on important issues. Your careful size-up lays the foundation for an organized and timely approach toward patient care and scene management.

REVIEW QUESTIONS

1. Which of the following is *not* a component of the scene size-up?
   a. Standard Precautions
   b. mechanism of injury
   c. primary assessment
   d. location of all patients

2. The HEPA mask is designed to protect you from _____.
   a. tuberculosis
   b. AIDS
   c. hepatitis
   d. meningitis

3. The top priority in any emergency situation is _____.
   a. patient assessment
   b. bystander cooperation
   c. customer service
   d. your personal safety

4. As you approach a scene, something just does not seem right. It is not anything you can put your finger on, just a sense that something is wrong or is about to happen. What should you do about it?
   a. Wait until law enforcement arrives before entering.
   b. Ignore your feelings and enter the scene.
   c. Enter the scene with something with which to protect yourself.
   d. Call out for the patient to come outside.

5. You are responding to a shooting at a well-known bar. How should you approach the scene?
   a. Stage outside the bar until the police arrive.
   b. Wait for another ambulance or rescue crew before entering.
   c. Just enter the scene.
   d. Stage your ambulance a few blocks away until law enforcement arrives.

6. You arrive on the scene and see that a power line lies close to your pediatric patient. You are fairly sure the line is live and decide to move it with a dry piece of equipment. Which of the following should you use?
   a. a wooden-handled ax
   b. a fallen tree branch
   c. a nylon rope
   d. none of the above

7. When you and your partner arrive at a multiple-patient incident, you should _____.
   a. begin assessing and treating the first patient you encounter
   b. establish command and begin triage
   c. provide intensive emergency care to the most critical patient
   d. start at opposite ends and begin assessing patients

REVIEW QUESTIONS

These questions ask students to review and recall key information they have just learned.

REFERENCES

This listing is a compilation of source material providing the basis of updated data and research used in the preparation of each chapter.

REFERENCES

1. U.S. Department of Transportation/National Highway Traffic Safety Administration. *National EMS Scope of Practice Model.* Washington, DC, 2006.
2. National Registry of Emergency Medical Technicians. 2004 National EMS Practice Analysis. Columbus, OH: National Registry of EMTs, 2005.
3. American College of Surgeons. *Verified Trauma Centers.* [Available at: http://www.facs.org/trauma/verified.html]
4. Feldman, M. J., J. L. Lukins, P. R. Verbeek, et al. "Use of Treat-and-Release Directives for Paramedics at a Mass Gathering." *Prehosp Emerg Care* 9 (2005): 213–217.
5. American College of Emergency Physicians. "Interfacility Transportation of the Critical Care Patient and Its Medical Direction." *Ann Emerg Med* 47 (2006): 305.
6. Harkins, S. "Documentation: Why Is It So Important?" *Emerg Med Serv* 31 (2002): 93–94.
7. Lerner, E. B., A. R. Fernandez, and M. N. Shah. "Do Emergency Medical Services Professionals Think They Should Participate in Disease Prevention?" *Prehosp Emerg Care* 13 (2009): 64–70.
8. Polifico, F. "The Role of EMS in Public Access Defibrillation." *Emerg Med Serv* 32 (2003): 73.
9. Streger M. R. "Professionalism." *Emerg Med Serv* 32 (2003): 35.
10. Klugman, C. M. "Why EMS Needs Its Own Ethics. What's Good for Other Areas of Healthcare May Not Be Good for You." *Emerg Med Serv* 36 (2007): 114–122.
11. Touchstone, M. "Professional Development. Part 1: Becoming an EMS Leader." *Emerg Med Serv* 38 (2009): 59–60.
12. Bledsoe, B. E. "EMS Needs a Few More Cowboys." *JEMS* 28 (2003): 112–113.

FURTHER READING

This list features recommendations for books and journal articles that go beyond chapter coverage.

FURTHER READING

Bailey, E. D. and T. Sweeney. "Considerations in Establishing Emergency Medical Services Response Time Goals." *Prehosp Emerg Care* 7 (2003): 397–399.

Bledsoe, B. E. "Searching for the Evidence behind EMS." *Emerg Med Serv* 31 (2003): 63–67.

Heightman, A. J. "EMS Workforce. A Comprehensive Listing of Certified EMS Providers by State and How the Workforce Has Changed Since 1993." *JEMS* 5 (2000): 108–112.

Jaslow, D. J., J. Ufberg, and R. Marsh. "Primary Injury Prevention in an Urban EMS System." *J Emerg Med* 25 (2003): 167–170.

National Academy of Sciences, National Research Council. *Accidental Death and Disability: The Neglected Disease of Modern Society.* Washington, DC:

U.S. Department of Health, Education, and Welfare, 1966.

Page, J. O. *The Magic of 3 AM.* San Diego, CA: JEMS Publishing, 2002.

Page, J. O. *The Paramedics.* Morristown, NJ: Backdraft Publications, 1979. [No longer available for purchase except as a used book. Entire book can be viewed online at www.JEMS.com/Paramedics.]

Page, J. O. *Simple Advice.* San Diego, CA: JEMS Publishing, 2002.

Persse, D. E., C. B. Key, R. N. Bradley, et al. "Cardiac Arrest Survival as a Function of Ambulance Deployment Strategy in a Large Urban Emergency Medical Services System." *Resusc* 59 (2003): 97–104.

CASE STUDY

This feature at the start of each chapter draws students into the reading and creates a link between text content and real-life situations.

YOU MAKE THE CALL

A scenario at the end of each chapter promotes critical thinking by requiring students to apply principles to actual practice.

PROCEDURE SCANS

Visual skill summaries provide step-by-step support in skill instruction.

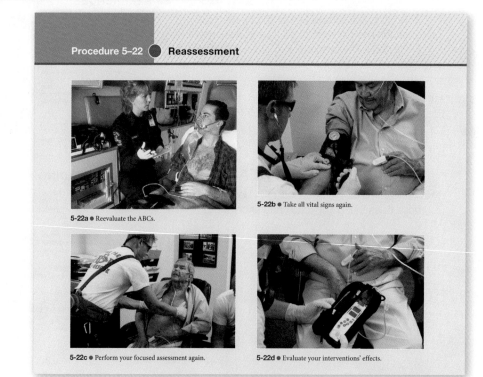

Procedure 5–22 ● Reassessment

5-22a ● Reevaluate the ABCs.

5-22b ● Take all vital signs again.

5-22c ● Perform your focused assessment again.

5-22d ● Evaluate your interventions' effects.

Special Features

PATHO PEARLS

Offer a snapshot of pathological considerations students will encounter in the field.

PATHO PEARLS

Patient assessment actually starts as soon as you approach the scene. Clues about the patient's underlying pathophysiology might be evident from such things as positioning of the vehicle, downed power lines, or the appearance and actions of bystanders. However, your safety, and that of your fellow rescuers, is always paramount. Never approach a scene that appears unsafe. With time, you will develop a "sixth sense" about emergency scenes and bystanders.

As you begin the patient encounter, process all that you see into your patient assessment and care. For example, consider this scenario: A car with two 16-year-old girls fails to negotiate a turn on a country road and overturns into a flowing creek adjacent to the road. Although the ambient temperature is in the 60s, you know that the temperature of the water in this area often is in the 40s. Thus, you should immediately suspect the possibility of hypothermia.

As the girls are removed from entrapment, no obvious injuries are noted. Vital signs are normal other than slight tachycardia. However, peripheral pulses are weak and the skin is pale and cool. Is it shock? Is it hypothermia? Is it both? Your index of suspicion is high for both hypothermia and blunt force trauma. You follow local protocols with regard to immobilization, fluid therapy, and monitoring. Once in the ambulance and wrapped in blankets, both girls start to show signs that blood flow to the skin is improving. By the time you reach the hospital, their skin has a normal color and their pulse rates are normal.

Following a comprehensive assessment in the emergency department, the girls are discharged to their parents with no apparent injuries. Thus, your instincts were right. The potential for shock was a greater risk to the girls than the potential for hypothermia, and you had to treat based on this risk. But hypothermia turned out to be the principal problem. Integrating information from the scene size-up, patient history, and patient examination gave you a clear picture of the patients' underlying pathophysiologic process.

CULTURAL CONSIDERATIONS

Provide an awareness of beliefs that might affect patient care.

CULTURAL CONSIDERATIONS

Eye contact is a major form of nonverbal communication. Short eye contact is often seen as friendly, whereas prolonged eye contact may be interpreted as threatening. Thus, timing is an important factor in how a person interprets eye contact.

One's culture also influences how eye contact is interpreted. Eye contact can mean respect in one culture and disrespect in another. Often, Asians will avoid eye contact even when they have nothing to hide. Eye contact between people of different sexes is problematic in Muslim cultures, in which a prolonged look in the face of a member of the opposite sex might be misinterpreted. Because of this, people in Middle Eastern countries might look a person of the same sex in the eye and not look into the eyes of a person of the opposite sex.

If you work in a culturally diverse community, you should learn the customs of eye contact and other forms of nonverbal communication of those you might encounter during the course of your work.

LEGAL NOTES

Present instances in which legal or ethical considerations should be evaluated.

LEGAL CONSIDERATIONS

Gatekeeper to the Health Care System. *The EMS system is often the initial point of contact for a person entering the health care system. Thus, to a certain extent, a paramedic frequently functions as a sort of gatekeeper to the health care system as a whole.*

Part of a paramedic's responsibility is to ensure that a patient is taken to a facility that can appropriately care for the patient's condition. Today, hospitals have become more specialized. That is, some hospitals have chosen to provide certain services and not provide others. For example, one hospital may elect to specialize in cardiac care, another in stroke care, another in burn care, and so on. This is especially true in communities with multiple hospitals. Because of this, it is essential that paramedics understand the capabilities of the hospitals in the system where they work. Also, with overcrowding in modern emergency departments, diversion of ambulances by hospitals whose emergency departments are full has become commonplace.

For all these reasons, local EMS system protocols must be available to guide prehospital personnel in ensuring that each patient is delivered to a facility that can adequately care for the patient's condition.

ASSESSMENT PEARLS

Offer tips, guidance, and information to aid in patient assessment.

ASSESSMENT PEARLS

Chest pain is a common reason that people summon EMS. However, the causes of chest pain are numerous. In emergency medicine or EMS, we often look to exclude the most serious causes before determining whether chest pain is of a benign origin. Internal organs do not have as many pain fibers as do such structures as the skin and other areas. Pain arising from an internal organ tends to be dull and vague. This is because nerves from various spinal levels innervate the organ in question. The heart, for example, is innervated by several thoracic spinal nerve segments. Thus, cardiac pain tends to be dull and is sometimes described as pressure. It also tends to cause referred pain (i.e., pain in an area somewhat distant to the organ), such as pain in the left arm and jaw. Dull pain that is hard to localize (or to reproduce with palpation) may be due to cardiac disease. One sign often seen with patients suffering cardiac disease is Levine's sign. With Levine's sign, the patient will subconsciously cle... pain. Levine's sign is a... (e.g., angina or acute c...

ASSESSMENT PEARLS

Assessing skin abnormalities in dark-skinned people can be a challenge. Try the following techniques:

Jaundice Look for a yellow color in the sclera and hard palate.

Erythema Look for an ashen color in the sclera, conjunctiva, mouth, tongue, lips, nail beds, palms, and soles.

Pallor Feel for warmth in the affected area.

Petechiae Look for tiny purplish dots on the abdomen.

Cyanosis Look for a dull, dark coloring in the mouth, tongue, lips, nail beds, palms, and soles.

Rashes Feel for abnormal skin texture.

Edema Look for decreased color and feel for tightness.

Student Workbook

A student workbook with review and practice activities accompanies each volume of the Paramedic Care series. The workbooks include multiple-choice questions, other exercises, case studies, and special projects, along with an answer key with text page references.

REVIEW OF CHAPTER OBJECTIVES

Tied to chapter objectives, content summaries review important information and concepts.

CASE STUDY REVIEW

An in-depth analysis at the start of each chapter highlights essential information and applied principles.

CONTENT SELF-EVALUATION

Multiple-choice, matching, and short-answer questions test reading comprehension.

SPECIAL PROJECTS

Experiences have been designed to help students remember information and principles.

PATIENT SCENARIO FLASHCARDS

Flashcards present scenarios with signs and symptoms and information to make field diagnoses.

DRUG FLASHCARDS

A special set of flashcards represents drugs commonly used in paramedic care.

MyBRADYLab™

www.mybradylab.com

WHAT IS MyBRADYLab?

MyBRADYLab is a comprehensive online program that gives you the opportunity to test yourself on basic information, concepts, and skills to see how well you know paramedic course material. From the test results, the program builds a self-paced, personalized study plan unique to your needs. Remediation in the form of e-text pages, illustrations, animations, exercises, and video clips is provided for those areas in which you may need additional instruction or reinforcement. You can then work through the program until material is learned and mastered. **MyBRADYLab** is available as a standalone program or with an embedded e-text.

  MyBRADYLab maps objectives created from the National EMS Education Standards for the Paramedic level to each learning module. With **MyBRADYLab**, you can track your own progress through the entire course. The personalized study plan material supports you as you work to achieve success in the classroom and on certification exams.

HOW DO STUDENTS BENEFIT?

MyBRADYLab helps you:

- Keep up with the new, complex information presented in the text and lectures.
- Save time by focusing study and review on just the content you need.
- Increase understanding of difficult concepts with study material for different learning styles.
- Remediate in areas in which you need additional review.

KEY FEATURES OF MyBRADYLab

Pre-Tests and Post-Tests Using questions aligned to Paramedic Standards, quizzes measure your understanding of topics and expected learning outcomes.

Personalized Study Material Based on the topic pre-test results, you will receive a personalized study plan highlighting areas where you may need improvement. Study tools include:

- Skills and animation videos
- Links to specific pages in the e-text
- Images for review
- Interactive exercises
- Audio glossary
- Access to full chapters of the e-text

HOW DO INSTRUCTORS BENEFIT?

- Save time by providing students with a comprehensive, media-rich study program
- Track student understanding of course content in the program Gradebook
- Monitor student activity with viewable student assignments

What Resources Are Available to Instructors?

Visit **www.bradybooks.com** to log onto Brady's Resource Central website for the Paramedic Care series. Your Brady sales representative will assist with access codes. At Resource Central instructors will find a wealth of curriculum management material to support class presentations, student assessment, and administrative functions.

Where Do I Get More Information?

Contact your local Brady representative for more information.

1

Gynecology

Bryan Bledsoe, DO, FACEP, FAAEM, EMT-P

STANDARD
Medicine (Gynecology)

COMPETENCY
Integrates assessment findings with principles of epidemiology and pathophysiology to formulate a field impression and implement a comprehensive treatment/disposition plan for a patient with a medical complaint.

OBJECTIVES

Terminal Performance Objective
After reading this chapter, you should be able to integrate patient assessment findings, patient history, and knowledge of anatomy, physiology, pathophysiology, and basic and advanced life support interventions to recognize and manage patients with gynecologic emergencies.

Enabling Objectives
To accomplish the terminal performance objective, you should be able to:

1. Define key terms introduced in this chapter.

2. Relate the anatomy and physiology of the female reproductive system to the assessment and management of patients with gynecologic disorders.

3. Use a process of clinical reasoning to guide and interpret the patient assessment and management process for patients with specific gynecologic complaints.

4. Adapt the scene size-up, primary assessment, patient history, secondary assessment, and use of monitoring technology to meet the needs of patients with complaints and presentations related to gynecologic disorders.

5. Adapt the scene size-up, primary assessment, patient history, secondary assessment, and use of monitoring technology to meet the needs of patients with complaints and presentations related to sexual assault.

6. Demonstrate concern for the psychosocial needs of patients with gynecologic emergencies and sexual assault.

7. Relate the pathophysiology of specific gynecologic disorders, including pelvic inflammatory disease, ovarian cysts, cystitis, mittelschmerz, endometritis, endometriosis, ectopic pregnancy, nontraumatic vaginal bleeding, and genital trauma to the priorities of patient assessment and management.

8. Observe special considerations for evidence preservation when dealing with a patient who has been sexually assaulted.

9. Observe special considerations in documentation of calls involving sexual assault.

KEY TERMS

CASE STUDY

It is near dusk on a warm summer evening when you and your partner, Sam Rusk, are dispatched from quarters to a nearby community park for an "assault." Within 4 minutes, you pull up to the park access gate near the security office, where you meet a police officer and the park security supervisor. The police officer tells you that your 28-year-old female patient was found wandering in the park by a security officer just as the park was closing. He tells you that the Crime Scene Unit is en route. The supervisor reports that the officer who found her is sitting with her in the office.

You enter the security office as Sam gets the stretcher and jump kit from the back of the medic unit. The patient is seated on a cot facing away from the door. The security officer is sitting on a chair next to the cot, talking quietly to her. The patient has a white cotton blanket, provided by the officer, wrapped tightly over her shoulders and around her body. You observe that her hair is tangled and matted, with leaves and small twigs sticking from it. As you approach her, you identify yourself, and introduce Sam, as paramedics who are there to help her. She turns her tear-stained, battered face toward you and nods, saying "I know" so quietly that you can barely hear her. The park officer stands and tells you that your patient's name is Stephanie. He then excuses himself, telling her that she is in good hands and that he will be right outside.

You pull up the chair that had been used by the officer and position it in front of Stephanie to complete your primary assessment. Although your priority is the assessment of her ABCs, you cannot ignore her obvious injuries. She has dried blood on her nose and mouth and her left eye is bruised and nearly swollen shut. You tell her that you need to perform some simple procedures to make sure that she is okay, and you ask her permission to do so. Again she nods, her eyes never leaving your face. In a soft hoarse voice, she says quietly, "He raped me, even though I begged him not to."

Stephanie's airway is open and her breathing is regular in rate and depth. You ask her if you can check her pulse, and she unwraps the blanket just enough to let her right forearm extend toward you. You find that her pulse is strong but rapid and her skin is cool and dry. You notice an abrasion around her wrist that makes you wonder if she had been tied down. You also observe that she has several broken nails on the trembling hand she extends toward you. Again with her permission, you gently unwrap the blanket to reveal a torn, dirty T-shirt that is splattered with blood. She is wearing nothing else. Her inner thighs are covered with dried blood, as well as with dirt and leaves. You limit your rapid trauma assessment to merely a search for life-threatening injuries, as Stephanie will undergo a thorough exam by the sexual assault nurse examiner (SANE). Stephanie's blood pressure is 108/70 mmHg. Her pulse is strong and regular at 110 beats per minute. Her breathing is quiet and nonlabored at a rate of 24 breaths per minute, with a pulse oximeter reading of 99 percent on room air.

Explaining exactly what you're going to do and asking her permission to do so, you and Sam help her stand and then pivot her onto the stretcher, leaving her wrapped in the blanket in which you found her. You move her to the medic unit. As you get her settled, and before beginning the short drive to the hospital, Sam contacts medical direction and requests that the SANE meet you at the hospital.

En route, you complete Stephanie's history. She denies allergies and reports that the only medication she takes is a multivitamin tablet daily. Stephanie denies any significant past medical history. She ate a chef's salad for lunch about mid-afternoon. Stephanie says that she was grabbed from behind while she was jogging and that she was dragged off the path and into the woods. You reassure her that she is safe now and no one will hurt her. Within minutes, you arrive at the hospital.

Emma Cannise, RN, the SANE coordinator, meets you at the emergency entrance to the hospital. You introduce Stephanie to Emma, who then accompanies you to the evaluation unit located behind the main emergency department. You give her a brief report, and she signs off on your patient care report.

Returning to quarters, you and Sam discuss how ironic it was that this month's continuing medical education (CME) program was a presentation by Emma Cannise on caring for victims of sexual assault.

INTRODUCTION

The term **gynecology** is derived from the Greek *gynaik,* meaning "woman." Gynecology is the branch of medicine that deals with the health maintenance and the diseases of women and primarily of their reproductive organs. **Obstetrics** is the branch of medicine that deals with the care of women throughout pregnancy. Most of the gynecologic emergency patients that you will encounter will be experiencing either abdominal pain or vaginal bleeding. This chapter focuses on the assessment and care of nonpregnant patients with problems of the reproductive system. The assessment and care of the obstetric patient is the subject of the next chapter.

ANATOMY AND PHYSIOLOGY

It is essential that you have a thorough understanding of the anatomy and physiology of the female reproductive system. This knowledge will allow you to better understand, recognize, and treat gynecologic emergencies when they arise.

Female Reproductive Organs

The most important female reproductive organs are internal and are located within the pelvic cavity. These include the ovaries, fallopian tubes, uterus, and vagina, which are essential to reproduction. The external genitalia have accessory functions, in that they protect body openings and play an important role in sexual functioning.

External Genitalia

The female external genitalia are known collectively as the *vulva,* or *pudendum* (Figure 1-1 ●).

Perineum   The *perineum* is a roughly diamond-shaped, skin-covered muscular tissue that separates the vagina and the anus. These tissues form a slinglike structure supporting the internal pelvic organs and are able to stretch during childbirth. This

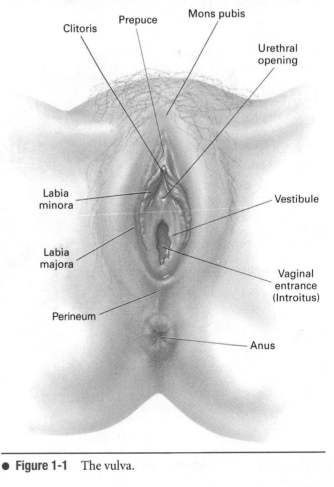

● **Figure 1-1**   The vulva.

area is sometimes torn as a result of sexual assault or during childbirth. An *episiotomy,* or incision of the perineum, may be done to facilitate delivery of the baby and to prevent spontaneous tearing, which may cause significant injury to the perineum and adjacent structures. Sometimes the term *perineum* is used to include the entire vulvar area.

Mons Pubis   The *mons pubis* is a fatty layer of tissue over the *pubic symphysis,* the junction of pubic bones. During puberty, the hormone *estrogen* causes fat to be deposited under the skin, giving it a moundlike shape. This serves as a cushion that protects the pubic symphysis during intercourse. Also during puberty, the mons becomes covered with pubic hair and its sebaceous and sweat glands become more active.

Labia   The *labia* are the structures that protect the vagina and the urethra. There are two distinct sets of labia. The *labia majora* are located laterally, whereas the *labia minora* are more medial. Both sets of labia are subject to injury during trauma to the vulvar area, such as that which occurs with sexual assault.

The *labia majora* are two folds of fatty tissue that arise from the mons pubis and extend to the perineum, forming a cleft. During puberty, pubic hair grows on the lateral surface, and sebaceous glands on the hairless medial surface begin to secrete lubricants. The labia majora serve to protect the inner structures of the vulva. The *labia minora,* lying medially within the labia majora, are two smaller, thinner folds of highly vascular tissue, well supplied with nerves and sebaceous glands, which secrete lubricating fluid. During sexual arousal the labia minora become engorged with blood.

The area protected by the labia minora is called the *vestibule.* The vestibule contains the urethral opening and the external opening of the vagina, called the vaginal orifice, or *introitus.* The secretions of two pairs of glands (Skene and Bartholin glands) lubricate these structures during sexual stimulation. Located within the vestibule is the *hymen,* a thin fold of mucous membrane that forms the external border of the vagina, partly closing it.

Clitoris   The *clitoris* is highly innervated and richly vascular erectile tissue that lies anterior to the labia minora. This cylindrical structure is a major site of sexual stimulation and orgasm in women. The *prepuce* is a fold of the labia minora that covers the clitoris.

Urethra   Although not truly a part of the female reproductive system, the *urethra,* which drains the urinary bladder, is superior and anterior to the vagina. In the human female, the urethra is only 2 to 3 centimeters in length, which enables bacteria to travel more easily to the bladder than in the male. For this reason, the female is more susceptible to bladder infections than the male. As a rule, bladder infections occur more often in females once they become sexually active. In fact, after periods of prolonged sexual activity, it is not uncommon for women to develop a bladder infection. Sometimes this is referred to as "honeymoon cystitis."

Internal Genitalia

The internal female reproductive organs are the vagina, the uterus, the fallopian tubes, and the ovaries (Figures 1-2 ● and 1-3 ●).

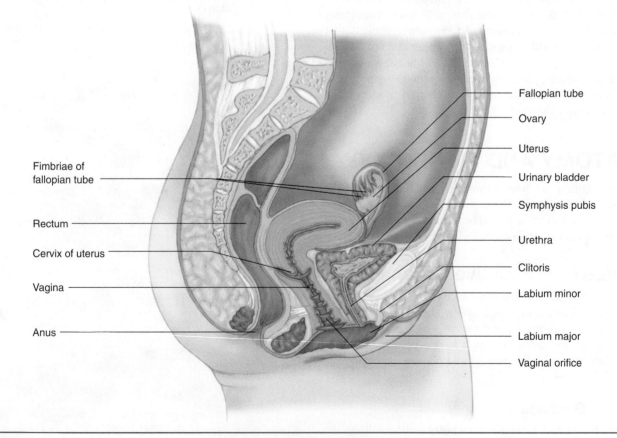

● **Figure 1-2**   Cross-sectional anatomy of the female reproductive system.

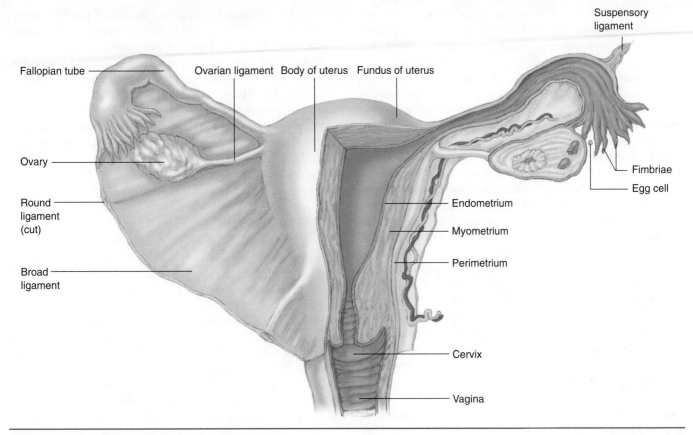

● **Figure 1-3**   The uterus, fallopian tubes, and ovaries.

Vagina   The *vagina* is an elastic canal of primarily smooth muscle, 9 to 10 centimeters in length, that connects the external genitalia to the uterus. It lies between the urethra/bladder and the anus/rectum. Lined with mucous membrane, the vagina extends up and back from the vaginal orifice to the lower end of the uterus (cervix). The vaginal walls are crisscrossed with ridges that allow it to stretch during childbirth, allowing passage of the fetus. The vagina's primary blood supply is the vaginal artery. The pudendal nerve innervates the lower third of the vagina and the external genitalia.

   The vagina has three functions:

● It is the female organ of copulation and receives the penis during sexual intercourse.

● Often called the birth canal, it forms the final passageway for the infant during childbirth.

● It provides an outlet for menstrual blood and tissue to leave the body.

Uterus   The *uterus* is a hollow, thick-walled, muscular, inverted-pear-shaped organ that connects with the vagina. It lies in the center of the pelvis and is flexed forward between the bladder and rectum above the vagina. Approximately 7.5 centimeters (3 inches) long and 5 centimeters (2 inches) wide, the uterus is held loosely in position by ligaments, peritoneal folds, and the pressure of adjacent abdominal structures. The primary function of the uterus is to provide a site for fetal development. During pregnancy, the uterus stretches to a size capable of containing the fetus, placenta, and the associated membranes

and amniotic fluid. At term, the gravid uterus measures approximately 40 centimeters (16 inches) in length. The uterus has an extensive blood supply, primarily from the uterine arteries which are branches of the internal iliac artery. The autonomic nervous system innervates the uterus. In a nonpregnant state, the uterine cavity is flat and triangular.

   The uterus has two major parts: the *body* (or corpus) and the *cervix,* or neck. The upper two-thirds of the uterus forms the body and consists of smooth muscle layers. The lower third is the cervix.

   The rounded uppermost portion of the body of the uterus is the *fundus,* which lies above the point at which the fallopian tubes attach. Measurement of fundal height (distance from the pubic symphysis to the fundus) may be used to estimate gestational age during pregnancy. The fundal height, measured in centimeters, is generally comparable to the weeks of gestation. For instance, if the fundal height is 30 centimeters, the gestational age is about 30 weeks. This method of assessing uterine size is most accurate from 22 to 34 weeks.

   The body of the uterus has three layers of tissue that make up the uterine wall. The innermost layer or lining is called the **endometrium.** Each month, stimulated by estrogen and progesterone, the endometrium builds up in preparation for the implantation of a fertilized ovum. If fertilization does not occur, the lining degenerates and sloughs off. This sloughing of the uterine lining is referred to as the *menses,* or menstrual period.

   The thick middle layer of the uterine wall, called the **myometrium,** consists of three distinct layers of smooth muscle fibers. In the outer layer, primarily over the fundus, the fibers run longitudinally, which allows expulsion of the fetus following cervical dilation. The middle (and thicker) layer is made up of figure-eight patterns of interlaced muscle fibers that surround large blood vessels. The contraction of these fibers helps control postdelivery bleeding. The myometrial fibers also contract during menstruation to maximize the sloughing of the endometrium. It has been suggested that menstrual cramps are due to fatigue of the myometrial fibers. The innermost layer of the myometrium consists of circular smooth muscle fibers that form sphincters at the point of fallopian tube attachment and at the internal opening of the cervix.

The outermost layer of the uterine wall is a serous membrane called the **perimetrium**, which partially covers the corpus of the uterus. The perimetrium, a layer of the visceral peritoneum that lines the abdominal cavity and abdominal organs, does not extend to the cervix. The most significant aspect of this partial coverage is that it allows surgical access to the uterus without the risk of infection that is associated with peritoneal incisions.

The cervix, or neck of the uterus, extends from the narrowest portion of the uterus to connect with the vagina. That distance forms the cervical canal and is only approximately 2.5 centimeters (1 inch) in length. Elasticity characterizes the cervix. During labor, it dilates to a diameter of approximately 10 centimeters to allow delivery of the fetus.

Ovaries The *ovaries* are the primary female gonads, or sex glands. Almond shaped, the ovaries are situated laterally on either side of the uterus in the upper portion of the pelvic cavity. The ovaries have two functions. One function is the secretion of the hormones estrogen and progesterone in response to stimulation from follicle-stimulating hormone (FSH) and luteinizing hormone (LH) secreted from the anterior pituitary gland. The second function of the ovaries is the development and release of eggs (ova) for reproduction.

Fallopian Tubes The two *fallopian tubes,* also called *uterine tubes,* are thin flexible tubes that extend laterally from the uterus and curve up and over each ovary on either side. Each tube is approximately 10 centimeters (4 inches) in length and about 1 centimeter in diameter (about the size of a pencil lead), except at its ovarian end, which is trumpet shaped. Each fallopian tube has two openings, a fimbriated (fringed) end that opens into the abdominal cavity in the area adjacent to the ovaries and a minute opening into the uterus. The function of the tubes is to conduct the egg from the space around the ovaries into the uterine cavity via peristalsis (wavelike muscular contractions). Fertilization usually occurs in the distal third of the fallopian tube.

The Menstrual Cycle

The woman undergoes a monthly hormonal cycle, generally every 28 days, that prepares the uterus to receive a fertilized egg. The onset of the menstrual cycle—that is, the onset of ovulation at puberty—establishes female sexual maturity. This onset, known as **menarche**, usually begins between the ages of 10 and 14. At first, the periods are irregular. Later they become more regular and predictable. The length of the menstrual cycle may vary from 21 to 32 days. A "normal" menstrual cycle is what is

normal for the woman in question. Because of this, it is important to inquire as to the normal length of the patient's menstrual cycle. Regardless of the length of the menstrual cycle, the period of time from ovulation to menstruation is always 14 days. Any variance in cycle length occurs during the preovulatory phase.

From puberty to menopause, the female sex hormones (estrogen and progesterone) control the ovarian–menstrual cycle, pregnancy, and lactation. These hormones are not produced at a constant rate, but rather their production surges and diminishes in a cyclical fashion. The secretion of estrogen and progesterone by the ovaries is controlled by the secretion of FSH and LH (Figure 1-4 ●).

Proliferative Phase

The first two weeks of the menstrual cycle, known as the *proliferative phase,* are dominated by estrogen, which causes the uterine lining (endometrium) to thicken and become engorged with blood. In response to a surge of LH at approximately day 14, **ovulation** (release of an egg) takes place.

At birth, each female's ovary contains some 200,000 ova within immature ovarian follicles known as *graafian follicles.* This is the woman's lifetime supply of ova, which are gradually "used up" through ovulation during her lifetime.

In response to FSH and increased estrogen levels, once during every menstrual cycle, a follicle reaches maturation and ruptures, discharging its egg through the ovary's outer covering into the fallopian tube. The ruptured follicle, under the influence of LH, develops the *corpus luteum,* a small yellowish body of cells, which produces progesterone during the second half of the menstrual cycle. If the egg is not fertilized, the corpus luteum will atrophy about three days prior to the onset of the menstrual phase. If the egg is fertilized, the corpus luteum will produce progesterone until the placenta takes over that function.

The cilia (fine, hairlike structures) on the fimbriated ends of the fallopian tubes draw the egg into the tube and sweep it toward the uterus. If the woman has had sexual intercourse within approximately 24 hours of ovulation, fertilization may take place. If the egg is fertilized, it normally implants in the thickened lining of the uterus, where the fetus subsequently develops. If it is not fertilized, it passes into the uterine cavity and is expelled.

Secretory Phase

The stage of the menstrual cycle immediately surrounding ovulation is referred to as the *secretory phase.* If the egg is not fertilized, the woman's estrogen level drops sharply while the progesterone level dominates. Uterine vascularity increases during this phase in anticipation of implantation of a fertilized egg.

Ischemic Phase

If fertilization does not occur, estrogen and progesterone levels fall. Vascular changes cause the endometrium to become pale and small blood vessels to rupture.

Menstrual Phase

During the menstrual phase, the ischemic endometrium is shed, along with a discharge of blood, mucus, and cellular debris, a process known as **menstruation**. A "normal" menstrual cycle

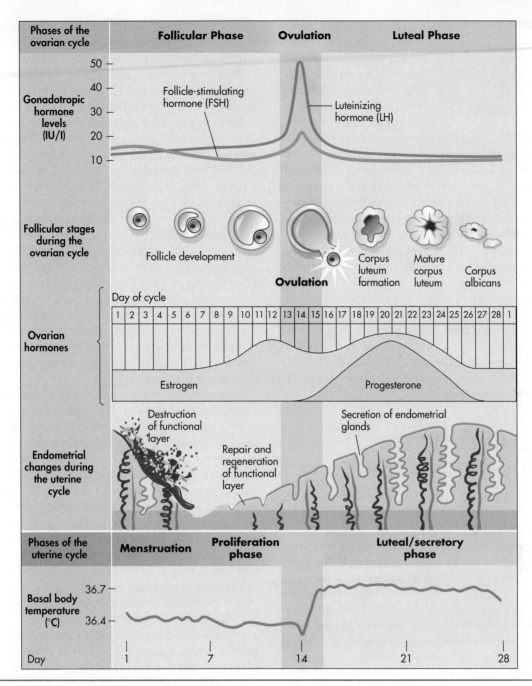

| Phases of the ovarian cycle | Follicular Phase | Ovulation | Luteal Phase |

Gonadotropic hormone levels (IU/I)

50
40
30
20
10

Follicle-stimulating hormone (FSH)

Luteinizing hormone (LH)

Follicular stages during the ovarian cycle

Follicle development

Ovulation

Corpus luteum formation

Mature corpus luteum

Corpus albicans

Ovarian hormones

Day of cycle

| 1 | 2 | 3 | 4 | 5 | 6 | 7 | 8 | 9 | 10 | 11 | 12 | 13 | 14 | 15 | 16 | 17 | 18 | 19 | 20 | 21 | 22 | 23 | 24 | 25 | 26 | 27 | 28 | 1 |

Estrogen

Progesterone

Endometrial changes during the uterine cycle

Destruction of functional layer

Repair and regeneration of functional layer

Secretion of endometrial glands

| Phases of the uterine cycle | Menstruation | Proliferation phase | Luteal/secretory phase |

Basal body temperature (°C)

36.7
36.4

| Day | 1 | 7 | 14 | 21 | 28 |

● **Figure 1-4**   Phases of the menstrual cycle.

depends on the regular pattern in the individual woman. The first day of the menstrual cycle is the day on which bleeding begins; the menstrual flow usually lasts from three to five days, although this varies from woman to woman. An average blood loss of about 50 mL is common. The absence of a menstrual period in any woman in the childbearing years (generally ages 12 to 55) who is sexually active and whose periods are usually regular should raise the suspicion of pregnancy.

Some women regularly experience marked physical signs and symptoms immediately prior to the onset of their menstrual period. These are collectively known as **premenstrual syndrome (PMS)**. Although you may hear crude jokes made about PMS, there is no denying the reality of the physical changes that accompany the changing hormonal levels. It is not uncommon for

women to report breast tenderness or engorgement, transient weight gain or bloating as a result of fluid retention, excessive fatigue, and/or cravings for specific foods. Women who are prone to migraine headaches may see them increase during the premenstrual period. Other women may have only minimal physical symptoms, but are more affected by emotional responses such as irritability, anxiety, or depression. The severity of PMS varies with each individual and may require treatment focused on relief of symptoms.[1]

Premenstrual dysphoric disorder (PMDD) is a similar condition in which a woman has severe symptoms of depression, irritability, and tension before menstruation. The symptoms of PMDD are more severe than those seen with premenstrual syndrome and include a wide range of physical or emotional symptoms that typically occur about 5 to 11 days before a woman starts her monthly menstrual cycle. The symptoms usually stop when her period begins or shortly thereafter.[2]

Menopause, the cessation of menses, marks the cessation of ovarian function and the cessation of estrogen secretion. Menstrual periods generally continue to occur until a woman is 45 to 55 years old, at which time they begin to decline in frequency and length until they ultimately stop. The end of reproductive life is also known as the *climacteric*, which is derived from Greek meaning "critical time of life." Occasionally, physicians use the term *surgical menopause*, which means that a woman's periods have stopped because of surgical removal of her uterus, ovaries, or both. The decrease in estrogen levels causes many women to experience hot flashes, night sweats, and mood swings during menopause. It is not uncommon for hormone replacement therapy (oral estrogen or estrogen and progesterone) to be prescribed to help relieve these complaints and to provide other health benefits associated with continuing adequate levels of these hormones.

ASSESSMENT OF THE GYNECOLOGIC PATIENT

Beyond labor and delivery, the most common emergency complaints of women in the childbearing years are abdominal pain and vaginal bleeding. Abdominal pain in women in the childbearing years is often due to problems of the reproductive organs. Complete the primary assessment in the usual manner. Then proceed with the secondary assessment. In addition to the usual history and physical assessment activities, you will need to ask specific questions pertinent to reproductive function and dysfunction. However, do not allow yourself to get distracted from getting complete past medical histories, including chronic medical problems, medications, and allergies.

You may feel uncomfortable asking a patient about her reproductive history, but remember that you are a health care professional who is trying to obtain pertinent information in order to provide the best possible care for your patient. If you conduct yourself in this manner, it should not be uncomfortable for you or your patient. Assess your patient's emotional state. If she is reluctant to discuss her complaint in detail, respect her wishes and transport her to the emergency department, where a more thorough assessment can be done.

History

Once you have completed your primary assessment, use a structured approach for obtaining additional information about the history of the present illness.

If the chief complaint is pain, then use the mnemonic OPQRST to gather more information. Is the patient's pain abdominal or in the pelvic region? Is it localized in a specific quadrant of the pelvis? Is she having her menstrual period? If so, how does the pain she is having now compare with the way she usually feels? Some women have severe discomfort during their menstrual periods. This is called **dysmenorrhea**. Others may experience **dyspareunia**, painful sexual intercourse. Does walking or defecation aggravate her pain? What, if anything, alleviates her pain? Does positioning herself on her back or side with her knees bent relieve her discomfort?

You need to determine whether there are any associated signs or symptoms that will be helpful in determining what is wrong with your patient. For instance, does your patient report a fever or chills? Is she reporting signs of gastrointestinal problems such as nausea, vomiting, diarrhea, or constipation? Is she complaining of urinary problems such as frequency, painful urination, or "colicky" urinary cramping? Does she report a vaginal discharge or bleeding? If so, obtain information about the color, amount, frequency, or odors associated with either vaginal bleeding or discharge. If she reports vaginal bleeding, how does the amount compare with the volume of her usual menstrual period? Does she report dizziness with changes in position (orthostatic hypotension), syncope, or diaphoresis?

You will need to obtain specific information about her obstetric history. Has she ever been pregnant? *Gravida (G)* is the term used to describe the number of times a woman has been pregnant, including this one if she is pregnant. How many of those pregnancies ended in the delivery of a viable infant? *Para* or *parity (P)* refers to the number of deliveries. *Abortion (Ab)* refers to any pregnancy that ends before 20 weeks of gestation, regardless of cause. You may see this information recorded in shorthand—for example, $G_3 P_2 Ab_1$, or gravida 3, para 2, ab 1. This means that the woman has been pregnant three times and had two prior deliveries and one pregnancy that ended before 20 weeks' gestation. These terms refer to the number of pregnancies and deliveries, not the number of infants delivered, so even twins or triplets count only as one pregnancy and one delivery.

You will also need to obtain a gynecologic history. Question the patient about previous ectopic pregnancies, infections, cesarean sections, pelvic surgeries such as tubal ligation, abortions (either elective or therapeutic), and dilation and curettage (D&C) procedures. Also ask the patient about any prior history of trauma to the reproductive tract. It is often helpful to find out whether the patient, if she is sexually active, has had pain or bleeding during or after sexual intercourse.

It is important to document the date of the patient's last menstrual period, commonly abbreviated LMP (or LNMP for "last normal menstrual period"). Ask whether the period was of a normal length and whether the flow was heavier or lighter than usual. An easy way for women to estimate menstrual flow is by the number of pads or tampons used. The patient can easily compare this number to her routine usage. It is also important to inquire how regular the patient's periods tend to be. Ask her what form of birth control, if any, she uses. Also, find out whether she uses it regularly. Direct questions such as "Could you be pregnant?" are generally unlikely to get an accurate response. Indirect questioning is often more helpful in determining the likelihood of pregnancy, such as "When did your last menstrual period start?" If you suspect pregnancy, inquire about other signs, including a late or missed period, breast tenderness, bloating, urinary frequency, or nausea and vomiting. Until proven otherwise, you should assume that any missed or late period is due to pregnancy even though your patient may deny it.

Contraception, or the prevention of pregnancy, takes many forms, with variable degrees of effectiveness. You should have some familiarity with the various forms, their method of action, and their reliability (Table 1–1). Remember that many contraceptives are medications, so ask about their use. With the exception of oral contraceptives ("the pill") and intrauterine devices (IUDs), side effects caused by contraceptives are relatively rare. Oral contraceptives have been associated with hypertension, rare incidents of stroke and heart attack, and possibly pulmonary embolism. IUDs can cause perforation of the uterus, uterine infection, or irregular uterine bleeding. This is especially true for IUDs that have remained in place longer than the time recommended by the manufacturer, which rarely exceeds two years.

Physical Exam

Physical examination of the gynecologic patient is limited in the field. More than at any other time, the patient's comfort level should guide your actions. Respect your patient's modesty and maintain her privacy. This may mean that you need to exclude parents from the room when assessing adolescent patients or that you need to exclude spouses of married patients. Recognizing that most people are not comfortable discussing matters related to sexuality or reproductive organs, take your cues from the patient. Maintain a professional demeanor. Explain all procedures thoroughly so your patient can understand them before you initiate any care. Some women may feel more comfortable if they can be cared for by a female paramedic.

TABLE 1–1 | Contraceptives

Type of Contraceptive	Method of Action	Effectiveness
Rhythm method	Abstinence during fertile phase—follows six to eight months of monitoring the menstrual cycle to determine fertile phase	Effective if abstinent during fertile phase; however, this is difficult to judge with precision
Coitus interruptus (withdrawal)	Penis withdrawn prior to ejaculation	Oldest and least reliable form of contraception
Condom	Barrier prevents transport of sperm	Reliable if used consistently and properly; additional benefit is that latex condoms prevent disease transmission
Vaginal ring (NuvaRing)	Transparent, flexible ring that secretes hormones similar to birth control pills; placed deep in the vagina and left for three weeks, then removed for one week (to allow for menses) and another inserted	As effective as birth control pills (99%)
Diaphragm	Barrier covers cervix to prevent entry of sperm	Reliable if fit properly and used consistently
Spermicide	Destroys sperm or neutralizes vaginal secretions to immobilize sperm	Limited effectiveness, but increases when used with a barrier device
Intrauterine device (IUD)	Unclear; either prevents implantation of fertilized egg or affects sperm motility through cervix	Highly effective
Oral contraceptives (birth control pill)	Combination of estrogen and progesterone inhibits release of egg	Highly effective
Norplant	Progestin-containing capsules cause changes in cervical mucus to inhibit sperm penetration*	Highly effective and continuous (up to six years) but requires surgical implantation
Depo-Provera	Suppresses ovulation	Highly effective and continuous (three months)
Tubal ligation	Prevents egg from being fertilized by blocking tube	Highly effective but requires surgery

*No longer available in the United States.

The Gynecologic Physical Exam

Fortunately, paramedics seldom have to examine a woman's genitalia. Even when necessary, all that is required is a brief look at the external structures for injury and for any evidence of hemorrhage. Always have a chaperone when examining the genitalia of any person of the opposite sex, or even of the same sex. This will protect you from possible allegations of sexual assault or inappropriate touching. Always explain to the patient what you are planning to do and talk to her throughout the examination.

With the exception of emergent treatment for a breech birth (to maintain the infant's airway) or for a prolapsed cord (to keep the baby's head off the cord), there is no reason to perform an internal vaginal examination in the field. Even significant vaginal bleeding (unless caused by a tear in the labia or introitus) cannot be controlled with packing. These patients require immediate transport, treatment for shock, and rapid gynecologic examination at the hospital.

As always, the level of consciousness is the best indicator of your patient's status. Assess your patient's general appearance, paying particular attention to the color of her skin and mucous membranes. Cyanosis and pallor may indicate shock or a gas-exchange problem, whereas a flushed appearance is more indicative of fever.

Remember that vital signs are useful clues to the nature of your patient's problem. Pain and fever tend to cause an increase in pulse and respiratory rates along with a slight increase in blood pressure. Significant bleeding will cause increased pulse and respiratory rates as well as narrowing pulse pressures (the difference between systolic and diastolic pressures). Perform a tilt test to assess for orthostatic changes in her vital signs (a decrease in blood pressure and an increase in pulse rate when the patient rises from a supine or seated position), which again points to significant blood loss.

Assess your patient for evidence of vaginal bleeding or discharge. If possible, estimate blood loss. The use of more than two sanitary pads per hour is considered significant bleeding. If serious bleeding is reported or evident, it may be necessary to inspect the patient's perineum. Document the color and character of the discharge, as well as the amount, and the presence or absence of clots. *Do not perform an internal vaginal exam in the field.*

Pay particular attention to the abdominal examination. Auscultate the abdomen and note whether bowel sounds are absent or hyperactive. Gently palpate the abdomen. Document and report any masses, distention, guarding, localized tenderness, or rebound tenderness. In thin patients, a palpable mass in the lower abdomen may be an intrauterine pregnancy. At 3 months, the uterus is barely palpable above the symphysis pubis. At 4 months, the uterus is palpable midway between the umbilicus and the symphysis pubis. At 5 months (approximately 20 weeks), the uterus is palpable at the level of the umbilicus.

MANAGEMENT OF GYNECOLOGIC EMERGENCIES

In general, the management of the patient experiencing a gynecologic emergency is focused on supportive care. Rely on your primary assessment to guide your decision making about the need for oxygen therapy, intravenous access, and analgesia. If your patient's status warrants it, administer oxygen or assist ventilation as necessary. As a rule, intravenous access and fluid replacement are usually not indicated. However, if your patient has excessive bleeding or demonstrates signs of shock, then establish at least one large-bore IV and administer normal saline at a rate indicated by the patient's presentation. You may also want to initiate cardiac monitoring if your patient is unstable. Analgesics are often required for pain management.

Continue to monitor and evaluate serious bleeding. *Do not pack dressings in the vagina.* Discourage the use of tampons to absorb blood flow. If your patient is bleeding heavily, count and document the number of sanitary pads used. If shock is not a consideration, then position your patient for comfort in the left lateral recumbent position or supine with her knees bent, as this decreases tension on the peritoneum. Opiate analgesics can help to mitigate or alleviate moderate to severe pain.

Because it is not appropriate to perform an internal vaginal exam in the field, most patients with gynecologic complaints will be transported to be evaluated by a physician. Some problems may require surgical intervention, so you should consider emergency transport to the appropriate facility based on your local protocols.

Psychological support is particularly important when caring for patients with gynecologic complaints. Keep calm. Maintain your patient's modesty and privacy. Remember that this is likely to be a very stressful situation for your patient, and she will appreciate your gentle, considerate care.

SPECIFIC GYNECOLOGIC EMERGENCIES

Gynecologic emergencies can be generally divided into two categories—medical and traumatic.

Medical Gynecologic Emergencies

Gynecologic emergencies of a medical nature are often hard to diagnose in the field. The most common symptoms of a medical gynecologic emergency are abdominal pain and/or vaginal bleeding.

Gynecologic Abdominal Pain

Pelvic Inflammatory Disease Probably the most common cause of nontraumatic abdominal pain is **pelvic inflammatory disease (PID)**, an infection of the female reproductive tract that can be caused by a bacterium, virus, or fungus. The organs most commonly involved are the uterus, fallopian tubes, and ovaries (Figure 1-5 ●). Occasionally the adjoining structures,

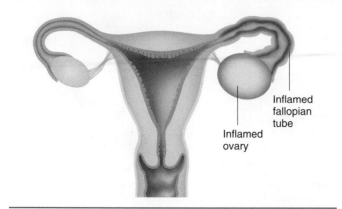

● **Figure 1-5** Pelvic inflammatory disease (PID). (© *Dorling Kindersley*)

such as the peritoneum and intestines, become involved. PID is the most common cause of abdominal pain in women in the childbearing years, occurring in 1 percent of that population. The highest rate of infection occurs in sexually active women ages 15 to 24. The most common causes of PID are gonorrhea (*Neisseria gonorrhoeae*) or chlamydia (*Chlamydia trachomatis*), although rarely streptococcus or staphylococcus bacteria may cause it. Commonly, gonorrhea or chlamydia progresses undetected in a woman until frank PID develops.

Predisposing factors include multiple sexual partners, prior history of PID, recent gynecologic procedure, or an IUD. Postinfection damage to the fallopian tubes is a common cause of infertility. PID may be either acute or chronic. If it is allowed to progress untreated, sepsis may develop. Additionally, PID may cause adhesions, in which the pelvic organs "stick together." Adhesions are a common cause of chronic pelvic pain and increase the frequency of infertility and ectopic pregnancies.

Although it is possible for a patient with PID disease to be asymptomatic, most patients with PID complain of abdominal pain, which is often diffuse and located in the lower abdomen. It may be moderate to severe, which occasionally makes it difficult to distinguish it from appendicitis. Pain may intensify either before or after the menstrual period. It may also worsen during sexual intercourse, as movement of the cervix tends to cause increased discomfort. Patients with PID tend to walk with a shuffling gait, as walking often intensifies their pain. In severe cases, fever, chills, nausea, vomiting, or even sepsis may accompany PID. Occasionally, patients have a foul-smelling vaginal discharge, often yellow in color, as well as irregular menses. It is common also to have midcycle bleeding.

Generally, on physical examination, the patient with PID appears acutely ill or toxic. The blood pressure is normal, although the pulse rate may be slightly increased. Fever may or may not be present. Palpation of the lower abdomen generally elicits moderate to severe pain. Occasionally, in severe cases, the abdomen will be tense with obvious rebound tenderness. Such cases may be impossible to distinguish from appendicitis in the prehospital setting.

The primary treatment for PID is antibiotics, often administered intravenously over an extended period. Once the causative organism is determined, the sexual partner may also require treatment. In the field, the primary goal is to make the patient as comfortable as possible. Place the patient on the ambulance stretcher in the position in which she is most comfortable.

She may wish to draw her knees up toward her chest, as this decreases tension on the peritoneum. *Do not perform a vaginal examination.* If your patient has signs of sepsis, administer oxygen (if hypoxic) and establish intravenous access.[3]

Ruptured Ovarian Cyst *Cysts* are fluid-filled pockets. When they develop in the ovary, they can rupture and be a source of abdominal pain. When an egg is released from the ovary, a cyst, known as a *corpus luteum cyst,* is often left in its place (Figure 1-6 ●). Occasionally, cysts develop independent of ovulation. When the cysts rupture, a small amount of blood is spilled into the abdomen. Because blood irritates the peritoneum, it can cause abdominal pain and rebound tenderness. Ovarian cysts may be found during a routine pelvic examination. However, in the field setting, your patient is likely to complain of moderate to severe unilateral abdominal pain, which may radiate to her back. She may also report a history of dyspareunia, irregular bleeding, or a delayed menstrual period. It is not uncommon for patients to rupture ovarian cysts during intercourse or physical activity. This often results in immediate, severe abdominal pain causing the patient to immediately stop intercourse or other physical activity. Ruptured ovarian cysts may be associated with vaginal bleeding.

Cystitis Urinary bladder infection, also called urinary tract infection (UTI) or **cystitis**, is a common cause of abdominal pain. Bacteria usually enter the urinary tract via the urethra, ascending into the bladder and ureters. The bladder lies anterior to the reproductive organs and, when inflamed, causes pain, generally immediately above the pubic symphysis. If untreated, the infection can progress to the kidneys. In addition to abdominal pain, your patient may report urinary frequency, pain or burning with urination (**dysuria**), and a low-grade fever. She may also complain of trouble starting and stopping her urinary stream (hesitancy). Occasionally the urine may be blood tinged.

Mittelschmerz Occasionally, ovulation is accompanied by midcycle abdominal pain known as **mittelschmerz**. It is thought that the pain is related to peritoneal irritation due to follicle rupture or bleeding at the time of ovulation. The unilateral lower quadrant pain is usually self-limited and may be accompanied by midcycle spotting. Although some women may report a low-grade fever, it should be noted that body temperature normally increases at the time of ovulation and remains elevated until the

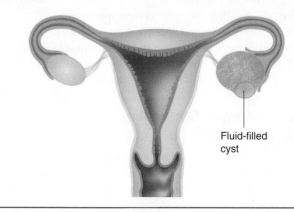

● **Figure 1-6** Large ovarian cyst. (© *Dorling Kindersley*)

day prior to the onset of the menstrual period. Treatment is symptomatic.

Endometritis An infection of the uterine lining called **endometritis** is an occasional complication of **miscarriage**, childbirth, or gynecologic procedures such as dilation and curettage (D&C). Commonly reported signs and symptoms include mild to severe lower abdominal pain; a bloody, foul-smelling discharge; and fever (101°F to 104°F). The onset of symptoms is usually 48 to 72 hours after the gynecologic procedure or miscarriage. These infections often mimic the presentation of PID and can be quite serious if not quickly treated with the appropriate antibiotics. Complications of endometritis may include sterility, sepsis, or even death.

Endometriosis **Endometriosis** is a condition in which endometrial tissue is found outside the uterus. Most commonly it is found in the abdomen and pelvis, although it has been found virtually everywhere in the body, including the central nervous system and lungs. Regardless of its site, the tissue responds to the hormonal changes associated with the menstrual cycle and thus bleeds in a cyclic manner. This bleeding causes inflammation, scarring of adjacent tissues, and the subsequent development of adhesions, particularly in the pelvic cavity.

Endometriosis is usually seen in women between the ages of 30 to 40 and is rarely seen in postmenopausal women. The exact cause is unknown. The most common symptom is dull, cramping pelvic pain that is usually related to menstruation. Dyspareunia and abnormal uterine bleeding are also commonly reported. Painful bowel movements have also been reported when the endometrial tissue has invaded the gastrointestinal tract. It is not uncommon for endometriosis to be diagnosed when the patient is being evaluated for infertility. Definitive treatment may include medical management with hormones, analgesics, and antiinflammatory drugs, and/or surgery to remove the excessive endometrial tissue or adhesions from other organs.

Ectopic Pregnancy An **ectopic pregnancy** is the implantation of a fetus outside the uterus. The most common site is within the fallopian tubes. This is a surgical emergency, because the tube can rupture, triggering a massive hemorrhage (Figure 1-7 ●). Patients with ectopic pregnancy often have severe unilateral abdominal pain that may radiate to the shoulder on the affected side, a late or missed menstrual period, and, occasionally, vaginal bleeding. Additional discussion of ectopic pregnancy is presented in the next chapter.[4]

Management of Gynecologic Abdominal Pain

Any woman with significant abdominal pain should be treated and transported to the hospital for evaluation. Administer oxygen (if the patient is hypoxic) and establish intravenous access if indicated. Refer to the earlier section on management of gynecologic emergencies for additional information.

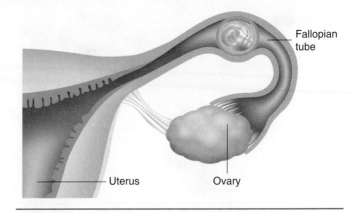

● **Figure 1-7** Ectopic (tubal) pregnancy shown in the fallopian tube. (© *Dorling Kindersley*)

Nontraumatic Vaginal Bleeding

Nontraumatic vaginal bleeding, often called *dysfunctional uterine bleeding,* is rarely seen in the field unless it is severe. Refer to the earlier section in this chapter on completing a patient history. You should not presume that vaginal bleeding is due to normal menstruation. Occasionally a woman will experience **menorrhagia**, or excessive menstrual flow, but rarely is it the cause for a 911 call. Hemorrhage, regardless of cause, is always potentially life threatening, so be alert for signs of impending shock.

The most common cause of nontraumatic vaginal bleeding is a spontaneous abortion (miscarriage). If it has been more than 60 days since your patient's LMP, you should assume that this is the cause. Vaginal bleeding due to miscarriage is often associated with cramping abdominal pain and the passage of clots and tissue. The loss of a pregnancy, even at a very early phase, is a significant emotional event for your patient, so your kind and considerate care is important. Spontaneous abortion and other causes of bleeding in the obstetric patient will be discussed further in the next chapter.

Another common cause of vaginal bleeding in the nonpregnant woman is the presence of uterine fibroids. Uterine fibroids—or, more correctly, *leiomyomas*—are noncancerous tumors that develop in the uterus. They are the most common pelvic tumor and can be found in 1 in 5 women of childbearing age. They typically affect women in their 30s (fourth decade of life) and are more common in African Americans than in those of Caucasian descent. The signs and symptoms of uterine fibroids include vaginal bleeding (usually between periods), heavy periods (menorrhagia), abdominal fullness or swelling, and pain during intercourse (dyspareunia). Fibroids often shrink when a woman goes through menopause and the estrogen effect is lost. Other potential causes of vaginal bleeding include cancerous lesions, PID, or the onset of labor.

Management of Nontraumatic Vaginal Bleeding

Your field management of patients suffering nontraumatic vaginal bleeding will depend on the severity of the situation and your assessment of the patient's status. Absorb the blood flow. *Do not pack the vagina.* If your patient is passing clots or tissue, save these for evaluation by a physician. Transport your patient in a position of comfort. The initiation of oxygen therapy (if the patient is hypoxic) and intravenous access should be guided by the patient's condition.

Traumatic Gynecologic Emergencies

Most cases of vaginal bleeding result from obstetric problems or are related to the menstrual period. However, trauma to the vagina and perineum can also cause bleeding and abdominal pain.

Causes of Gynecologic Trauma

The incidence of genital trauma is increasing, with vaginal injury occurring far more commonly than male genital injury. Gynecologic trauma may occur at any age. Blunt trauma occurs more frequently than penetrating trauma. Straddle injury (such as that which may occur while riding a bicycle) is the most common form of blunt trauma. Vaginal injuries are most often lacerations due to sexual assault. Other causes of gynecologic trauma include blunt force to the lower abdomen due to assault or seat belt injuries, direct blows to the perineal area, foreign bodies inserted into the vagina, self-attempts at abortion, and lacerations following childbirth.

Management of Gynecologic Trauma

Injuries to the external genitalia should be managed by direct pressure over the laceration or a chemical cold pack applied to a hematoma. In most cases of vaginal bleeding, the source is not readily apparent. If bleeding is severe or your patient demonstrates signs of shock, establish IV access to maintain intravascular volume and monitor vital signs closely. Blunt force may cause organ rupture, leading to the development of peritonitis or sepsis. *Never* pack the vagina with any material or dressing, regardless of the severity of the bleeding. Expedite transport to the emergency department because surgical intervention is often required.

Sexual Assault

Sexual assault continues to represent the most rapidly growing violent crime in America. More than 700,000 women are sexually assaulted annually. Unfortunately, it is estimated that more than 60 percent of all sexual assaults are never reported to authorities. Male victims represent 5 percent of reported sexual assaults. Sexual abuse of children is reported even less frequently. It is estimated that the incidence of sexual abuse in children ranges from 50,000 to 350,000 per year. There is no "typical victim" of sexual assault. No one, from small children to elderly adults, is immune.

Most victims of sexual assault know their assailants. Friends, acquaintances, intimates, and family members commit the vast majority (80 percent) of sexual assaults against women. Acquaintance rape is particularly common among adolescent victims. Sexual assault is a crime of violence, not passion, that is motivated by aggression and a need to control, humiliate, or inflict pain. There are very few predictors of who is capable of committing sexual assault, as age, economic status, and ethnic origins vary widely. Common behavioral characteristics found among rapists include poor impulse control, the need to achieve sexual satisfaction within the context of violence, and immaturity.

The definition of sexual assault varies from state to state. The common element of any definition is sexual contact without consent. Generally, rape is defined as penetration of the vagina or rectum of an unwilling female or the rectum in an unwilling male. In most states, penetration must occur for an act to be classified as rape. Sexual assault also includes oral–genital sex. Regardless of the legal definition, sexual assault is a crime of violence with serious physical and psychological implications.

Assessment   The victim of sexual assault is a unique patient with unique needs. Your patient needs emergency medical treatment and psychological support. Your patient also needs to have legal evidence gathered. *Your* objectivity is essential, as your attitude may affect long-term psychological recovery. As a rule, victims of sexual abuse *should not* be questioned about the incident in the field. Do not ask questions about specific details of the assault. It is not important, from the standpoint of prehospital care, to determine whether penetration took place. Do not inquire about the patient's sexual practices. Confine your questions to the physical injuries the patient received. Even well-intentioned questions may lead to guilt feelings in the patient. Do not ask questions, for instance, such as "Why did you go with him or get in his car?"

The psychological response of sexual assault victims is widely variable. The victim of sexual assault may be withdrawn or hysterical. Some use denial, anger, or fear as defense mechanisms. Approach the patient calmly and professionally. Allay the patient's fear and anxiety. Respond to the patient's feelings but be aware of your own. If the patient is incompletely dressed, a cover should be offered. Respect the patient's modesty. Explain all procedures and obtain the patient's permission before beginning them. Avoid touching the patient other than to take vital signs or examine other physical injuries. *Do not* examine the genitalia unless there is life-threatening hemorrhage.

In some instances, the patient may have been drugged. Flunitrazepam (Rohypnol) is the classic "date rape" drug, but any medication that alters mental status, including alcohol, can be used.[5] More recently, some of the "designer drugs," including gamma-hydroxybutyric acid (GHB), have been associated with rape. These can be placed in the victim's drink—often without the victim's knowledge.[6] Paramedics should always be concerned about the possibility of medication ingestion in any rape.

Management   In most situations, psychological and emotional support is the most important help you can offer. Maintain a nonjudgmental attitude and assure the patient of confidentiality. If the patient is female, allow her to be cared for by a female EMT or paramedic (if available). If the patient desires, have a woman accompany her to the hospital. Provide a safe environment, such as the back of a well-lit ambulance. Respond to the patient's feelings and respect the patient's wishes. Unless your patient is unconscious, do not touch the patient unless given permission. Even when your patient appears to have an altered level of consciousness, explain what is going to be done before initiating any treatment.

Preservation of physical evidence is important. When the patient arrives at the hospital, a physician or sexual assault nurse examiner will complete a sexual assault examination to gather physical evidence. To protect this evidence, it is important that you adhere to the following guidelines:

- Consider the patient a crime scene and protect that scene.
- Handle clothing as little as possible, if at all.
- If you must remove clothing, bag separately each item that must be bagged.
- Do not cut through any tears or holes in the clothing.
- Place bloody articles in brown paper bags.
- Do not examine the perineal area.
- If the assault took place within the hour or the patient is bleeding, put an absorbent underpad (e.g., Chux) under the patient's hips to collect that evidence.
- If you cover the patient with a sheet or blanket, turn that over to the hospital as evidence.

- Do not allow patients to change their clothes, bathe, or douche (if female) before the medical examination.
- Do not allow patients to comb their hair, brush their teeth, or clean their fingernails.
- Do not clean wounds, if at all possible.
- If you must initiate care on scene, avoid disruption of the crime scene.

Documentation When completing your patient care report, keep the following documentation guidelines in mind:

- State the patient's remarks accurately.
- Objectively state your observations of the patient's physical condition, environment, or torn clothing.
- Document any evidence (e.g., clothing, sheets) turned over to the hospital staff and the name of the individual to whom you gave it.
- Do *not* include your opinions as to whether rape occurred.

■ SUMMARY

The vast majority of gynecologic emergency patients will present with abdominal pain, vaginal bleeding, or both. Even though it may be uncomfortable for the patient, it is beneficial to obtain a detailed history including whether the patient is sexually active. Because of women's short urethras, urinary tract infections are commonplace in women, especially following periods of prolonged sexual activity.

Additional causes of abdominal pain in sexually active females can include pelvic inflammatory disease and ectopic pregnancy. In either case, the treatment for the patient remains predominantly the same, including supportive care and IV therapy as necessary to maintain normotension. If the patient does not want to divulge information, treat her for the worst-case scenario. Keep in mind that many times, especially in young teens, patients will deny having a sexual relationship even though they may have indeed had one.

When dealing with nontraumatic vaginal bleeding, the best historian will be the patient. Menarche occurs as early as the age of 10 and is the beginning of further development into sexual maturity. Initial cycles may have a slight variation to the dates and eventually lead to a regular 28-day cycle. The patient should be able to tell you where she is in her cycle and whether this type of bleeding is normal. Remember that you should *never* pack anything into the vagina, but use 5 × 9 or trauma dressings to absorb the blood flow and keep any tissue or clots that are passed. Keep the patient comfortable and treat hypotension with IV and oxygen therapy (if the patient is hypoxic).

There are few differences between the treatment of traumatic vaginal bleeding and any other traumatic bleeding. Here, again, do not pack the vagina, but apply pressure to the injury site. If the injury is secondary to an assault, keep in mind the importance of preservation of evidence, but remember to make patient care your number-one priority. Here again, treatment with IV and oxygen therapy will be largely symptom based.

Unfortunately, a paramedic can do very few things for gynecologic emergencies. General supportive care and basic IV therapy are the primary weapons for paramedics transporting patients with these types of emergencies. The patient should be placed in a position of comfort, which may include a position in which she is able to draw her knees up.

There are a variety of etiologies for female abdominal pain or vaginal bleeding. It is more important that the patient be treated symptomatically with dignity and respect than it is to have a definitive field diagnosis of endometriosis or ruptured ovarian cysts. Remember that patient care is the paramedic's top priority beyond self-safety.

YOU MAKE THE CALL

Late one evening in early winter, you are dispatched to a dormitory at the local university for a female patient with abdominal pain. When you arrive, the resident assistant escorts you to the room of your 17-year-old patient. There, the resident assistant introduces you to your patient and tells her that she will wait in the other room. Your patient is a slightly built young female who appears to be acutely ill. She is lying on her left side with her knees drawn up to her chest, crying quietly. Her skin is slightly flushed and diaphoretic. The tearful patient complains of excruciating lower abdominal pain that has increased in intensity over the past several hours. She says that she has not eaten today because she was too nauseated, but she denies vomiting or diarrhea.

The patient's blood pressure is 82/64 mmHg. Her pulse is 116 and thready. Respirations are 24 per minute with a pulse oximetry reading of 95 percent. Her temperature is 104°F. Lung sounds are clear and equal bilaterally. The abdominal exam reveals diffuse tenderness over both lower quadrants. She denies any past medical problems and says that she takes no medications, including birth control pills. She denies any allergies. Her LMP was seven weeks ago, but reports that earlier that evening she noticed a foul-smelling, bloody discharge. After questioning, she admits that she found out she was pregnant a week ago, but when she told her boyfriend, he told her to "get rid of it." She reports that three days ago she had an abortion at a local clinic. Her obstetric history is gravida 1, para 0, ab 1.

1. What is your first priority?

2. What else should you do?

3. What do you suspect is the likely cause of her signs and symptoms?

4. Because your patient is a minor, do you have any legal requirements to notify her parents or obtain their consent before treating her?

See Suggested Responses at the back of this book.

REVIEW QUESTIONS

1. The female external genitalia are known collectively as the _____.
   a. labia
   b. vulva
   c. mons pubis
   d. perineum

2. The _____ are two folds of fatty tissue that arise from the mons pubis and extend to the perineum, forming a cleft.
   a. pudendum
   b. labia minora
   c. labia majora
   d. sebaceous glands

3. The serous membrane that forms the outermost layer of the uterine wall is the _____.
   a. myometrium
   b. endometrium
   c. perimetrium
   d. ectometrium

4. Regardless of the length of the menstrual cycle, the period of time from ovulation to menstruation is always _____ days.
   a. 10
   b. 14
   c. 18
   d. 20

5. _____ is the term used to describe the number of times a woman has been pregnant.
   a. Para (Pa)   c. Gravida (G)
   b. Parity (P)   d. Abortion (Ab)

6. Abdominal pain associated with ovulation is called _____.
   a. dysuria   c. mittelschmerz
   b. endometritis   d. endometriosis

7. The most common cause of nontraumatic vaginal bleeding is _____.
   a. pelvic inflammatory disease
   b. the onset of labor
   c. spontaneous abortion
   d. cancerous lesions

8. In the case of sexual assault, the paramedic should _____.
   a. determine whether any life-threatening physical injuries exist
   b. respect the patient's wishes and offer emotional support
   c. make every effort to preserve physical evidence
   d. do all of the above

See Answers to Review Questions at the back of this book.

REFERENCES

1. Futterman, A. and A. J. Rapkin. "Diagnosis of Pre-menstrual Disorders." *J Reprod Med* 51 (2006) (2 Suppl): 349–358.

2. DiGiulo, G. and E. D. Reissing. "Premenstrual Dysphoric Disorder: Prevalence, Diagnostic Considerations, and Controversies." *J Psychosom Obstet Gyneacol* 27 (2006): 201–210.

3. Crossman, S. H. "The Challenge of Pelvic Inflammatory Disease." *Am Fam Physician* 73 (2006): 859–864.

4. Kruszka, P. S. and S. J. Kruszka. "Evaluation of Acute Pelvic Pain in Women." *Am Fam Physician* 82 (2010): 141–147.

5. Schwartz, R. H., R. Milteer, and M. A. LeBeau. "Drug-Facilitated Sexual Assault ('Date Rape')." *South Med J* 93 (2000): 558–561.

6. Nemeth, Z., B. Kun, and Z. Demetrovics. "The Involvement of Gamma-Hydroxybutyrate in Reported Sexual Assaults: A Systematic Review of the Literature." *J Psychopharmacol* 24 (2010): 1281–1287.

FURTHER READING

Greenspan, F. S. and G. J. Strewler. *Basic & Clinical Endocrinology.* 7th ed. Stamford, CT: Appleton & Lange, 2004.

Ladewig, P. W., M. L. London, and S. B. Olds. *Contemporary Maternal-Newborn Maternal Care.* 5th ed. Menlo Park, CA: Addison Wesley Longman, 2001.

McCance, K. L. and S. E. Huether. *Pathophysiology: The Biologic Basis for Disease in Adults and Children.* 4th ed. St. Louis: C.V. Mosby, 2001.

2

Obstetrics

Bryan Bledsoe, DO, FACEP, FAAEM, EMT-P

STANDARD
Special Patient Populations (Obstetrics)

COMPETENCY
Integrates assessment findings with principles of epidemiology and pathophysiology and knowledge of psychosocial needs to formulate a field impression and implement a comprehensive treatment/disposition plan for patients with special needs.

OBJECTIVES

Terminal Performance Objective
After reading this chapter, you should be able to integrate patient assessment findings, patient history, and knowledge of anatomy, physiology, pathophysiology, and basic and advanced life support interventions to recognize and manage patients with obstetric presentations.

Enabling Objectives
To accomplish the terminal performance objective, you should be able to:

1. Define key terms introduced in this chapter.

2. Relate the anatomy and physiology of pregnancy and fetal development to the assessment and management of patients with obstetric presentations.

3. Use a process of clinical reasoning to guide and interpret the patient assessment and management process for patients with specific obstetric presentations.

4. Adapt the scene size-up, primary assessment, patient history, secondary assessment, and use of monitoring technology to meet the needs of patients with complaints and presentations related to obstetric conditions.

5. Demonstrate concern for the psychosocial needs of patients with obstetric conditions.

6. Identify indications of imminent obstetric delivery.

7. Perform the steps of caring for the mother and newborn in complicated and uncomplicated newborn delivery.

8. Recognize abnormal deliveries that cannot be managed in the prehospital setting.

9. Relate the pathophysiology of specific obstetric disorders, including trauma in pregnancy, abortion, ectopic pregnancy, preterm labor, placenta previa, abruptio placenta, hypertensive disorders of pregnancy, abnormal fetal presentations in labor, and postpartum complications, to the priorities of patient assessment and management.

10. Communicate all relevant information about obstetric patients orally and in writing when transferring care to hospital personnel.

KEY TERMS

abortion, p. 27
afterbirth, p. 19
amniotic fluid, p. 19
amniotic sac, p. 19
crowning, p. 26
effacement, p. 32

estimated date of
  confinement (EDC), p. 22
labor, p. 33
lochia, p. 34
neonate, p. 38
ovulation, p. 19

placenta, p. 19
puerperium, p. 33
tocolysis, p. 33
umbilical cord, p. 19

CASE STUDY

The crew members of Fire Station 32 are relaxing in the television room when, suddenly, they hear an automobile screech to a halt at the station door. The captain rushes to the door and finds an old station wagon parked out front with a man standing beside it yelling, "Help! My wife needs help!"

The whole crew spills out the door. In the back seat of the station wagon, they see a pregnant female. She keeps saying, "The baby is coming! The baby is coming!" The ambulance normally based at Station 32 has gone out for gas. The captain notifies fire dispatch, which orders the ambulance to return. Meanwhile, the paramedics assigned to the engine learn that the patient is 29 years old and that this is her sixth pregnancy. She exclaims that she feels as if she has to move her bowels.

Now the patient begins to scream. "I've got to push! I've got to push!" she yells. The paramedics take Standard Precautions and the senior paramedic checks for crowning. He easily spots the top of the baby's head during a contraction. One member of the crew retrieves an OB kit and an oxygen bottle from the medic box on the fire engine. Shortly thereafter, the patient gives birth to a baby girl in the back of the station wagon.

At the time of delivery, the ambulance crew arrives. They assist the engine crew in cutting the cord, then dry and wrap the baby in a warming blanket. APGAR scores are 8 at 1 minute and 9 at 5 minutes. The mother receives fundal massage and an IV of normal saline solution. The paramedics then transport both mother and daughter to the hospital without incident. The father follows in the station wagon.

The next morning, as the Station 32 crewmembers are walking to their cars, they see a stork artfully painted on the window of the car belonging to the paramedic who delivered the baby.

INTRODUCTION

Pregnancy, childbirth, and the potential complications of each are the focus of this chapter. Pregnancy is a normal, natural process of life that results from ovulation and fertilization. Complications of pregnancy are uncommon, but when they do occur, you must be prepared to recognize them quickly and manage them appropriately. Complications such as hypertension or eclampsia may result from the pregnancy itself. In addition, complications such as diabetes or cardiac diseases may result from the body's responses to the pregnancy. In some cases, complications are a consequence of trauma.

Childbirth occurs daily, usually requiring only the most basic assistance, although childbirth complications do occasionally occur. These include preterm labor, multiple births, abnormal presentations, bleeding, or distressed neonates, to name but a few.

This chapter will prepare you to assess and care for the female patient throughout her pregnancy and delivery of her child.

THE PRENATAL PERIOD

The *prenatal period* (literally, "prebirth period") is the time from conception until delivery of the fetus. During this period, fetal development takes place. In addition, significant physiologic changes occur in the mother. Health care visits during pregnancy are referred to as "prenatal visits" or "prenatal care."

Anatomy and Physiology of the Obstetric Patient

As you learned in the previous chapter, the first two weeks of the menstrual cycle are dominated by the hormone estrogen, which causes the endometrium (the inner lining of the uterus) to thicken and become engorged with blood. In response to a surge of luteinizing hormone (LH) and follicle-stimulating hormone (FSH), **ovulation**, or release of an egg (ovum) from the ovary, takes place. The egg travels down the fallopian tube to the uterus. If the egg has been fertilized, it becomes implanted in the uterus and pregnancy begins. If the egg has not been fertilized, menstruation (discharge of blood, mucus, and cellular debris from the endometrium) takes place 14 days after ovulation. (The time from ovulation to menstruation is always exactly 14 days. However, the time from menstruation to the next ovulation may vary by several days from the average of 14 days, which is why it can be difficult for couples to find the optimum time of the month to conceive, or to avoid conceiving, a baby.)

If the woman has had intercourse within 24 to 48 hours before ovulation, fertilization may occur. The man's seminal fluid, carrying numerous spermatozoa, or male sex cells, enters the vagina and uterus and travels toward the fallopian tubes. Fertilization, which usually takes place in the distal third of the fallopian tube, occurs when a male spermatozoon fuses with the female ovum (Figure 2-1 ●). After fertilization, the ovum begins cellular division immediately, which continues as it moves through the fallopian tube to the uterus. The ovum then becomes a *blastocyst* (a hollow ball of cells). The blastocyst normally implants in the thickened uterine lining, which has been prepared for implantation by the hormone progesterone, where the fetus and placenta subsequently develop.

Approximately three weeks after fertilization, the placenta develops on the uterine wall at the site where the blastocyst attached (Figure 2-2 ●). The **placenta**, known as the "organ of pregnancy," is a temporary, blood-rich structure that serves as the lifeline for the developing fetus. It transfers heat while exchanging oxygen and carbon dioxide; delivering nutrients, such as glucose, potassium, sodium, and chloride; and carrying away wastes, such as urea, uric acid, and creatinine. The placenta also serves as an endocrine gland throughout pregnancy, secreting hormones necessary for fetal survival as well as the estrogen and progesterone required to maintain the pregnancy. Additionally, the placenta serves as a protective barrier against harmful substances. (However, some drugs, such as narcotics, steroids, and some antibiotics, are able to cross the placental membrane from the mother to the fetus.) When expelled from the uterus following birth of the child, the placenta and accompanying membranes are called the **afterbirth**.

The placenta is connected to the fetus by the **umbilical cord**, a flexible, ropelike structure approximately 2 feet (0.6 m) in length and 0.75 inch (1.9 cm) in diameter. Normally, the umbilical cord contains two arteries and one vein. The umbilical vein transports oxygenated blood to the fetus, and the umbilical arteries return relatively deoxygenated blood to the placenta.

The fetus develops within the **amniotic sac**, sometimes called the "bag of waters" (BOW). This thin-walled membranous covering holds the **amniotic fluid** that surrounds and protects the fetus during intrauterine development. The amniotic fluid increases in volume throughout the course of the pregnancy. After the 20th week of gestation, the volume varies from 500 to 1,000 mL. The presence of amniotic fluid allows for fetal movement within the uterus and serves to cushion and protect the fetus from trauma. The volume changes constantly as amniotic fluid moves back and forth across the placental membrane. During the latter part of the pregnancy, the fetus contributes to the volume by secretions from the lungs and urination. Although it may rupture earlier, the amniotic sac usually breaks during labor, and the amniotic fluid or "water" flows out of the vagina. This is called *rupture of the membranes* (ROM). This is what has happened when the pregnant woman says, "My water has broken."

Physiologic Changes of Pregnancy

The physiologic changes associated with pregnancy are due to an altered hormonal state, the mechanical effects of the enlarging uterus and its significant vascularity, and the increasing metabolic demands on the maternal system. It is important for you to understand the physiologic changes associated with pregnancy so that you can better assess your pregnant patients.

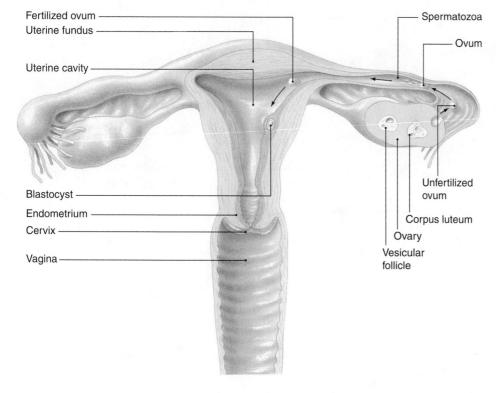

Labels: Fertilized ovum, Uterine fundus, Uterine cavity, Spermatozoa, Ovum, Blastocyst, Endometrium, Cervix, Vagina, Unfertilized ovum, Corpus luteum, Ovary, Vesicular follicle

● **Figure 2-1** Fertilization and implantation of the ovum.

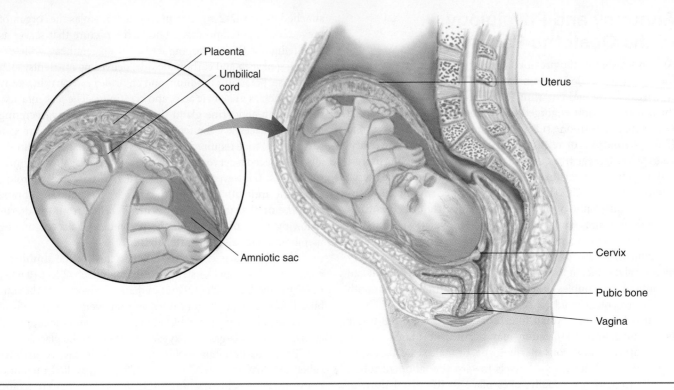

● **Figure 2-2** Anatomy of the placenta.

Reproductive System It is understandable that the most significant pregnancy-related changes occur in the uterus. In its nonpregnant state, the uterus is a small pear-shaped organ weighing about 60 g (2 oz) with a capacity of approximately 10 mL. By the end of pregnancy, its weight has increased to 1,000 g (slightly more than 2 pounds), whereas its capacity is now approximately 5,000 mL (Figure 2-3 ●). Another notable change is that during pregnancy the vascular system of the uterus contains about one-sixth (16 percent) of the mother's total blood volume.

Other changes occurring in the reproductive system include the formation of a mucus plug in the cervix that protects the developing fetus and helps to prevent infection. This plug will be expelled when cervical dilation begins prior to delivery. Estrogen causes the vaginal mucosa to thicken, vaginal secretions to increase, and the connective tissue to loosen to allow for delivery.

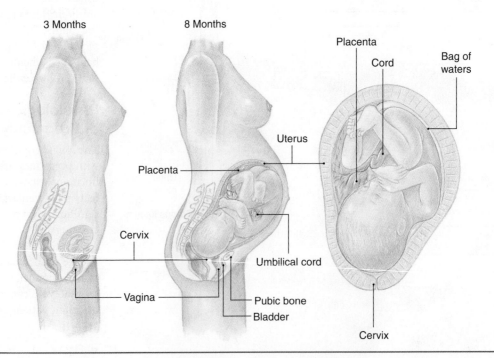

● **Figure 2-3** Uterine changes associated with pregnancy.

The breasts enlarge and become more nodular as the mammary glands increase in number and size in preparation for lactation.

Respiratory System   During pregnancy, maternal oxygen demands increase. To meet this need, progesterone causes a decrease in airway resistance. This results in a 20 percent increase in oxygen consumption and a 40 percent increase in tidal volume. There is only a slight increase in respiratory rate. The diaphragm is pushed up by the enlarging uterus, resulting in flaring of the rib margins to maintain intrathoracic volume.

Cardiovascular System   Various changes take place in the cardiovascular system during pregnancy (Figure 2-4 ●). Cardiac output increases throughout pregnancy, peaking at 6 to 7 liters/minute by the time the fetus is fully developed. The maternal blood volume increases by 45 percent and, although both red blood cells and plasma increase, there is slightly more plasma, resulting in a relative anemia. To combat this anemia, pregnant women receive supplemental iron to increase the oxygen-carrying capacity of their red blood cells. Because of the increase in blood volume, the pregnant female may suffer an acute blood loss of 30 to 35 percent without a significant change in vital signs. The maternal heart rate increases by 10 to 15 beats/minute. Blood pressure decreases slightly during the first two trimesters of pregnancy and then rises to near nonpregnant levels during the third trimester.

Supine hypotensive syndrome occurs when the gravid uterus compresses the inferior vena cava when the mother lies

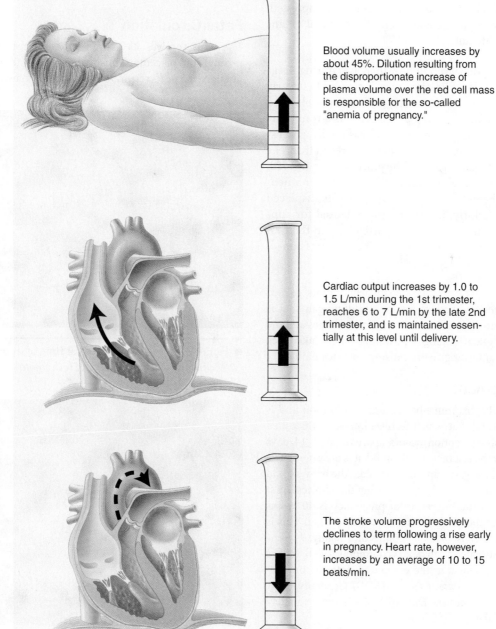

Blood volume usually increases by about 45%. Dilution resulting from the disproportionate increase of plasma volume over the red cell mass is responsible for the so-called "anemia of pregnancy."

Cardiac output increases by 1.0 to 1.5 L/min during the 1st trimester, reaches 6 to 7 L/min by the late 2nd trimester, and is maintained essentially at this level until delivery.

The stroke volume progressively declines to term following a rise early in pregnancy. Heart rate, however, increases by an average of 10 to 15 beats/min.

● **Figure 2-4**   The hemodynamic changes of pregnancy.

in a supine position, causing decreased venous return to the right atrium, which lowers blood pressure. Current research suggests that the abdominal aorta may also be compressed. The enlarging uterus also may press on the pelvic and femoral vessels, causing impaired venous return from the legs and venous stasis. This may lead to the development of varicose veins, dependent edema, and postural hypotension. Some patients are predisposed to this problem because of an overall decrease in circulating blood volume or because of anemia. Assessment and management of supine hypotensive syndrome will be discussed later in this chapter.

Gastrointestinal System   Nausea and vomiting are common in the first trimester as a result of hormone levels and changed carbohydrate needs. Peristalsis is slowed, so delayed gastric emptying is likely and bloating or constipation is common. As the uterus enlarges, abdominal organs are compressed, and the resulting compartmentalization of abdominal organs makes assessment difficult.

Urinary System   Renal blood flow increases during pregnancy. The glomerular filtration rate increases by nearly 50 percent in the second trimester and remains elevated throughout the remainder of the pregnancy. As a result, the renal tubular absorption also increases. Occasionally, glucosuria (large amounts of sugar in the urine) may result from the kidney's inability to reabsorb all of the glucose being filtered. Glucosuria may be normal or may indicate the development of gestational diabetes. The urinary bladder gets displaced anteriorly and superiorly, increasing the potential for rupture. Urinary frequency is common, particularly in the first and third trimesters, as a result of uterine compression of the bladder.

Musculoskeletal System   Loosened pelvic joints caused by hormonal influences account for the waddling gait that is often associated with pregnancy. As the uterus enlarges and the mother's center of gravity changes, postural changes take place to compensate for anterior growth, causing low back pain.

Fetal Development

Fetal development begins immediately after fertilization and is quite complex. The time at which fertilization occurs is called *conception*. Because conception occurs approximately 14 days after the first day of the last menstrual period, it is possible to calculate, with fair accuracy, the approximate date the baby should be born. This estimate is usually made during the mother's first prenatal visit. The normal duration of pregnancy is 40 weeks from the first day of the mother's last menstrual period. This is equal to 280 days, which is 10 lunar months or, roughly, 9 calendar months. This estimated birth date is commonly called the *due date*. Medically, it is known as the **estimated date of confinement (EDC)** or *estimated date of delivery (EDD)*. Generally, pregnancy is divided into *trimesters*. Each trimester is approximately 13 weeks, or 3 calendar months, long.

During the course of pregnancy, several different terms are used to describe the stages of development. The *preembryonic stage* covers the first 14 days following conception. The *embryonic stage* begins at day 15 and ends at approximately 8 weeks (Figures 2-5 ● and 2-6 ●). The period from 8 weeks until delivery is known as the *fetal stage*. As a paramedic, you should be familiar with some of the significant developmental milestones that occur during these three periods (Table 2–1).

During normal fetal development, the sex of the infant can usually be determined by 16 weeks' gestation. By the 20th week, *fetal heart tones (FHTs)* can be detected by stethoscope. The mother also has generally felt fetal movement. By 24 weeks, the baby may be able to survive if born prematurely. Fetuses born after 28 weeks have an excellent chance of survival (Figure 2-7 ●). By the 38th week the baby is considered *term*, or fully developed.

Most of the fetus's organ systems develop during the first trimester. Therefore, this is when the fetus is most vulnerable to the development of birth defects.

Fetal Circulation

The fetus receives its oxygen and nutrients from its mother through the placenta. Thus, while in the uterus, the fetus does not need to use its respiratory system or its gastrointestinal tract.

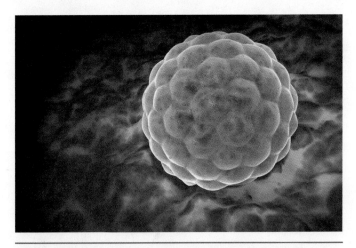

● **Figure 2-5**   Human embryo at time of implantation. *(© MedicalRF/Custom Medical Stock Photo)*

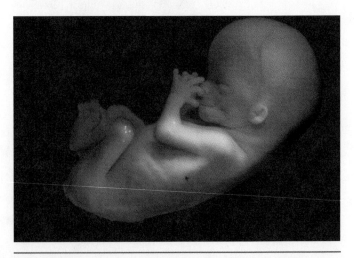

● **Figure 2-6**   Human fetus at 9 weeks of development. *(© C. Meitchik/Custom Medical Stock Photo)*

TABLE 2–1 | Significant Fetal Development Milestones

	Preembryonic Stage
2 Weeks	Rapid cellular multiplication and differentiation
	Embryonic Stage
4 Weeks	Fetal heart begins to beat
8 Weeks	All body systems and external structures are formed
	Size: approximately 3 cm (1.2 inches)
	Fetal Stage
8–12 Weeks	Fetal heart tones audible with Doppler
	Kidneys begin to produce urine
	Size: 8 cm (3.2 in.), weight about 1.6 oz
	Fetus most vulnerable to toxins
16 Weeks	Sex can be determined visually
	Swallowing amniotic fluid and producing meconium
	Looks like a baby, although thin
20 Weeks	Fetal heart tones audible with stethoscope
	Mother able to feel fetal movement
	Baby develops schedule of sucking, kicking, and sleeping
	Hair, eyebrows, and eyelashes present
	Size: 19 cm (8 in.), weight approximately 16 oz
24 Weeks	Increased activity
	Begins respiratory movement
	Size: 28 cm (11.2 in.), weight 1 lb 10 oz
28 Weeks	Surfactant necessary for lung function is formed
	Eyes begin to open and close
	Weighs 2–3 lb
32 Weeks	Bones are fully developed but soft and flexible
	Subcutaneous fat being deposited
	Fingernails and toenails present
	Weighs 3–4 lb
38–40 Weeks	Considered to be full term
	Baby fills uterine cavity
	Baby receives maternal antibodies

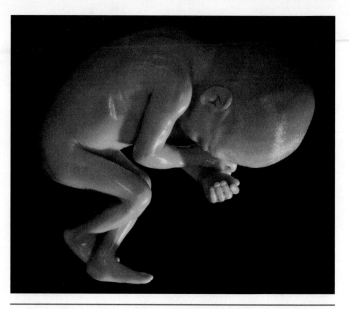

● **Figure 2-7** Mature human fetus at 7 to 8 months development (near-term). (© *A. Bartel/Custom Medical Stock Photo*)

Because of this, the fetal circulation shunts blood around the lungs and gastrointestinal tract.

The infant receives his blood from the placenta by means of the umbilical vein (Figure 2-8 ●). The umbilical vein connects directly to the inferior vena cava by a specialized structure called the *ductus venosus*. Blood then travels through the inferior vena

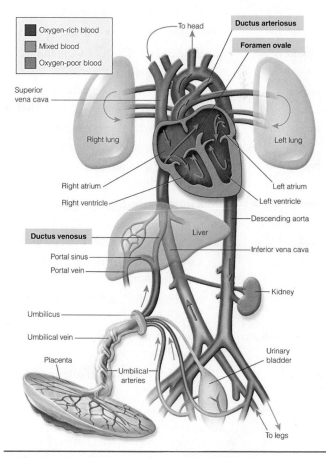

● **Figure 2-8** The maternal-fetal circulation.

cava to the heart. The blood enters the right atrium and passes through the tricuspid valve into the right ventricle. It then exits the right ventricle and travels through the pulmonic valve, into the pulmonary artery. The fetus's heart has a hole between the right and left atria, termed the *foramen ovale,* which allows mixing of the oxygenated blood in the right atrium with that leaving the left ventricle bound for the aorta. This serves to aid in blood flow bypassing the lungs.

At this time, the blood is still oxygenated. Once in the pulmonary artery, the blood enters the *ductus arteriosus,* which connects the pulmonary artery with the aorta. The ductus arteriosus causes blood to bypass the uninflated lungs. Once in the aorta, blood flow is basically the same as in extrauterine life. Deoxygenated blood containing waste products

---

Obstetric Terminology

The field of obstetrics has its own unique terminology. You should be familiar with this terminology, as patient documentation and communications with other health care workers and physicians often require it.

antepartum	the time interval prior to delivery of the fetus
postpartum	the time interval after delivery of the fetus
prenatal	the time interval prior to birth, synonymous with antepartum
natal	relating to birth or the date of birth
gravidity*	the number of times a woman has been pregnant
parity*	number of pregnancies carried to full term
primigravida	a woman who is pregnant for the first time
primipara	a woman who has given birth to her first child
multigravida	a woman who has been pregnant more than once
nulligravida	a woman who has not been pregnant
multipara	a woman who has delivered more than one baby
nullipara	a woman who has yet to deliver her first child
grand multiparity	a woman who has delivered at least seven babies
gestation	period of time for intrauterine fetal development

*The gravidity and parity of a woman is expressed in the following "shorthand": G4P2. "G" refers to the gravidity, and "P" refers to the parity. The woman in this example would have had four pregnancies and two births.

---

exits the fetus, after passage through the liver, via the umbilical arteries.

The fetal circulation changes shortly after birth. As soon as the baby takes his first breath, the lungs inflate, greatly decreasing pulmonary vascular resistance to blood flow. Also, the ductus arteriosus closes, diverting blood to the lungs. In addition, the ductus venosus closes, stopping blood flow from the placenta. The foramen ovale also closes as a result of pressure changes in the heart, which stops blood flow from the right to left atrium.

GENERAL ASSESSMENT OF THE OBSTETRIC PATIENT

Primary Assessment

The initial approach to the obstetric patient should be the same as for the nonobstetric patient, with special attention paid to the developing fetus. Complete the primary assessment quickly and then obtain essential obstetric information.

History

The SAMPLE history will allow you to gain specific information about the mother's situation as well as her pertinent medical history.

General Information

You will want to obtain information about the pregnancy, such as the mother's gravidity and parity, the length of gestation, and the estimated due date, if known. In addition, you should determine whether the patient has had any cesarean sections or any gynecologic or obstetric complications in the past. It is also important to ascertain whether the patient has had any prenatal care. Determine what type of health care professional (physician or nurse midwife) is providing her care and when she was last evaluated. Ask the patient whether a sonogram examination was done. A sonogram reveals the age of the fetus, the presence of more than one fetus, abnormal presentations, and certain birth defects. A general overview of the patient's current state of health is important. Pay particular attention to current medications and drug and/or medication allergies.

Preexisting or Aggravated Medical Conditions

Pregnancy aggravates many preexisting medical conditions and may trigger new ones.

Diabetes   Previously diagnosed diabetes can become unstable during pregnancy owing to altered insulin requirements. Diabetics are at increased risk of developing preeclampsia and hypertension (discussed later in this chapter). Pregnancy may also accelerate the progression of vascular disease complications of diabetes. It is not uncommon for pregnant diabetics to have problems with fluctuating blood sugar levels, causing hypoglycemic or hyperglycemic episodes. In addition, many patients develop diabetes during pregnancy (*gestational diabetes*). Pregnant diabetics cannot be managed with oral hypoglycemic agents because these drugs tend to cross the placenta and affect the fetus. Therefore, all pregnant diabetics are placed on insulin if their blood sugar levels cannot be controlled by diet alone. It has been shown that maintaining careful control of the mother's blood sugar between 70 and 120 mg/dL reduces risks to the mother and fetus.[1]

Diabetes also affects the infant. Infants of diabetic mothers, especially those with poorly controlled blood sugar levels, tend to be large. This complicates delivery. Such infants also may have trouble maintaining body temperature after birth and may be subject to hypoglycemia. Babies born to diabetic mothers are also at increased risk of congenital anomalies (birth defects).

Heart Disease   During pregnancy, cardiac output increases up to 30 percent. Patients who have serious preexisting heart disease may develop congestive heart failure in pregnancy. When confronted by a pregnant patient in obvious or suspected heart failure, inquire about preexisting heart disease or murmurs. It is important to be aware, however, that most patients develop a quiet systolic flow murmur during pregnancy. This is caused by increased cardiac output and is rarely a source of concern.

Hypertension   Hypertension is also aggravated by pregnancy. Generally, blood pressure is lower in pregnancy than in the nonpregnant state. However, women who were borderline hypertensive before becoming pregnant may become dangerously hypertensive when pregnant. Furthermore, many common blood pressure medications cannot be used during pregnancy. In addition, preeclampsia (discussed later in this chapter) may contribute to maternal hypertension. Persistent hypertension may adversely affect the placenta, thus compromising the fetus as well as placing the mother at increased risk for stroke, seizure, or renal failure.

Seizure Disorders   Most women with a history of seizure disorders controlled by medication have uneventful pregnancies and deliver healthy babies. However, women who have poorly controlled seizure disorders are likely to have increased seizure activity during pregnancy. Medications to control seizures are commonly administered throughout the pregnancy.

Neuromuscular Disorders   Disabilities associated with neuromuscular disorders, such as multiple sclerosis, may be aggravated by pregnancy. However, it is more common that pregnant women enjoy remission of symptoms during pregnancy and a slight increase in relapse rate during the postpartum period. The strength of uterine contractions is not diminished in these patients. Also, their subjective sensation of pain is often less than that seen in other patients.

Pain

If the patient is in pain, try to determine when the pain started and whether its onset was sudden or slow. Also, attempt to define the character of the pain—its duration, location, and radiation, if any. It is especially important to determine whether the pain is occurring on a regular basis.

Vaginal Bleeding

The presence of vaginal bleeding or spotting is a major concern in an obstetric patient. Ask about events immediately prior to the start of bleeding. You also need to gain information about the color, amount, and duration of bleeding. To assess the amount of bleeding, count the number of sanitary pads or tampons used. If your patient is passing clots or tissue, save this material for evaluation. In addition, question the patient about the presence of other vaginal discharges, as well as the color, amount, and duration.

Active Labor

When confronted with a patient in active labor, assess whether the mother feels the need to push or has the urge to move her bowels. Determine whether the patient thinks her membranes have ruptured. Patients often sense this as a dribbling of water or, in some cases, a true gush of water.

Physical Examination

Physical examination of the obstetric patient is essentially the same as that for any emergency patient. However, you should be particularly careful to protect the patient's modesty as well as to maintain her dignity and privacy.

When examining a pregnant patient, first estimate the date of the pregnancy by measuring the *fundal height*. The fundal height is the distance from the pubic symphysis to the top of the uterine fundus. Each centimeter of fundal height roughly corresponds to a week of gestation. For example, a woman with a fundal height of 24 centimeters has a gestational age of approximately 24 weeks. If the fundus is just palpable above the pubic symphysis, the pregnancy is about 12 to 16 weeks' gestation. When the uterine fundus reaches the umbilicus, the pregnancy is about 20 weeks. As pregnancy reaches term, the fundus is palpable near the xiphoid process. If fetal movement is felt when the abdomen is palpated, the pregnancy is at least 20 weeks. Fetal heart tones can be heard by stethoscope at approximately 18 to 20 weeks. The normal fetal heart rate ranges from 140 to 160 beats per minute.

Generally, vital signs in the pregnant patient should be taken with the patient lying on her left side. As noted earlier, as pregnancy progresses, the uterus increases in size. Ultimately, when the patient is supine, the weight of the uterus compresses the inferior vena cava, severely compromising venous blood return from the lower extremities. Turning the patient to her left side alleviates this problem. Occasionally, it may be helpful to perform orthostatic vital signs. First, obtain the blood pressure and pulse rate after the patient has rested for 5 minutes in the left lateral recumbent position. Then repeat the vital signs with the patient sitting up or standing. A drop in the blood pressure level of 15 mmHg or more, or an increase in the pulse rate of 20 beats per minute or more, is considered significant and should be reported and documented. When performing this maneuver, it is always important to be alert for syncope. This procedure should *not* be performed if the patient is in obvious shock.

You may need to examine the genitals to evaluate any vaginal discharge, the progression of labor, or the presence of a *prolapsed cord,* an umbilical cord that comes out of the uterus ahead of the fetus. This can be accomplished simply by looking at the perineum. If, during the physical examination, the patient reports that she feels the need to push, or if she feels as though she must move her bowels, examine her for crowning. **Crowning** is the bulging of the fetal head past the opening of the vagina during a contraction. Crowning is an indication of impending delivery. Examine for crowning only during a contraction. *Do not perform an internal vaginal examination in the field.*

GENERAL MANAGEMENT OF THE OBSTETRIC PATIENT

The first consideration for managing emergencies in obstetric patients is to remember that you are, in fact, caring for two patients, the mother and the fetus. Fetal well-being is dependent on maternal well-being. Also keep in mind that your calm, professional demeanor and caring attitude will go a long way in reducing the emotional stress during any obstetric emergency. Remember to protect your patient's privacy and maintain her modesty.

The physiologic priorities for obstetric emergencies are identical to those for any other emergency situation. Focus your efforts on maintaining the airway, breathing, and circulation. Administer oxygen, if needed, to correct hypoxia. Initiate intravenous access by using a large-bore catheter in a large vein and consider fluid resuscitation based on your local protocols. If your patient is bleeding or showing signs of shock, establish two IV lines. Cardiac monitoring is also appropriate. Place your

patient in a position of comfort, but remember that the left lateral recumbent position is preferred after the 24th week.

If pain is the primary complaint, administer analgesics such as morphine. However, analgesics should be used with caution, as they can alter your ability to assess a deteriorating condition as well as other changes in patient status and may negatively affect the fetus. Nitrous oxide is the preferred analgesic in pregnancy, but narcotics are acceptable.

When transport is indicated, transport immediately to a hospital that is capable of managing emergency obstetric and neonatal care. Report the situation to the receiving hospital prior to your arrival, as emergency department personnel may want to summon obstetrics department staff to assist with patient care.

COMPLICATIONS OF PREGNANCY

Pregnancy is a normal process. However, women who are pregnant are not immune from injury or other health problems. There may also be complications associated with the pregnancy itself.

Trauma

Paramedics frequently receive calls to help a pregnant woman who has been in a motor vehicle accident or who has sustained a fall. In pregnancy, syncope occasionally occurs (studies show that between 5 and 30 percent of pregnant women experience syncope). The syncope of pregnancy often results from compression of the inferior vena cava, as described earlier, or from normal changes in the cardiovascular system associated with pregnancy. Also, the weight of the gravid uterus alters the patient's balance, making her more susceptible to falls.

Pregnant victims of major trauma are more susceptible to life-threatening injury than are nonpregnant victims because of the increased vascularity of the gravid uterus. Trauma is the most frequent nonobstetric cause of death in pregnant women. Some form of trauma, usually a motor vehicle crash or a fall and even physical abuse, can occur in 6 to 7 percent of all pregnancies. Because the primary cause for fetal mortality is maternal mortality, the pregnant trauma patient presents a unique challenge. The later in the pregnancy, the larger the uterus and the greater the likelihood of injury. All patients at 20 weeks' (or more) gestation with a history of direct or indirect injury should be transported for evaluation by a physician.

Paramedics should *anticipate* the development of shock based on the mechanism of injury rather than waiting for overt signs and symptoms. Because of the cardiovascular changes of pregnancy, overt signs of shock are late and inconsistent. Trauma significant enough to cause maternal shock is associated with a 70 to 80 percent fetal mortality. In the face of acute blood loss, significant vasoconstriction will occur in response to catecholamine release, resulting in maintenance of a normotensive state for the mother. However, this causes significant uterine hypoperfusion (20 to 30 percent decrease in cardiac output) and fetal bradycardia.

Generally, the amniotic fluid cushions the fetus from blunt trauma fairly well. However, in direct abdominal trauma, the pregnant patient may suffer premature separation of the placenta from the uterine wall, premature labor, abortion, uterine rupture, and possibly fetal death. The presence of vaginal bleeding or a tender abdomen in a pregnant patient should increase your suspicion of serious injury. Fetal death may result from death of the mother, separation of the placenta from the uterine wall, maternal shock, uterine rupture, or fetal head injury. Any pregnant patient who has suffered trauma should be immediately transported to the emergency department and evaluated by a physician. Trauma management essentials include the following:

- Apply a C-collar to provide cervical stabilization and immobilize on a long backboard.
- Administer oxygen if the patient is hypoxic.
- Initiate two large-bore IVs for crystalloid administration per protocol.
- Transport tilted to the left to minimize supine hypotension.
- Reassess frequently.
- Monitor the fetus.

Medical Conditions

The pregnant patient is subject to all the medical problems that occur in the nonpregnant state. Abdominal pain is a common complaint. It is often caused by the stretching of the ligaments (e.g., round ligament) that support the growing uterus. However, appendicitis and cholecystitis can also occur. Pregnant women are at increased risk of developing gallstones as a result of hormonal influences that delay emptying of the gallbladder. In pregnancy, the abdominal organs are displaced because of the increased mass of the gravid uterus in the abdomen, which makes assessment more difficult. The pregnant patient with appendicitis may complain of right upper quadrant pain or even back pain. The symptoms of acute cholecystitis may also differ from those in nonpregnant patients. Any pregnant patient with abdominal pain should be evaluated by a physician.

Bleeding in Pregnancy

Vaginal bleeding may occur at any time during pregnancy. Bleeding is usually due to abortion, but can also occur with ectopic pregnancy, placenta previa, or abruptio placentae. Generally, the exact etiology of vaginal bleeding during pregnancy cannot be determined in the field. Refer to the earlier discussion in this chapter and your own local protocols for management of obstetric emergencies. Vaginal bleeding is associated with potential fetal loss. Keep in mind that this is an emotional and stressful situation for your patient, so a professional, caring demeanor is imperative.

Abortion

Abortion, the expulsion of the fetus prior to 20 weeks' gestation, is the most common cause of bleeding in the first and second trimesters of pregnancy. The terms *abortion* and *miscarriage* can be used interchangeably. Generally, abortion is considered to be termination of pregnancy at maternal request and miscarriage is considered to be an accident of nature. Medically, the term *abortion* applies to both kinds of fetal loss. Spontaneous abortion, the naturally occurring termination of pregnancy that is often called miscarriage, is most commonly seen between 12 and 14 weeks' gestation. It is estimated that 10 to 20 percent of all pregnancies end in spontaneous abortion. If the pregnancy has not yet been confirmed, the mother often assumes she is merely having a period with unusually heavy flow.

About half of all abortions are the result of fetal chromosomal anomalies. Other causes include maternal reproductive system abnormalities, maternal use of drugs, placental defects, or maternal infections. Although many people believe that trauma and psychological stress can cause abortion, research does not support that belief.

Assessment

The patient experiencing an abortion is likely to report cramping abdominal pain and a backache. She is also likely to report vaginal bleeding, which is often accompanied by the passage of clots and tissue. If the abortion was not recent, then frank signs and symptoms of infection may be present. In addition to your routine emergency assessments, assess for orthostatic vital sign changes and ascertain the amount of vaginal bleeding.

Management Place the patient who is experiencing an abortion in a position of comfort. Treat for shock with oxygen therapy (if hypoxic) and IV access for fluid resuscitation. As mentioned earlier, any tissue or large clots should be retained and given to emergency department personnel. If the abortion occurs during the late first trimester or later, a fetus may be passed. Often, the placenta does not detach, and the fetus is suspended by the umbilical cord. In such a case, place the umbilical clamps from the OB kit on the cord and cut it. Carefully wrap the fetus in linen or other suitable material and transport it to the hospital with the mother.

An abortion is generally a very sad occurrence. Provide emotional support to the parents. This can be a devastating psychological experience for the mother, so avoid saying trite but inaccurate phrases meant to provide comfort. Inappropriate remarks include "You can always get pregnant again" or "This is nature's way of dealing with a defective fetus." Parents who wish to view the fetus should be allowed to do so. Occasionally, Roman Catholic parents may request baptism of the fetus. You can perform this by making the sign of a cross and stating, "I baptize you in the name of the father, the son, and the holy spirit. Amen."

Ectopic Pregnancy

As you learned earlier, the fertilized egg normally is implanted in the endometrial lining of the uterine wall. The term *ectopic pregnancy* refers to the abnormal implantation of the fertilized egg outside the uterus. Approximately 95 percent are implanted in the fallopian tube. Occasionally (< 1 percent), the egg is

CONTENT REVIEW

▶ Causes of Bleeding during Pregnancy

- Abortion
- Ectopic pregnancy
- Placenta previa
- Abruptio placentae

Classifications of Abortion

Because you will be interacting with other health care professionals, you must be familiar with the variety of terms used to describe the classifications of abortion.

Complete abortion	An abortion in which all the uterine contents, including the fetus and placenta, have been expelled.
Incomplete abortion	An abortion in which some, but not all, fetal tissue has been passed. Incomplete abortions are associated with a high incidence of infection.
Threatened abortion	A potential abortion characterized by unexplained vaginal bleeding during the first half of pregnancy in which the cervix is slightly open and the fetus remains in the uterus and is still alive. In some cases of threatened abortion, the fetus still can be saved.
Inevitable abortion	A potential abortion, characterized by vaginal bleeding accompanied by severe abdominal cramping and cervical dilation, in which the fetus has not yet passed from the uterus, but the fetus cannot be saved.
Spontaneous abortion	Naturally occurring expulsion of the fetus prior to viability, generally as a result of chromosomal abnormalities. Most spontaneous abortions occur before week 12 of pregnancy. Many occur within two weeks after conception and are mistaken for menstrual periods. Commonly called a *miscarriage.*
Elective abortion	An abortion in which the termination of pregnancy is desired and requested by the mother. Elective abortions during the first and second trimesters of pregnancy have been legal in the United States since 1973. Most elective abortions are performed during the first trimester. Some clinics perform second-trimester abortions. Second-trimester abortions have a higher complication rate than first-trimester abortions. Third-trimester elective abortions are generally illegal in this country.
Criminal abortion	Intentional termination of a pregnancy under any condition not allowed by law. It is usually the attempt to destroy a fetus by a person who is not licensed or permitted to do so. Criminal abortions often are attempted by amateurs and they are rarely performed in aseptic surroundings.
Therapeutic abortion	Termination of a pregnancy deemed necessary by a physician, usually to protect maternal health and well-being.
Missed abortion	An abortion in which fetal death occurs but the fetus is not expelled. This poses a potential threat to the life of the mother if the fetus is retained beyond six weeks.
Habitual abortion	Spontaneous abortions that occur in three or more consecutive pregnancies.

implanted in the abdominal cavity. Current research indicates that the incidence of ectopic pregnancy is 1 in 44 live births. Improved diagnostic technology is credited with an increased incidence, as most are detected between the 2nd and 12th week. Ectopic pregnancy accounts for approximately 10 percent of maternal mortality.

Predisposing factors in the development of ectopic pregnancy include scarring of the fallopian tubes due to pelvic inflammatory disease (PID), a previous ectopic pregnancy, or previous pelvic or tubal surgery, such as a tubal ligation. Other factors include endometriosis or use of an intrauterine device (IUD) for birth control.[2]

Assessment Ectopic pregnancy most often presents as abdominal pain, which starts out as diffuse tenderness and then localizes as a sharp pain in the lower abdominal quadrant on the affected side. This pain is due to rupture of the fallopian tube when the fetus outgrows the available space. The woman often reports that she missed a period or that her LMP occurred four to six weeks earlier, but with decreased menstrual flow that was brownish in color and of shorter duration than usual. As the intraabdominal bleeding continues, the abdomen becomes rigid and the pain intensifies and is often referred to the shoulder on the affected side. The pain is often accompanied by syncope, vaginal bleeding, and shock.

Assume that any woman of childbearing age with lower abdominal pain is experiencing an ectopic pregnancy.

Management Ectopic pregnancy poses a significant life threat to the mother. Transport this patient immediately, as surgery is often required to resolve the situation. Interim care measures should include oxygen therapy (if the patient is hypoxic) and IV access for fluid resuscitation.

Placenta Previa

Placenta previa occurs as a result of abnormal implantation of the placenta on the lower half of the uterine wall, resulting in partial or complete coverage of the cervical opening

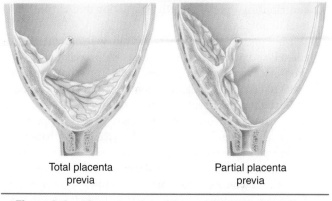

Total placenta
previa

Partial placenta
previa

● **Figure 2-9** Placenta previa (abnormal implantation).

(Figure 2-9 ●). Vaginal bleeding, which may initially be intermittent, occurs after the 7th month of the pregnancy as the lower uterus begins to contract and dilate in preparation for the onset of labor. This process pulls the placenta away from the uterine wall, causing bright red vaginal bleeding. Placenta previa occurs in about 1 in 250 live births. It is classified as complete, partial, or marginal, depending on whether the placenta covers all or part of the cervical opening or is merely in close proximity to the opening.

Although the exact cause of placenta previa is unknown, certain predisposing factors are commonly seen. These factors include a previous history of placenta previa, multiparity, or increased maternal age. Other factors include the presence of uterine scars from cesarean sections, a large placenta, or defective development of blood vessels in the uterine wall.

Assessment The patient with placenta previa is usually a multigravida in her third trimester of pregnancy. She may have a history of prior placenta previa or of bleeding early in the current pregnancy. She may report a recent episode of sexual intercourse or vaginal examination just before vaginal bleeding began, or she may not bleed until the onset of labor. The onset of painless bright red vaginal bleeding, which may occur as spotting or recurrent hemorrhage, is the hallmark of placenta previa. In fact, any painless bleeding in pregnancy is considered placenta previa until proven otherwise. The bleeding may or may not be associated with uterine contractions. The uterus is usually soft, and the fetus may be in an unusual presentation. *Vaginal examination should never be attempted, as an examining finger can puncture the placenta, causing fatal hemorrhage.*

The presence of placenta previa may already have been diagnosed with an ultrasound during prenatal care, in which case the mother is anticipating the onset of symptoms. The prognosis for the fetus is dependent on the extent of the previa. Obviously, in profuse hemorrhage the fetus is at risk of severe hypoxia and the viability

of the placenta is compromised. You should perform your assessment and physical exam as discussed earlier in this chapter.

Management If the placenta previa was previously diagnosed, your patient may already have been managed by placing her on bed rest. Because of the potential for profuse hemorrhage, you should treat for shock. Administer oxygen as needed and initiate intravenous access. Additionally, continue to monitor the maternal vital signs and fetal heart tones (FHTs). Because the definitive treatment is delivery of the fetus by cesarean section, it is imperative to transport the patient to a hospital with obstetric surgical capability.

Abruptio Placentae

Abruptio placentae, or the premature separation (abruption) of a normally implanted placenta from the uterine wall, poses a potential life threat for both mother and fetus (Figure 2-10 ●). The incidence of abruptio placentae is 1 in 120 live births. It is associated with 20 to 30 percent fetal mortality, which rises to 100 percent in cases in which the majority of the placenta has separated. Maternal mortality is relatively uncommon, although it rises markedly if shock is inadequately treated. Abruptio placentae is classified as marginal (or partial), central (severe), or complete, as explained next.

Although the cause of abruptio placentae is unknown, predisposing factors include multiparity, maternal hypertension, trauma, cocaine use, increasing maternal age, and history of abruption in a previous pregnancy.

Assessment The presenting signs and symptoms of abruptio placentae vary depending on the extent and character of the abruption. Partial abruptions can be marginal or central. Marginal abruption is characterized by vaginal bleeding but no increase in pain. In central abruption, the placenta separates centrally and the bleeding is trapped between the placenta and the uterine wall, or "concealed," so there is no vaginal bleeding. However, there is a sudden sharp, tearing pain and development of a stiff, boardlike abdomen. In complete abruptio placentae there is massive vaginal

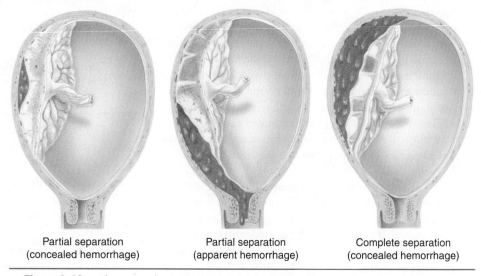

Partial separation
(concealed hemorrhage)

Partial separation
(apparent hemorrhage)

Complete separation
(concealed hemorrhage)

● **Figure 2-10** Abruptio placentae (premature separation).

CONTENT REVIEW

▶ Medical Complications of Pregnancy

• Hypertensive disorders of pregnancy
• Supine hypotensive syndrome
• Gestational diabetes

bleeding and profound maternal hypotension. If the patient is in labor at the time of the abruption, separation of the placenta from the uterine wall will progress rapidly, with fetal distress versus fetal demise dependent on percentage of separation.

Management Abruptio placentae is a life-threatening obstetric emergency. Immediate intervention to maintain maternal oxygenation and perfusion is imperative. Immediately place two large-bore intravenous lines and begin fluid resuscitation. Position your patient in the left lateral recumbent position. Transport immediately to a hospital with available surgical obstetric and high-risk neonatal care.

Medical Complications of Pregnancy

As discussed earlier, pregnancy can exacerbate preexisting medical conditions such as diabetes, heart disease, hypertension, and seizure or neuromuscular disorder.

Hypertensive Disorders of Pregnancy

The American College of Obstetricians and Gynecologists has identified four classifications of *hypertensive disorders of pregnancy* (formerly called "toxemia of pregnancy").[3] They are:

● *Preeclampsia and eclampsia.* Hypertensive disorders of pregnancy (HDP), which include preeclampsia and eclampsia, occur in approximately 5 percent of all pregnancies. Preeclampsia is the most common hypertensive disorder seen in pregnancy. There is a higher incidence among primigravidas, particularly if they are teenagers or over age 35. Others at increased risk are diabetics, women with a history of preeclampsia, and those who are carrying multiple fetuses.

Preeclampsia is a progressive disorder that is usually categorized as mild or severe. Seizures (or coma) develop in its most severe form, known as eclampsia. Preeclampsia is defined as an increase in systolic blood pressure by 30 mmHg and/or a diastolic increase of 15 mmHg over baseline on at least two occasions at least 6 hours apart. Remember that maternal blood pressure normally drops during pregnancy, so a woman may be hypertensive at 120/80 if her baseline in early pregnancy was 90/66. If there is no baseline blood pressure available, a reading of 140/90 or higher is considered to be hypertensive.

Preeclampsia is most commonly seen in the last 10 weeks of gestation, during labor, or in the first 48 hours postpartum. The exact cause of preeclampsia is unknown. It is thought to be caused by abnormal vasospasm, which results in increased maternal blood pressure and other associated symptoms. Additionally, the vasospasm causes decreased placental perfusion,

contributing to fetal growth retardation and chronic fetal hypoxia.

Mild preeclampsia is characterized by hypertension, edema, and protein in the urine. Severe preeclampsia progresses rapidly, with maternal blood pressures reaching 160/110 or higher, while the edema becomes generalized and the amount of protein in the urine increases significantly. Other commonly seen signs and symptoms in the severe state include headache, visual disturbances, hyperactive reflexes, and the development of pulmonary edema, along with a dramatic decrease in urine output.

Patients who are preeclamptic have intravascular volume depletion, because a great deal of their body fluid is in the third space. Those who develop severe preeclampsia and eclampsia are at increased risk for cerebral hemorrhage, pulmonary embolism, abruptio placentae, disseminated intravascular coagulopathy (DIC), and the development of renal failure.

Eclampsia, the most serious manifestation of the hypertensive disorders of pregnancy, is characterized by generalized tonic-clonic (major motor) seizure activity. Eclampsia is often preceded by visual disturbances, such as flashing lights or spots before the eyes. The development of epigastric pain or pain in the right upper abdominal quadrant often indicates impending seizure. Eclampsia can often be distinguished from epilepsy by the history and physical appearance of the patient. Patients who become eclamptic are usually grossly edematous and have markedly elevated blood pressure, whereas epileptics usually have a prior history of seizures and are usually taking anticonvulsant medications. If eclampsia develops, death of the mother and fetus frequently results. The risk of fetal mortality increases by 10 percent with each maternal seizure.

● *Chronic hypertension.* Hypertension is considered chronic when the blood pressure is 140/90 or higher before pregnancy or prior to the 20th week of gestation, or if it persists for more than 42 days postpartum. As a general rule, if the diastolic pressure exceeds 80 mmHg during the second trimester, chronic hypertension is likely. The cause of chronic hypertension is unknown. The goal of management is to prevent the development of preeclampsia.

● *Chronic hypertension superimposed with preeclampsia.* It is not uncommon for the chronic hypertensive patient who develops preeclampsia to progress rapidly to eclampsia even prior to the 30th week of gestation. The same diagnostic criteria for preeclampsia are used (systolic blood pressure increases > 30 mmHg over baseline, edema, and protein in the urine).

● *Transient hypertension.* Transient hypertension is defined as a temporary rise in blood pressure that occurs during labor or early in postpartum and normalizes within 10 days.

Assessment Obtaining an accurate history is extremely important when you suspect one of the hypertensive disorders of pregnancy (HDP). Question the patient about excessive weight gain, headaches, visual problems, epigastric or right upper quadrant abdominal pain, apprehension, or seizures. On physical exam, patients with HDP or preeclampsia are usually markedly edematous. They are often pale and apprehensive. The reflexes are hyperactive. The blood pressure, which is usually elevated, should be taken after the patient has rested for 5 minutes in the left lateral recumbent position.

Management Definitive treatment of the hypertensive disorders of pregnancy is delivery of the fetus. However, in the field, use the following management tactics to prevent dangerously high blood pressures or seizure activity.

- *Hypertension.* Closely monitor the patient who is pregnant and has elevated blood pressure without edema or other signs of preeclampsia. Record the fetal heart tones and the mother's blood pressure level.

- *Preeclampsia.* The patient who is hypertensive and shows other signs and symptoms of preeclampsia, such as edema, headaches, and visual disturbances, should be treated quickly. Keep the patient calm and dim the lights. Place the patient in the left lateral recumbent position and quickly carry out the primary assessment. Begin an IV of normal saline. Transport the patient rapidly, without lights or sirens. If the blood pressure is dangerously high (diastolic > 110), medical direction may request the administration of hydralazine (Apresoline) or similar antihypertensives that are safe for use in pregnancy. If the transport time is long, the administration of magnesium sulfate may also be ordered.

- *Eclampsia.* If the patient has already suffered a seizure or a seizure appears to be imminent, then, in addition to the preceding measures, administer oxygen (if the

patient is hypoxic) and manage the airway appropriately. Administer a bolus dose of magnesium sulfate (2 to 5 g diluted in 50 to 100 mL slow IV push) to control the seizures. If you are unable to control the seizures with magnesium sulfate, consider diazepam (Valium) or another sedative. It is important to keep calcium gluconate available for use as an antidote to magnesium sulfate. Also monitor your patient closely for signs (vaginal bleeding or abdominal rigidity) of abruptio placentae or developing pulmonary edema. Transport immediately to a hospital with surgical obstetric and neonatal care availability.

CONTENT REVIEW

▶ Hypertensive Disorders of Pregnancy

- Chronic hypertension
- Pregnancy-induced hypertension
- Preeclampsia
- Eclampsia

Supine Hypotensive Syndrome

Supine hypotensive syndrome usually occurs in the third trimester of pregnancy. Also known as *vena caval syndrome*, supine hypotensive syndrome occurs when the gravid uterus compresses the inferior vena cava when the mother lies in a supine position (Figure 2-11 ●).

Assessment Supine hypotensive syndrome usually occurs in a patient late in her pregnancy who has been supine for a period of time. The patient may complain of dizziness, which results from the decrease in venous return to the right atrium and consequent lowering of the patient's blood pressure. Question the patient about prior episodes of a similar nature and

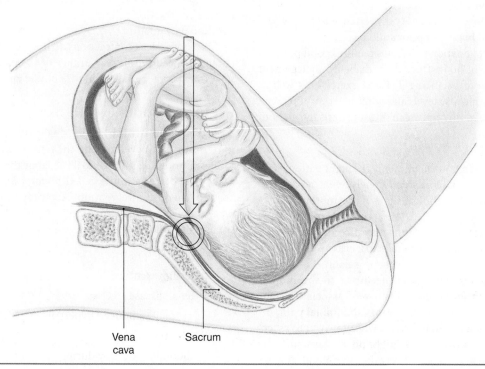

Vena cava

Sacrum

● **Figure 2-11** Supine hypotensive syndrome results from compression of the inferior vena cava by the gravid uterus.

about any recent hemorrhage or fluid loss. Direct the physical examination at determining whether the patient is volume depleted.

Management   If there are no indications of volume depletion, such as decreased skin turgor or thirst, place the patient in the left lateral recumbent position or elevate her right hip. Monitor the fetal heart tones and maternal vital signs frequently. If there is clinical evidence of volume depletion, administer oxygen (if the patient is hypoxic) and start an IV of normal saline. Check for orthostatic changes (a decrease in blood pressure and increase in heart rate when rising from the supine position) and place electrodes for cardiac monitoring. Transport the patient promptly in the left lateral recumbent position.

Gestational Diabetes

Diabetes mellitus occurs in approximately 4 percent of all pregnancies. Hormonal influences cause an increase in insulin production as well as an increased tissue response to insulin during the first 20 weeks of gestation. However, during the last 20 weeks, placental hormones cause an increased resistance to insulin and a decreased glucose tolerance. This causes catabolism (the "breaking down" phase of metabolism) between meals and during the night. At these times, ketones may be present in the urine because fats are metabolized more rapidly. Further, maternal glucose stores are used up, as they are the sole source of glucose to meet the energy needs of the growing fetus. This is known as the *diabetogenic* (diabetes-causing) *effect of pregnancy*. Gestational diabetes usually subsides after pregnancy.

Routine prenatal care includes screening to detect diabetes throughout the pregnancy. Women who are considered to be at high risk for developing gestational diabetes are given a glucose tolerance test at their first prenatal visit. High risk is associated with maternal age (over 35), obesity, hypertension, family history of diabetes, and history of prior stillbirth.

Management of gestational diabetes requires good prenatal care. The mother will be instructed on diabetes management and the importance of balancing diet and exercise, as well as how to monitor her glucose levels and administer insulin. Fetal development will be monitored on an ongoing basis throughout the pregnancy.

Assessment   When you encounter a pregnant patient with an altered mental status, consider hypoglycemia as a likely cause. Remember that the clinical signs and symptoms of hypoglycemia are many and varied. An abnormal mental status is the most important. Physical signs may include diaphoresis and tachycardia. If the blood sugar falls to a critically low level, the patient may sustain a hypoglycemic seizure or become comatose, which poses a potential life threat to the mother and fetus. Obtaining an accurate history of associated signs and symptoms, such as nausea, vomiting, abdominal pain, increased urination, or a recent infection, will allow you to ascertain whether diabetic ketoacidosis might be the cause of your patient's altered mental status. Determine the blood glucose level in addition to obtaining baseline vital signs and FHTs.

Management   If the blood glucose level is noted to be less than 60 mg/dL, draw a red-top tube of blood and start an IV of normal saline. Next, administer 50 to 100 mL (25–50 g) of 50 percent dextrose intravenously. If the patient is conscious and able to swallow, complete glucose administration with orange juice, sugared soft drinks, or commercially available glucose pastes.

If the blood glucose level is in excess of 200 mg/dL, draw a red-top tube (or the tube specified by local protocols) of blood and then establish IV access to administer 1 to 2 L of 0.9 percent sodium chloride per protocol. If transport time is lengthy, medical direction may request intravenous or subcutaneous administration of regular insulin.

Braxton-Hicks Contractions

It is occasionally difficult to determine the onset of labor. As early as the 13th week of gestation, the uterus contracts intermittently, thus conditioning itself for the birth process. It is also believed that these contractions enhance placental circulation. These painless, irregular contractions are known as *Braxton-Hicks contractions*. As the EDC approaches, these contractions become more frequent. Ultimately, the contractions become stronger and more regular, signaling the onset of labor. Labor consists of uterine contractions that cause the dilation and **effacement** (thinning and shortening) of the cervix. The contractions of labor are firm, fairly regular, and quite painful. Prior to the onset of labor Braxton-Hicks contractions, occasionally called *false labor*, increase in intensity and frequency but do not cause cervical changes.

It is virtually impossible to distinguish false labor from true labor in the field. Distinguishing the two requires repeated vaginal examinations, over time, to determine whether the cervix is effacing and dilating. *Remember: Internal vaginal exams should not be performed in the field.* Therefore, all patients with uterine contractions should be transported to the hospital for additional evaluation.

Braxton-Hicks contractions do not require treatment by the paramedic aside from reassurance of the patient and, if necessary, transport for evaluation by a physician.

Preterm Labor

As you have already learned, normal gestation is 40 weeks and, in terms of fetal development, the fetus is not considered to be full term until the 38th week. True labor that begins before the 38th week of gestation is called *preterm labor* and frequently requires medical intervention. A variety of maternal, fetal, or placental factors may cause this potentially life-threatening situation for the mother and fetus.

- Maternal factors
  - Cardiovascular disease
  - Renal disease
  - Pregnancy-induced hypertension (PIH)
  - Diabetes
  - Abdominal surgery during gestation
  - Uterine and cervical abnormalities

- ○ Maternal infection
- ○ Trauma, particularly blows to the abdomen
- ○ Contributory factors: history of preterm birth, smoking, and cocaine abuse
- Placental factors
  - ○ Placenta previa
  - ○ Abruptio placentae
- Fetal factors
  - ○ Multiple gestation
  - ○ Excessive amniotic fluid
  - ○ Fetal infection

In many cases, physicians attempt to stop preterm labor to give the fetus additional time to develop in the uterus. Prematurity is the primary neonatal health problem in the nation and occurs in 7 to 10 percent of all live births. All of the preterm infant's organ systems are immature to some degree, but lung development is of greatest concern. Although technological advances in the care of preterm infants have improved the prognosis dramatically, the consequences of a preterm birth can last a lifetime.

Assessment When confronted by a patient with uterine contractions, first determine the approximate gestational age of the fetus. If it is less than 38 weeks, then suspect preterm labor. If gestational age is greater than 38 weeks, treat the patient as a term patient, as described later in this chapter.

After determining gestational age, obtain a brief obstetric history. Then question the mother about the urge to push or the need to move her bowels or urinate. Also ask if her membranes have ruptured. Any sensation of fluid leakage or "gushing" from the vagina should be interpreted as ruptured membranes until proven otherwise. Next, palpate the contractions by placing your hand on the patient's abdomen. Note the intensity and length of the contractions, as well as the interval between contractions.

Commonly reported signs and symptoms of preterm labor include contractions that occur every 10 minutes or less, low abdominal cramping that is similar to menstrual cramps, or a sensation of pelvic pressure. Other complaints, such as low backache, changes in vaginal discharge, and abdominal cramping with or without diarrhea, may also be reported. Rupture of the membranes is confirmatory for preterm labor.

Management Preterm labor, especially if quite early in the pregnancy, should be stopped if possible. The process of stopping labor, or **tocolysis**, is frequently practiced in obstetrics. However, it is infrequently done in the field.

There are three general approaches to tocolysis. The first is to sedate the patient, often with narcotics or barbiturates, thus allowing her to rest. Often, after a period of rest, the contractions stop on their own. The second approach is to administer a fluid bolus intravenously. The administration of approximately 1 liter of fluid intravenously increases the intravascular fluid volume, thus inhibiting ADH secretion from the posterior pituitary. Because oxytocin and ADH are secreted from the same area of the pituitary gland, the inhibition of

ADH secretion also inhibits oxytocin release, often causing cessation of uterine contractions. Ultimately, if the previous methods fail, magnesium sulfate or a beta-agonist, such as terbutaline or ritodrine, may be administered to stop labor by inhibiting uterine smooth muscle contraction. Current research in tocolysis includes the administration of calcium channel blockers, such as nifedipine, and prostaglandin inhibitors, such as indomethacin. You may also find that a patient with preterm labor has been given corticosteroids to accelerate fetal lung maturity.

As a rule, tocolysis in the field is limited to sedation and hydration, especially if transport time is long. Paramedics may, however, transport a patient from one medical facility to another with beta-agonist administration under way. You should therefore be familiar with its use. Commonly associated side effects include being jittery, tachycardia usually described by the patient as palpitations, and occasionally abdominal pain. You will, of course, want to transport your patient to the nearest facility that has neonatal intensive care capabilities. Careful and frequent monitoring of maternal vital signs and FHTs is imperative during tocolysis.

THE PUERPERIUM

The **puerperium** is the time period surrounding birth of the fetus. Childbirth generally occurs in a hospital or similar facility with appropriate equipment. Occasionally, prehospital personnel may be called on to attend a delivery in the field. Therefore, you should be familiar with the birth process and some of the complications that may be associated with it.

Labor

Childbirth, or the delivery of the fetus, is the culmination of pregnancy. The process by which delivery occurs is called **labor**, the physiologic and mechanical process in which the baby, placenta, and amniotic sac are expelled through the birth canal. The duration of labor is widely variable.

Prior to the onset of true labor, the head of the fetus descends into the bony pelvis area. The frequency and intensity of the Braxton-Hicks contractions increase in preparation for true labor. Increased vaginal secretions and softening of the cervix occur. Bloody show—pink-tinged secretions—is generally considered a sign of imminent labor as the mucus plug is expelled from the cervix. Labor then usually begins within 24 to 48 hours. Many people also consider the rupture of the membranes as a sign of impending labor. If labor does not begin spontaneously within 12 to 24 hours after rupture, labor will likely require induction because of the risk of infection.

Pressure exerted by the fetus on the cervix causes changes that lead to the subsequent expulsion of the fetus. Muscular uterine contractions increase in frequency, strength, and duration. You can assess the frequency and duration of contractions by placing one hand on the fundus of the uterus. Time contractions from the beginning of one contraction until the beginning of the next. It is important to note whether the uterus relaxes

CONTENT REVIEW

► Stages of Labor

  • Stage one: dilation
  • Stage two: expulsion
  • Stage three: placental

completely between contractions. It is also desirable to monitor fetal heart tones during and between contractions. Occasional fetal bradycardia occurs during contractions, but the heart rate should increase to a normal rate (120–160) after the contraction ends. Failure of the heart rate to return to normal between contractions is a sign of fetal distress.

Labor is generally divided into three stages (Figure 2-12 ●):

● *Stage one (dilation stage).* The first stage of labor begins with the onset of true labor contractions and ends with the complete dilation and effacement of the cervix. Early in pregnancy the cervix is quite thick and long, but after complete *effacement* it is short and paper thin. Effacement usually begins several days before active labor ensues. *Dilation* is the progressive stretching of the cervical opening. The cervix dilates from its closed position to 10 centimeters, which is considered complete dilation. This stage lasts approximately 8 to 10 hours for the woman in her first labor, the nullipara, and about 5 to 7 hours in the woman who has given birth previously, the multipara. Early in this stage the contractions are usually mild, lasting for 15 to 20 seconds with a frequency of 10 to 20 minutes. As labor progresses, the contractions increase in intensity and occur approximately every 2 to 3 minutes with duration of 60 seconds.

● *Stage two (expulsion stage).* The second stage of labor begins with the complete dilation of the cervix and ends with the delivery of the fetus. In the nullipara, this stage lasts 50 to 60 minutes, whereas it takes about half that amount of time for the multipara. The contractions are very strong, occurring every 2 minutes and lasting for 60 to 75 seconds. Often, the patient feels pain in her lower back as the fetus descends into the pelvis. The urge to push or "bear down" usually begins in the second stage. The membranes usually rupture at this time, if they have not ruptured previously. Crowning during contractions is evident as the delivery of the fetus nears. Crowning occurs when the head (or other presenting part of the fetus) is visible at the vaginal opening during a contraction and is the definitive sign that birth is imminent. The most common presentation is for the infant to be delivered headfirst, face down (vertex position).

● *Stage three (placental stage).* The third and final stage of labor begins immediately after the birth of the infant and ends with the delivery of the placenta. The placenta generally delivers within 5 to 20 minutes. There is no need to delay transport to wait for its delivery. Classic signs of placental separation include a gush of blood from the vagina; a change in size, shape, or consistency of the uterus; lengthening of the umbilical cord protruding from the vagina; and the mother's report that she has the urge to push. There will be a continued vaginal discharge called **lochia** that contains blood, mucus, and placental tissue. It will often continue for four to six weeks after delivery.

First stage: beginning of contractions to full cervical dilation

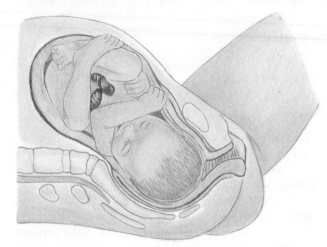

Second stage: baby enters birth canal and is born

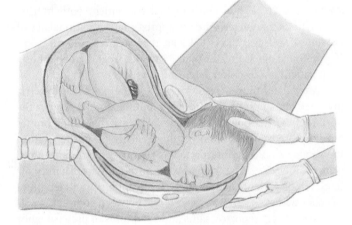
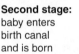

Third stage: delivery of the placenta

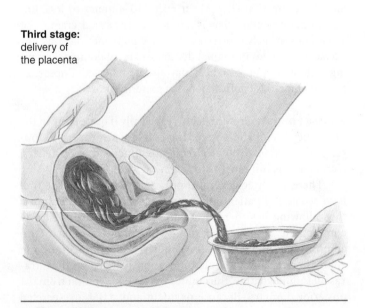

● **Figure 2-12** Stages of labor.

Management of a Patient in Labor

Probably one of the most important decisions you must make with a patient in labor is whether to attempt to deliver the infant at the scene or to transport the patient to the hospital (Figure 2-13 ●). It is generally preferable to transport the mother unless delivery is imminent. Several factors must be taken into consideration when making this decision. They include the patient's number of previous pregnancies, the length of labor during the previous pregnancies, the frequency of contractions, the maternal urge to push, and the presence of crowning. Some women have rapid labors and may be completely dilated in a short period of time. Also, as mentioned, multiparas generally have shorter labors than nulliparas. The maternal urge to push or the presence of crowning indicates that delivery is imminent. In such cases, the infant should be delivered at the scene or in the ambulance.

Traditionally, a woman who had previously delivered by a cesarean section was advised to deliver all subsequent infants by cesarean sections. However, current thinking encourages women to attempt vaginal birth after cesarean (VBAC). If your patient has had prenatal care during this pregnancy she has probably already discussed this with her health care provider. The only absolute contraindication for VBAC is a classic vertical uterine incision. However, most cesarean sections done today are done using a low transverse uterine incision. (Note that a horizontal skin incision does not ensure that the uterine incision is horizontal.) A labor patient who is opting for VBAC requires no more special care than any other labor patient does.

However, certain factors should prompt immediate transport, despite the threat of delivery. These include prolonged rupture of membranes (>24 hours), as prolonged time between rupture and delivery often leads to fetal infection; abnormal presentation, such as breech or transverse; prolapsed cord; or fetal distress, as evidenced by fetal bradycardia or meconium staining (the presence of meconium, the first fetal stools, in the amniotic fluid). The presence of multiple fetuses may also contribute to your decision to transport. You will read more about these conditions later in this chapter.

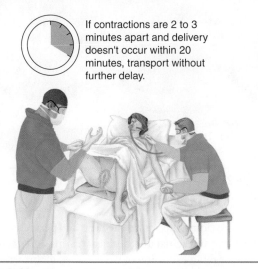

If contractions are 2 to 3 minutes apart and delivery doesn't occur within 20 minutes, transport without further delay.

● **Figure 2-13**   The decision to deliver at the scene or to attempt transport is often a difficult one.

Field Delivery

If delivery is imminent, you can assist the mother to deliver the baby in the field (Procedure 2–1 and Figures 2-14 ● through 2-21 ●). Equipment and facilities must be prepared quickly. Set up a delivery area. This should be out of public view, such as in a bedroom or the back of the ambulance. Administer oxygen to the mother (if she is hypoxic) via nasal cannula or nonrebreather mask. If time permits, establish intravenous access and administer normal saline at a keep-open rate. Place the patient on her back with knees and hips flexed and buttocks slightly elevated. It should be noted that this position is easier on you than on the mother. She may prefer to squat or lie in a semi-Fowler's position with her knees and hips flexed. Either of these positions enables gravity to facilitate the delivery. If time permits, drape the mother with toweling from the OB kit. Place one towel under the buttocks, another below the vaginal opening, and another across the lower abdomen.

Until delivery, the fetal heart rate should be monitored frequently. A drop in the fetal heart rate to less than 90 beats per minute indicates fetal distress and requires prompt immediate transport with the mother in the left lateral recumbent position. Coach the mother to breathe deeply between contractions and to push with contractions. If the baby does not deliver after

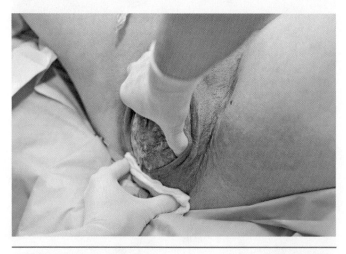

● **Figure 2-14**   Crowning.

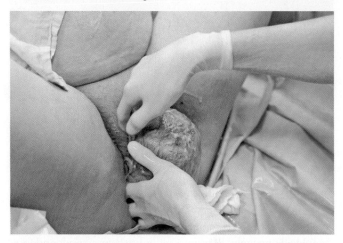

● **Figure 2-15**   Delivery of the head.

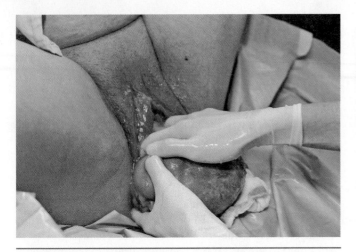

● **Figure 2-16** External rotation of the head.

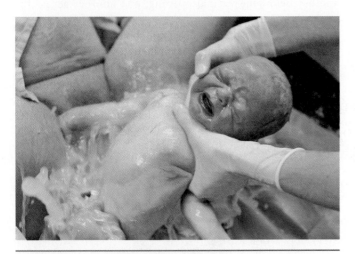

● **Figure 2-17** Delivery of the torso.

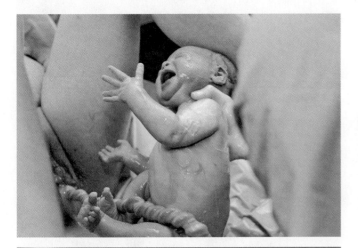

● **Figure 2-18** Complete delivery of the infant.

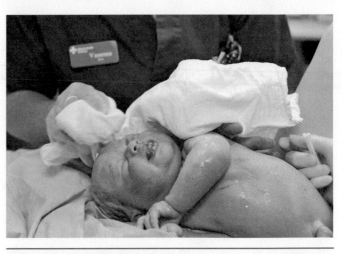

● **Figure 2-19** Dry the infant.

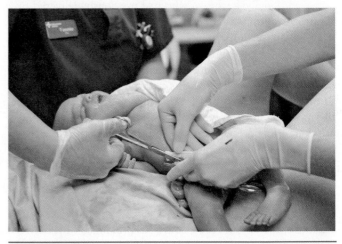

● **Figure 2-20** Place the infant on the mother's stomach and cut the umbilical cord.

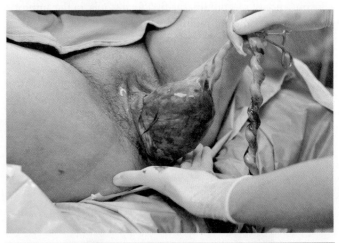

● **Figure 2-21** Deliver the placenta and save it for transport with the mother and infant.

20 minutes of contractions every 2 to 3 minutes, *transport immediately*.

Prepare the OB equipment and don sterile gloves, gown, and face shield or goggles. If time permits, wash your hands and forearms prior to gloving. As the head crowns, control it with gentle

pressure. Providing support to the head and perineum decreases the likelihood of vaginal and perineal tearing and decreases the potential for rapid expulsion of the baby's skull through the birth canal, which may cause intracranial injury. Support the head as it emerges from the vagina and begins to turn. If it is still enclosed

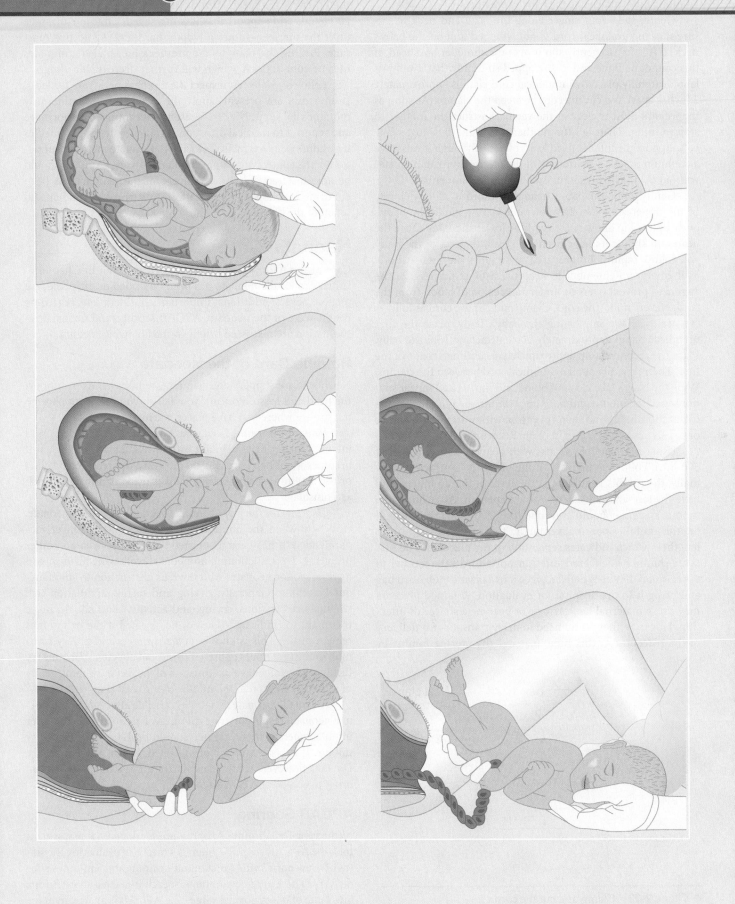

in the amniotic sac, tear the sac open to permit escape of the amniotic fluid and enable the baby to breathe.

Gently slide your finger along the head and neck to ensure that the umbilical cord is not wrapped around the baby's neck. If it is, try to gently slip it over the shoulder and head. If this cannot be done and it is wrapped so tightly that it inhibits labor, carefully place two umbilical cord clamps approximately 2 inches apart and cut the cord between the clamps. As soon as the infant's head is clear of the vagina, instruct the mother to stop pushing. Then tell the mother to resume pushing, while you support the infant's head as it rotates. Although it was once a common practice, suctioning of the nasopharynx in neonates without obvious obstruction is no longer recommended.

Gently guide the baby's head downward to allow delivery of the upper shoulder. Do not pull! Gently guide the baby's body upward to allow delivery of the lower shoulder. Once the head and shoulders have been delivered, the rest of the body will follow rapidly. Be prepared to support the infant's body as it emerges. Remember to keep the baby at the level of the vagina to prevent over- or undertransfusion of blood from the cord. Never "milk" the cord. Clamp and cut the cord as follows (Figure 2-22 ●): Supporting the baby's body, place the first umbilical clamp approximately 10 centimeters from the baby. Place the second clamp approximately 5 centimeters above the first. Then carefully cut the umbilical cord between the clamps. Wipe the baby's face clean of blood and mucus and repeat suctioning of the mouth and nose until the airway is clear. Dry the infant thoroughly and then cover him with warm, dry blankets or towels, and position on his side. Record the time of birth.

Usual maternal blood loss with delivery is 1 pint (about 500 mL). Following delivery, if the uterus is contracting normally, the fundus should be at the level of the umbilicus and have the size and consistency of a grapefruit. After birth, the mother's vagina should continue to ooze blood. Do not pull on the umbilical cord. Eventually, the cord will appear to lengthen, which indicates separation of the placenta. The placenta should be delivered and transported with the mother to the hospital. If it does deliver, place it in a plastic biohazard bag and bring it to the hospital for evaluation. Retained placenta may cause maternal hemorrhage or become a source of infection. However, there is no need to delay transport for delivery of the placenta. At this time, massage the uterine fundus by

placing one hand immediately above the pubic symphysis and the other on the uterine fundus. Cup the uterus between the two hands and support it as it is massaged. Continue massage until the uterus assumes a woody hardness. Avoid overmassage. Putting the baby to the mother's breast also stimulates uterine contractions, which will further decrease bleeding.

Following delivery, inspect the mother's perineum for tears. If any tears are present, apply direct pressure. Continuously monitor vital signs. Note the presence of continued hemorrhage and report it to medical direction. In some systems, paramedics may administer oxytocin (Pitocin) to facilitate uterine contraction in the control of postpartum hemorrhage. Oxytocin should be administered only *after* delivery of the placenta has been confirmed. Following stabilization, transport the mother and infant to the hospital.

Neonatal Care

Care of the **neonate** will be discussed in detail in Chapter 3. Initial care of the neonate has been described in the preceding section. Several additional important considerations regarding routine care of the neonate, APGAR scoring, and neonatal resuscitation are discussed briefly in the following sections.

Routine Care of the Neonate

Newborns are slippery and will require both hands to support the head and torso. Position yourself so you can work close to the surface where you have placed the infant.

Maintain warmth! Cold infants rapidly become distressed infants. Quickly dry the infant with towels, discarding each as it becomes wet. Then cover the infant with a dry receiving blanket or use a commercial warming blanket made of a material such as Thinsulate™.

Clearing the airway. Routine suctioning of the neonate, especially when the amniotic fluid is clear, is no longer recommended. It has been associated with bradycardia and other problems. Thus, suctioning immediately following birth should be reserved for neonates with obvious obstruction to spontaneous breathing. Generally, drying and tactile stimulation will stimulate respirations, crying, and activity.[4] This should cause the infant to "pink up." (Do not be alarmed if the extremities remain dusky. This is known as *acrocyanosis* and is very common in the first hours of life.) If this is not effective, you may try flicking your finger against the soles of the feet or rubbing gently in a circular motion in the middle of the back (Figure 2-23 ●).

Assess the neonate as soon as possible after birth. The normal neonatal respiratory rate should average 30 to 60 breaths per minute, whereas the heart rate should be 100 to 180 beats per minute. If resuscitation is not indicated, assign APGAR scores. Do not, however, delay resuscitative efforts and transport in order to complete APGAR scoring.

APGAR Scoring

Named for Dr. Virginia Apgar, who developed the assessment tool, the APGAR scoring system is a means of evaluating the status of a newborn's vital functions at 1 minute and 5 minutes after delivery. There are five parameters; each is given a score from a low value of 0 to a normal value of 2. APGAR is an acronym for

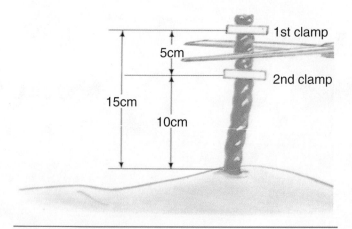

● **Figure 2-22** Clamp and cut the cord.

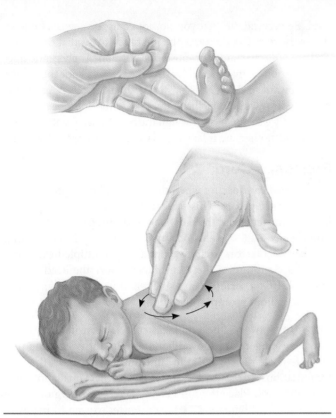

● **Figure 2-23** Stimulate the infant as required.

the names of the five parameters, which are **a**ppearance (skin color), **p**ulse rate, **g**rimace (irritability), **a**ctivity (muscle tone), and **r**espiratory effort (Table 2–2).

The majority of infants are healthy and active and have total scores between 7 and 10, requiring only routine care. Infants scoring between 4 and 6 are moderately depressed and require oxygen and stimulation to breathe. Infants scoring 0 to 3 are severely depressed and require immediate ventilatory and circulatory assistance. By repeating the score at 1 and 5 minutes, it is possible to determine whether intervention has caused a change in infant status.

Neonatal Resuscitation

It is estimated that approximately 6 percent of all neonates born in a hospital require resuscitation. It is likely that this percentage is higher for out-of-hospital deliveries, although the exact numbers are not available. Factors that contribute to the need for resuscitation include prematurity, pregnancy and delivery complications, maternal health problems, or inadequate prenatal care.

If tactile stimulation does not increase the neonate's respiratory rate, immediately assist ventilations using a pediatric bag-valve mask with room air initially. If the respiratory rate is now within normal limits, assess the heart rate. If not, continue ventilations.

Assess the heart rate using a stethoscope to auscultate the apical pulse, by feeling the pulse at the base of the umbilical cord, or by palpating the brachial or femoral artery. The heart rate should normally be between 100 and 180 beats per minute, with a range of 140 to 160 beats per minute being optimal. If the pulse is 100 or greater with spontaneous respirations, continue your assessment. If the rate is less than 100, continue positive pressure ventilations. Initiate chest compressions if the heart rate is less than 60 beats per minute and is not responding to ventilations. Continue to reassess respiratory status and heart rate frequently.

Make every effort to expedite transport to a facility capable of providing neonatal intensive care while you continue resuscitative efforts. If you have a long transport time, it may be necessary to initiate vascular access to administer medications or fluid resuscitation. The most logical (and easiest) access is the umbilical vein. If this is not feasible, consider peripheral veins or an intraosseous access. During transport, continue to maintain warmth while supporting ventilations, oxygenation, and circulation. Refer to Chapter 3 for more information regarding neonatal resuscitation.

Abnormal Delivery Situations
Breech Presentation

Most infants present head first and face down, which is called the *vertex position*. *Breech presentation* is the term used to describe the situation in which either the buttocks or both feet present first. This occurs in approximately 4 percent of all

CONTENT REVIEW

▶ Abnormal Deliveries

• Breech presentation
• Prolapsed cord
• Limb presentation
• Occiput posterior

TABLE 2–2	The APGAR Score				
Element	**0**	**1**	**2**	**Score**	
Appearance (skin color)	Body and extremities blue, pale	Body pink, extremities blue	Completely pink		
Pulse Rate	Absent	Below 100/min	100/min or above		
Grimace (irritability)	No response	Grimace	Cough, sneeze, cry		
Activity (muscle tone)	Limp	Some flexion of extremities	Active motion		
Respiratory Effort	Absent	Slow and irregular	Strong cry		
			TOTAL SCORE =		

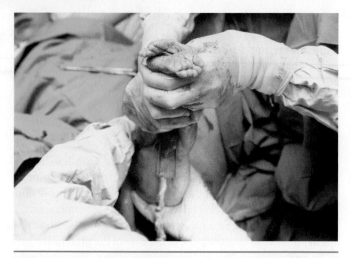

● **Figure 2-24** Breech delivery. (© *Science Photo Library/ Custom Medical Stock Photo*)

live births. In such presentations, there is an increased risk for delivery trauma to the mother, as well as an increased potential for cord prolapse, cord compression, or anoxic insult for the infant. Although the cause is unknown, breech presentations are most commonly associated with preterm birth, placenta previa, multiple gestation, and uterine and fetal anomalies.

Management   Because cesarean section is often required, delivery of the breech presentation is best accomplished at the hospital. However, if field delivery is unavoidable, the following maneuvers are recommended. First, position the mother with her buttocks at the edge of a firm bed. Ask her to hold her legs in a flexed position. She will often require assistance in doing this. As the infant delivers, do not pull on the infant's legs. Simply support them. Allow the entire body to be delivered with contractions while you merely continue to support the infant's body (Figure 2-24 ●).

As the head passes the pubis, apply gentle upward traction until the mouth appears over the perineum. If the head does not deliver, and the baby begins to breathe spontaneously with its face pressed against the vaginal wall, place a gloved hand in the vagina with the palm toward the infant's face. Form a "V" with the index and middle fingers on either side of the infant's nose, and push the vaginal wall away from the infant's face to allow unrestricted respiration (Figure 2-25 ●). If necessary, continue during transport.

Alternatively, you may find that the shoulders, not the head, are the most difficult part to deliver. In that case, allow the body to deliver to the level of the umbilicus. Support the infant's body in your palm while gently extracting approximately 4 to 6 inches of umbilical

cord. Be very careful that you do not compress the cord during this extraction. Gently rotate the infant's body so that the shoulders are now in an anterior–posterior position. Apply gentle traction to the body until the axillae become visible. Guide the infant's body upward to deliver the posterior shoulder. Then, guide the neonate downward to facilitate delivery of the anterior shoulder. Now gently ease the head through the birth canal. Continue your care of the mother and infant as you would with a normal delivery.

Prolapsed Cord

A *prolapsed cord* occurs when the umbilical cord precedes the fetal presenting part. This causes the cord to be compressed between the fetus and the bony pelvis, shutting off fetal circulation (Figure 2-26 ●). This occurs once in every 250 deliveries. Predisposing factors include prematurity, multiple births, and premature rupture of the membranes before the head is fully engaged. It is a serious emergency, and fetal death will occur quickly without prompt intervention.

Management   If the umbilical cord is seen in the vagina, insert two fingers of a gloved hand to raise the presenting part of the fetus off the cord. At the same time, gently check the cord for pulsations, but take great care to ensure that you do not compress the cord. Place the mother in a Trendelenburg or knee–chest position (Figure 2-27 ●). Administer oxygen (if hypoxic) and transport her immediately, with the fingers continuing to hold the presenting part off the umbilical cord. If assistance is available, apply a dressing moistened with sterile saline to the exposed cord. *Do not attempt delivery. Do not pull on the cord. Do not attempt to push the cord back into the vagina.*

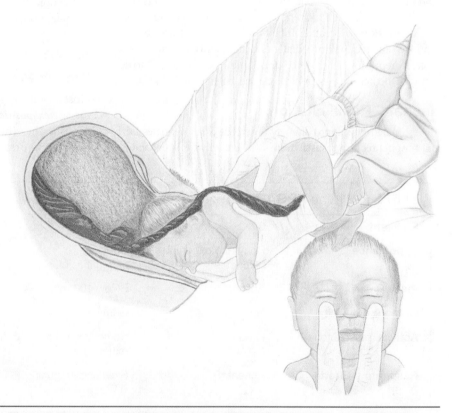

● **Figure 2-25**   Placement of the fingers to maintain the airway in a breech birth.

Limb Presentation

Sometimes, if the baby is in a transverse lie across the uterus, an arm or leg is the presenting part protruding from the vagina. This is seen in less than 1 percent of births and is more commonly associated with preterm birth and multiple gestation.

Management When examination of the perineum reveals a single arm or leg protruding from the birth canal, a cesarean section is necessary. Under no circumstance should you attempt a field delivery. Do not touch the extremity, as to do so may stimulate the infant to gasp, risking inhalation and aspiration of amniotic fluid. *Do not pull on the extremity or attempt to push it back into the vagina.*

Assist the mother into a knee–chest position, as is also done when there is a prolapsed cord, and administer oxygen (if the mother is hypoxic). Provide reassurance to the mother. Transport immediately (still in knee–chest position) for emergency cesarean section.

Other Abnormal Presentations

Other abnormal presentations can complicate delivery. One of the most common is the *occiput posterior position.* Normally, as the infant descends into the pelvis, its face is turned posteriorly. This is important, as extension of the head assists delivery. However, if the infant descends facing forward, or occiput posterior, its passage through the pelvis is delayed. This presentation occurs most frequently in primigravidas. In multigravidas it usually resolves spontaneously.

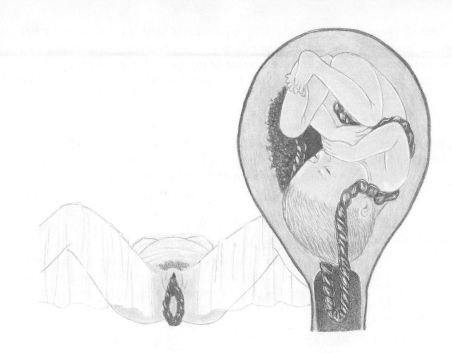

- Elevate hips, administer oxygen, and keep warm
- Keep baby's head away from cord
- Do not attempt to push cord back
- Wrap cord in sterile moist towel
- Transport mother to hospital, continuing pressure on baby's head

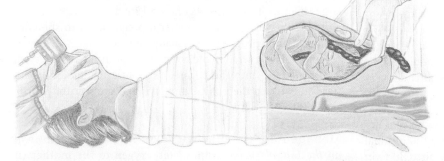

● **Figure 2-26** Prolapsed cord.

● **Figure 2-27** Patient positioning for prolapsed cord.

The presenting part may also be the face or brow, rather than the crown of the head. Occasionally, during these presentations, the face or brow can be seen high in the pelvis during a contraction. Usually, vaginal delivery is impossible in these cases.

As described earlier for a limb presentation, the fetus can lie transversely in the uterus. In such a case, the fetus cannot enter the pelvis for delivery. If the membranes rupture, the umbilical cord can prolapse, or an arm or leg can enter the vagina. Vaginal delivery is impossible.

Management Early recognition of an abnormal presentation is important. If one is suspected, the mother should be reassured, placed on oxygen (if hypoxic), and transported immediately, as forceps or cesarean delivery is often required.

Other Delivery Complications

Although most deliveries proceed without incident, complications can arise. Therefore, you should be prepared to deal with them.

Multiple Births

Multiple births are fairly rare, with twins occurring in approximately 1 in 90 deliveries, about 40 percent of those being preterm. Usually, the mother knows of, or at least suspects, the presence of more than one fetus. Multiple births should also be suspected if the mother's abdomen remains large after delivery of one baby and labor continues.

Management Manage this situation with the normal delivery guidelines, recognizing that you will need additional personnel and equipment to manage a multiple birth. In twin births, labor often begins earlier than expected, and the infants are generally smaller than babies born singly. Usually, one twin presents vertex and the other breech. There may be one shared placenta or two placentas. After delivery of the first baby, clamp and cut the cord. Then deliver the second baby. Because prematurity is common in multiple births, low birth weight is common and prevention of hypothermia is even more crucial.

Cephalopelvic Disproportion

Cephalopelvic disproportion occurs when the infant's head is too big to pass through the maternal pelvis easily. This may be caused by an oversized fetus. Large fetuses are associated with diabetes, multiparity, or postmaturity. Fetal abnormalities such as hydrocephalus, conjoined twins, or fetal tumors may make vaginal delivery impossible. Women of short stature or women with contracted pelvises are at increased risk for this problem. If cephalopelvic disproportion is not recognized and managed appropriately, fetal demise or uterine rupture may occur.

Cephalopelvic disproportion tends to develop most frequently in the primigravida. There may be strong contractions for an extended period of time. On physical examination, the fetus may feel large. Also, labor generally does not progress. The fetus may be in distress, as evidenced by fetal bradycardia or meconium staining.

Management The usual management of cephalopelvic disproportion is cesarean section. Administer oxygen to the mother (if she is hypoxic) and establish intravenous access. Transport should be immediate and rapid.

Precipitous Delivery

A *precipitous delivery* is a delivery that occurs after less than 3 hours of labor. This type of delivery occurs most frequently in the grand multipara and is associated with a higher-than-normal incidence of fetal trauma, tearing of the umbilical cord, or maternal lacerations.

Management The best way to handle precipitous delivery is to be prepared. Do not turn your attention from the mother. Be ready for a rapid delivery, and attempt to control the infant's head. Once delivered, the baby may have some difficulty with temperature regulation and must be kept warm.

Shoulder Dystocia

A *shoulder dystocia* occurs when the infant's shoulders are larger than its head. This occurs most frequently with diabetic and obese mothers and in postterm pregnancies. In shoulder dystocia, labor progresses normally and the head is delivered routinely. However, immediately after the head is delivered, it retracts back into the perineum because the shoulders are trapped between the pubic symphysis and the sacrum ("turtle sign") (Figure 2-28 ●).

Management If a shoulder dystocia occurs, *do not pull on the infant's head*. Administer oxygen to the mother (if she is hypoxic) and have her drop her buttocks off the end of the bed. Then flex her thighs upward to facilitate delivery and apply firm pressure with an open hand immediately above the pubic symphysis (McRobert's maneuver). If delivery does not occur, transport the patient immediately (Figure 2-29 ●).

Meconium Staining

Meconium staining occurs when the fetus passes feces into the amniotic fluid. Between 10 and 30 percent of all deliveries have meconium-stained fluid. It is always indicative of a fetal hypoxic incident. Hypoxia causes an increase in fetal peristalsis along with relaxation of the anal sphincter, causing meconium to pass into the amniotic fluid. In addition to the stress that caused the incident, there is a risk of aspiration of the meconium-stained fluid.

Meconium staining is often associated with prolonged labor but may be seen in term, postterm, and low-birth-weight infants. The incident may occur a few days prior to delivery or during labor. Some meconium staining is virtually

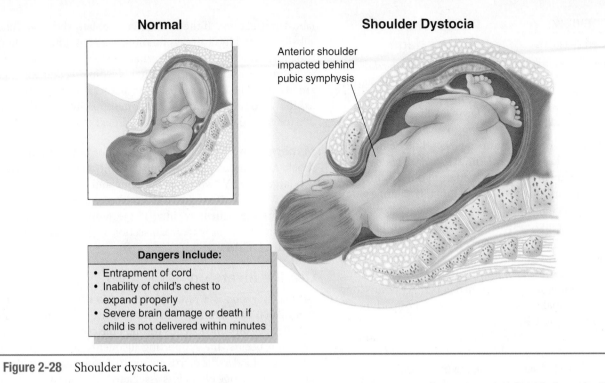

Normal

Shoulder Dystocia

Anterior shoulder impacted behind pubic symphysis

Dangers Include:
• Entrapment of cord
• Inability of child's chest to expand properly
• Severe brain damage or death if child is not delivered within minutes

● **Figure 2-28**   Shoulder dystocia.

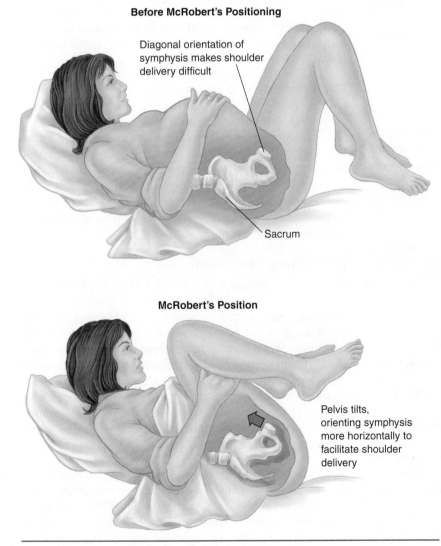

Before McRobert's Positioning

Diagonal orientation of symphysis makes shoulder delivery difficult

Sacrum

McRobert's Position

Pelvis tilts, orienting symphysis more horizontally to facilitate shoulder delivery

● **Figure 2-29**   McRobert's maneuver for shoulder dystocia.

always associated with breech deliveries as a result of vagal stimulation, which occurs as a result of the pressure of the contracting uterus on the fetus's head.

Evidence of meconium staining is readily observable. Normally the amniotic fluid is clear or possibly light-straw colored. When meconium is present, the color varies from a light yellowish-green to light green or, worst case, dark green, which is sometimes described as "pea soup." As a rule, the thicker and darker the color, the higher the risk of fetal morbidity.

Management   As noted earlier, bulb suctioning is no longer recommended. If the meconium is thin and light colored, no further treatment is generally required and you should continue with the delivery and routine care. However, if the meconium is thick, visualize the glottis and suction the hypopharynx and trachea using an endotracheal tube until you have cleared all of the meconium from the newborn's airway. Failure to do so will cause the meconium to be pushed farther into the airway and down into the lungs during the delivery process.

Maternal Complications of Labor and Delivery

Several maternal problems can arise during and after delivery. These include postpartum hemorrhage, uterine rupture, uterine inversion, and pulmonary embolism.

CONTENT REVIEW

► Maternal Complications

- Postpartum hemorrhage
- Uterine rupture
- Uterine inversion
- Pulmonary embolism

Postpartum Hemorrhage

Postpartum hemorrhage is the loss of more than 500 mL of blood immediately following delivery. It occurs in approximately 5 percent of deliveries. The most common cause of postpartum hemorrhage is *uterine atony,* or lack of uterine muscle tone. This tends to occur most frequently in the multigravida and is most common following multiple births or births of large infants. Uterine atony also occurs after precipitous deliveries and prolonged labors. In addition to uterine atony, postpartum hemorrhage can be caused by placenta previa, abruptio placentae, retained placental parts, clotting disorders in the mother, or vaginal and cervical tears. Occasionally, the uterus fails to return to its normal size during the postpartum period, and postpartum hemorrhage occurs long after the birth, potentially as much as two weeks postpartum.

Assessment of the patient with postpartum hemorrhage should focus on the history and the predisposing factors as described. You must rely heavily on the clinical appearance of the patient and her vital signs. Often, the uterus will feel boggy and soft on physical examination. Vaginal bleeding is usually obvious as a steady, free flow of blood. Counting the number of sanitary pads used is a good way to monitor the bleeding. When postpartum bleeding takes place in the hospital setting the pads are often weighed, as 500 mL of blood weighs approximately 1 pound. You should also examine the perineum for evidence of traumatic injury, which may be the source of the bleeding.

Management When confronted by a patient with postpartum hemorrhage, complete the primary assessment immediately. Administer oxygen (if the patient is hypoxic) and begin fundal massage. Establish at least one, preferably two, large-bore IVs of normal saline. Never attempt to force delivery of the placenta or pack the vagina with dressings. In severe cases, medical direction may request the administration of oxytocin (Pitocin). The usual dose is 10 to 20 USP units (20 mg) oxytocin in 1 liter of normal saline to run at 125 mL/hour titrated to response. If IV access cannot be obtained, an alternative therapy is to administer 10 USP units intramuscularly.

Uterine Rupture

Uterine rupture is the actual tearing, or rupture, of the uterus. It usually occurs with the onset of labor. However, it can also occur before labor as a result of blunt abdominal trauma. During labor, it often results from prolonged uterine contractions or a surgically scarred uterus, such as that which occurs from previous cesarean sections, especially in those with the classic vertical incision. It can also occur following a prolonged or obstructed labor, as in the case of cephalopelvic disproportion or in conjunction with abnormal presentations. Although it is a rare occurrence, it carries with it an extremely high maternal and fetal mortality rate.

The patient with uterine rupture will complain of excruciating abdominal pain and will often be in shock. Uterine rupture is virtually always associated with the cessation of labor contractions. If the rupture is complete, the pain usually subsides. On physical examination, there is often profound shock without evidence of external hemorrhage, although it is sometimes associated with vaginal bleeding. Fetal heart tones are absent. The abdomen is often tender and rigid and may exhibit rebound tenderness. It is often possible to palpate the uterus as a separate hard mass found next to the fetus.

Management Management is the same as for any patient in shock. Administer oxygen at high concentration. Next, establish two large-bore IVs with normal saline and begin fluid resuscitation. Monitor vital signs and fetal heart tones continuously. Transport the patient rapidly. If the fetus is still viable, the definitive treatment is cesarean section with subsequent repair or removal of the uterus.

Uterine Inversion

Uterine inversion is a rare emergency, occurring only once in every 2,500 live births. It occurs when the uterus turns inside out after delivery and extends through the cervix. When uterine inversion occurs, the supporting ligaments and blood vessels supplying blood to the uterus are torn, usually causing profound shock. The average blood loss associated with uterine inversion ranges from 800 to 1,800 mL. Uterine inversion usually results from pulling on the umbilical cord while awaiting delivery of the placenta or from attempts to express the placenta when the uterus is relaxed.

Management If uterine inversion occurs, you must act quickly. First, place the patient in a supine position and begin oxygen administration (if the patient is hypoxic). *Do not* attempt to detach the placenta or pull on the cord. Initiate two large-bore IVs of normal saline and begin fluid resuscitation. Make one attempt to replace the uterus, using the following technique. With the palm of the hand, push the fundus of the inverted uterus toward the vagina. If this single attempt is unsuccessful, cover the uterus with towels moistened with saline and transport the patient immediately.

Pulmonary Embolism

Pulmonary embolism is the presence of a blood clot in the pulmonary vascular system (see Volume 5, Chapter 1). It can occur after pregnancy, usually as a result of venous thromboembolism. It is one of the most common causes of maternal death and appears to occur more frequently following cesarean section than vaginal delivery. Pulmonary embolism may occur at any time during pregnancy. There is usually a sudden onset of severe dyspnea accompanied by sharp chest pain. Some patients also report a sense of impending doom. On physical examination, the patient may show tachycardia, tachypnea, jugular vein distention, and, in severe cases, hypotension.

Management Management of pulmonary embolism consists of administration of high-concentration oxygen and ventilatory support as needed. Also establish an IV of normal saline at a keep-open rate. Initiate cardiac monitoring and carefully monitor the patient's vital signs and oxygen saturation while transporting her immediately.

SUMMARY

Childbirth is a normal process and obstetric emergencies are fairly uncommon. However, all pregnant patients are at risk for developing complications, and it is impossible to predict which ones will actually occur. It is therefore important to recognize these complications and act accordingly. Luckily for us, if the mother has been seeing her obstetrician regularly for prenatal care, she will have a good idea of her situation and can provide important information about the placenta's location and baby positioning. Unfortunately, though, the vast majority of EMS responses for obstetric emergencies are to a population of patients who do not seek prenatal care and wait until the last minute to summon EMS for help. In these cases, you will barely have enough time to introduce yourself before being presented with the second patient.

Keep in mind that in all obstetric calls, you are caring for two patients, including one whom you are unable to monitor until birth. Whenever possible, it is always best to deliver in a facility that has the ability to monitor the baby and protect him. However, there will be times when a field delivery is necessary.

One of the most important things you can do following delivery is to keep the baby warm. A general rule of thumb is that you should be sweating in the back of the ambulance. Remember, the average room temperature is 68°F to 72°F and the baby should be kept at a balmy 98°F.

Field delivery can be an exciting and nerve-racking experience. As long as you remember the priorities of patient care, the situation should go smoothly. Relax and enjoy the opportunity to help bring a new life into the world. This is one of the few times when paramedics get to participate in a positive medical scenario.

YOU MAKE THE CALL

It is 9 A.M. and you and your partner are participating in an in-station drill when you are dispatched for a "possible stroke." You soon arrive at a garden apartment, where you are met by a very anxious man. He reports that he just arrived home from working the night shift and found his pregnant wife semiconscious on the living room floor. He says that he talked to her about an hour earlier and she was "fine."

Your assessment reveals a 25-year-old pregnant woman who responds to verbal stimuli with incoherent muttering. Her airway is patent and her respirations are nonlabored at a rate of 20 per minute. Lung sounds are clear bilaterally. Her pulse is strong and regular at 96 per minute. Her flushed skin is warm to the touch. She is diaphoretic. You observe that her ankles are markedly edematous. Her blood pressure is 158/100. There are no obvious signs of traumatic injury.

Your partner places a saline lock. He also checks her blood glucose level and finds that it is >120 mg/dL. You obtain her obstetric history, learning that she is a G1P0 who is at 32 weeks' gestation. She has had good prenatal care and is scheduled for an appointment today at 4 P.M. Her husband tells you that she has been taking prenatal vitamins with iron throughout her pregnancy. He denies any other medical problems other than the fact that her doctor has been "watching" her blood pressure for the past couple of months. He denies any alcohol or recreational drug use by his wife.

1. What is your first priority?

2. What do you suspect is the likely cause of the patient's signs and symptoms?

3. Your patient's husband is very concerned about the well-being of his wife and baby. What should you tell him?

4. How should this patient be transported to the hospital?

See Suggested Responses at the back of this book.

REVIEW QUESTIONS

1. The first two weeks of the menstrual cycle are dominated by the hormone _____, which causes the endometrium to thicken and become engorged with blood.
   a. pitocin
   b. estrogen
   c. epinephrine
   d. progesterone

2. During normal fetal development, the sex of the infant can usually be determined by _____ weeks' gestation.
   a. 10
   b. 12
   c. 14
   d. 16

3. A woman who has given birth to her first child is termed _____.
   a. multipara
   b. primipara
   c. primigravida
   d. multigravida

4. Generally, vital signs in the pregnant patient should be taken with the patient _____.
   a. sitting upright
   b. lying on her right side
   c. lying on her left side
   d. lying flat on her back

5. _____ is the preferred analgesic in pregnancy.
   a. Aspirin
   b. Ibuprofen
   c. Morphine sulfate
   d. Propoxyphene

6. Intentional termination of a pregnancy under any condition not allowed by law is termed _____.
   a. missed abortion
   b. elective abortion
   c. criminal abortion
   d. therapeutic abortion

7. _____ occurs as a result of abnormal implantation of the placenta on the lower half of the uterine wall, resulting in partial or complete coverage of the cervical opening.
   a. Placenta previa
   b. Ectopic pregnancy
   c. Abruptio placentae
   d. Incomplete abortion

8. An abortion in which fetal death occurs but the fetus is not expelled is termed _____.
   a. missed abortion
   b. criminal abortion
   c. habitual abortion
   d. incomplete abortion

9. The _____ stage of labor begins with the complete dilation of the cervix and ends with the delivery of the fetus.
   a. first   c. second
   b. third   d. dilation

10. Infants scoring _____ on the APGAR scoring system are moderately depressed and require oxygen and stimulation to breathe.
    a. 7–10   c. 6–9
    b. 0–3   d. 4–6

See Answers to Review Questions at the back of this book.

REFERENCES

1. American Diabetes Association. "Executive Summary: Standards of Medical Care in Diabetes—2011." *Diabetes Care* 34 (Suppl 1) (2011): S4–S10.
2. Nama, V. and I. Manyonda. "Tubal Ectopic Pregnancy: Diagnosis and Management." *Arch Gynecol Obstet* 279 (2009): 443–453.
3. Leeman, L. and P. Fontaine. "Hypertensive Disorders of Pregnancy." *Am Fam Physician* 78 (2008): 93–100.
4. Kattwinkel, J., J. M. Perlman, K. Aziz, et al. "Part 15: Neonatal Resuscitation: 2010 American Heart Association Guidelines for Cardiopulmonary Resuscitation and Emergency Cardiovascular Care." *Circulation* 122 (2010): S909–S919.

FURTHER READING

Cunningham, F., K. Loveno, S. Bloom, J. Hauth, D. Rouse, and C. Spong. *Williams Obstetrics.* 23rd ed. New York: McGraw Hill, 2009.

Gruenber, B. N. *Essentials of Prehospital Maternity Care.* Upper Saddle River, NJ: Pearson/Prentice Hall, 2006.

3

Neonatology

Bryan Bledsoe, DO, FACEP, FAAEM, EMT-P

STANDARD
Special Patient Populations (Neonatal Care)

COMPETENCY
Integrates assessment findings with principles of epidemiology and pathophysiology and knowledge of psychosocial needs to formulate a field impression and implement a comprehensive treatment/disposition plan for patients with special needs.

OBJECTIVES

Terminal Performance Objective
After reading this chapter, you should be able to integrate patient assessment findings, patient history, and knowledge of anatomy, physiology, pathophysiology, and basic and advanced life support interventions to recognize and manage problems in neonatal patients.

Enabling Objectives
To accomplish the terminal performance objective, you should be able to:

1. Define key terms introduced in this chapter.

2. Relate the anatomy and physiology of the neonate to the assessment and management of patients one month of age and younger.

3. Use a process of clinical reasoning to guide and interpret the patient assessment and management process for normal and distressed neonatal patients.

4. Adapt the scene size-up, primary assessment, patient history, secondary assessment, and use of monitoring technology to meet the needs of normal and distressed neonatal patients.

5. Demonstrate concern for the psychosocial needs of the parents of normal and distressed neonates.

6. Recognize specific problems in neonates, including meconium aspiration, apnea, respiratory distress, cyanosis, cardiac arrest, bradycardia, prematurity, seizures, fever, hypothermia, hypoglycemia, dehydration, and birth injuries.

7. Relate the pathophysiology of specific neonatal problems to the priorities of patient assessment and management.

8. Communicate relevant patient information orally and in writing when transferring care of the neonatal patient to hospital personnel.

KEY TERMS

CASE STUDY

A storm rages outside, making travel dangerous. Around midnight you receive a call from the dispatcher. A woman has just gone into labor. She lives about 20 minutes from the hospital, but her husband is worried about the weather conditions and requests help from your EMS unit.

On arrival, you find a 24-year-old woman who is about to deliver her second baby. You quickly determine that there is not enough time to transport the patient to the hospital. You and your partner begin to prepare the equipment needed for a field delivery.

The delivery goes beautifully, and you announce the arrival of the couple's new daughter. Following the birth, however, the baby remains blue and limp—even after you quickly dry the baby and then wrap her in a dry blanket. You stimulate the baby by rubbing her back and flicking the soles of her feet gently.

When the baby stays blue and limp, you push aside a very normal urge to panic and deliver breaths using a bag-valve-mask unit and room air. The baby "pinks up" almost immediately and begins to cry.

Using the pulse oximeter, you determine that the oxygen saturation is 95 percent and increasing. You prepare the baby for transport, making sure her head is covered. You ask the mother to hold her new daughter and then load both of your patients into the ambulance.

En route to the hospital, you continue to monitor the infant and assign a 5-minute APGAR score of 9. The trip is uneventful. The baby leaves the hospital only one day after the mother. The parents later pay a surprise visit to your EMS unit. They proudly introduce a healthy baby daughter!

INTRODUCTION

Babies pass through stages of physical and emotional development. This chapter concerns itself with babies 1 month old and under. Babies less than 1 month old are called **neonates**. Recently born neonates—those in the first few hours of their lives—may also be called **newborns** or *newly born infants* (Figure 3-1 ●).

After an unscheduled delivery in the field, you have two patients to manage—the mother and the baby. You can review information on care of the mother in Chapter 2 of this volume. The present chapter will describe the initial care of newborns, focusing on the special needs of distressed and premature newborns.

GENERAL PATHOPHYSIOLOGY, ASSESSMENT, AND MANAGEMENT

The care of newborns follows the same priorities as for all patients. Complete the primary assessment first. Correct any problems detected during the primary assessment before proceeding to the next step. The vast majority of newborns require no resuscitation beyond suctioning the airway, mild stimulation, and maintenance of body temperature. However, for newborns who require additional care, your quick actions can make the difference between life and death.

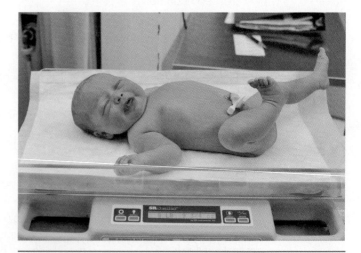

● **Figure 3-1** Term newborn.

Epidemiology

Approximately 10 percent of newborns require some assistance to begin breathing at birth, whereas less than 1 percent require extensive resuscitative measures.[1,2] Medications are rarely indicated in newborn resuscitation. The incidence of complications increases as the birth weight decreases. About 80 percent of newborns weighing less than 1,500 grams (3 pounds, 5 ounces) at birth require resuscitation. Determine whether newborns are at risk by considering the **antepartum** and **intrapartum** factors that may indicate complications at the time of delivery (Table 3–1).

Your success in resuscitating at-risk infants increases with training, ongoing practice, and proper stocking of equipment on board the ambulance. Make sure your ambulance carries a basic OB kit and resuscitation equipment for newborns of various sizes. (See the list in the Resuscitation section later in this chapter.)

Plan transport in advance. Know the types of facilities available in your locality and local protocols governing use of these facilities. A nearby neonatal intensive care unit (NICU) makes the best choice for at-risk newborns. However, if you must transport to a distant NICU, determine whether it might be in the best interests of the infant to transport him to the nearest facility for stabilization. Follow local protocols and consult medical direction as needed.

Pathophysiology

Upon birth, dramatic changes occur within the newborn to prepare it for **extrauterine** life. The respiratory system, which is essentially nonfunctional when the fetus is in the uterus, must suddenly initiate and maintain respirations. While in the uterus, fetal lung fluid fills the fetal lungs. The capillaries and arterioles of the lungs are closed. Most blood pumped by the heart bypasses the nonfunctional respiratory system by flowing through the **ductus arteriosus**.

Approximately one-third of fetal lung fluid is removed through compression of the chest during vaginal delivery. Under normal conditions, the newborn takes his first breath within the first few seconds after delivery. The timing of the first breath is unrelated to the cutting of the umbilical cord. Factors that stimulate the baby's first breath include:

- Mild acidosis
- Initiation of stretch reflexes in the lungs
- Hypoxia
- Hypothermia

With the first breaths, the lungs rapidly fill with air, which displaces the remaining fetal fluid. The pulmonary arterioles and capillaries open, decreasing pulmonary vascular resistance. At this point, the resistance to blood flow in the lungs is now less than the resistance of the ductus arteriosus. Because of this pressure difference, blood flow is diverted from the ductus arteriosus to the lungs, where it picks up oxygen for transport to the peripheral tissues (Figure 3-2 ●).

Soon, there is no need for the ductus arteriosus, and it eventually closes and becomes the *ligamentum arteriosum*. However, if hypoxia or severe acidosis occurs, the pulmonary vascular bed may constrict again and the ductus may reopen. This will retrigger fetal circulation with its attendant shunting and ongoing hypoxia. (This condition is called **persistent fetal circulation**.) To help the newborn make the transition to extrauterine life, it is very important for the paramedic to facilitate the first few breaths and to prevent ongoing hypoxia and acidosis.

Remain alert at all times to signs of respiratory distress. Infants are susceptible to hypoxemia, which can lead to permanent brain damage. After initial hypoxia, the infant rapidly gasps for breath. If the asphyxia continues, respiratory movements cease altogether, the heart rate begins to fall, and neuromuscular tone gradually diminishes. The infant then enters a period of apnea known as *primary apnea*. In most cases, simple stimulation and exposure to oxygen will reverse bradycardia and assist in the development of pulmonary perfusion.

With ongoing asphyxia, however, the infant will enter a period known as *secondary apnea*. During secondary apnea, the infant takes several last deep gasping respirations. The heart rate, blood pressure, and oxygen saturation in the blood continue to fall. The infant becomes unresponsive to stimulation and will not spontaneously resume respiration on his own. Death will occur unless you promptly initiate resuscitation. For this reason, always assume that apnea in the newborn is secondary apnea and rapidly treat it with ventilatory assistance and, when appropriate, chest compressions.

Many of the structures necessary for intrauterine life change following birth. The ductus arteriosus becomes the ligamentum arteriosum. The *foramen ovale* closes and becomes the *fossa ovalis*. The *ductus venosus* becomes the *ligamentum venosum*. The umbilical vein becomes the *ligamentum teres*. The umbilical arteries constrict although the proximal portions persist (Figure 3-3 ●).

TABLE 3–1 | Risk Factors Indicating Possible Complications in Newborns

Antepartum Factors	Intrapartum Factors
Multiple gestation	Premature labor
Inadequate prenatal care	Meconium-stained amniotic fluid
Mother's age (<16 or >35)	Rupture of membranes more than 24 hours prior to delivery
History of perinatal morbidity or mortality	Use of narcotics within 4 hours of delivery
Post-term gestation	Abnormal presentation
Drugs/medications	Prolonged labor or precipitous delivery
Toxemia, hypertension, diabetes	Prolapsed cord or bleeding

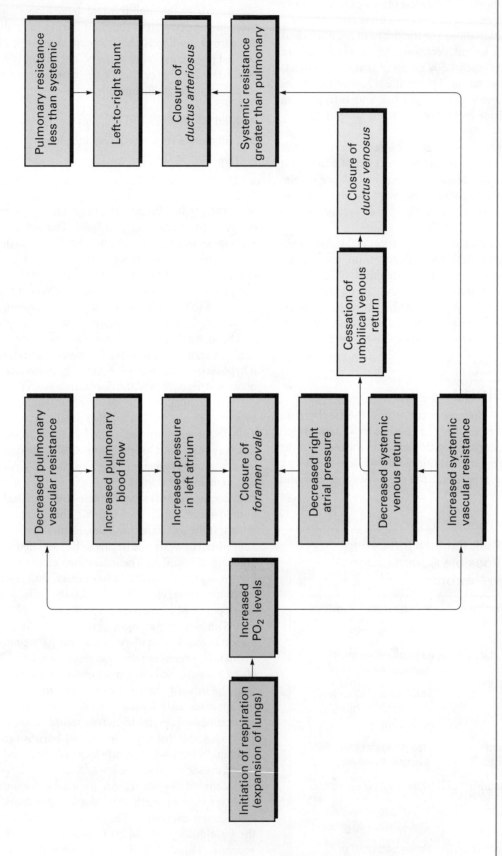

● **Figure 3-2** Hemodynamic changes in the newborn at birth.

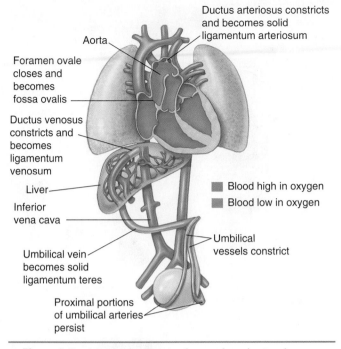

Aorta

Ductus arteriosus constricts and becomes solid ligamentum arteriosum

Foramen ovale closes and becomes fossa ovalis

Ductus venosus constricts and becomes ligamentum venosum

Liver

Inferior vena cava

Umbilical vein becomes solid ligamentum teres

Proximal portions of umbilical arteries persist

Umbilical vessels constrict

■ Blood high in oxygen
■ Blood low in oxygen

● **Figure 3-3**   Major changes in the newborn's circulatory system.

Congenital Anomalies

Approximately 2 percent of infants are born with some sort of congenital problem. Congenital problems typically arise from a problem in fetal development. Most fetal development occurs during the first trimester of pregnancy. It is during this time that the developing fetus is most sensitive to environmental factors and substances that can affect normal development.

There are many types of congenital anomalies. These may affect a single organ or structure or may affect many organs or structures. Congenital anomalies are the leading cause of death in infants, causing approximately one-quarter of infant deaths. Several recognized patterns, called *syndromes*, occur. It is not within the scope of this text to discuss all of the various congenital anomalies. However, a few of the congenital anomalies may make resuscitation of the neonate more difficult.

Among the congenital anomalies encountered, congenital heart defects are among the most common. The cause of these is largely unknown. Congenital heart defects are often classified by whether or not they increase pulmonary blood flow, decrease pulmonary blood flow, or obstruct blood flow.

Some congenital heart problems result in increased pulmonary blood flow. These include cases where the ductus arteriosus fails to close, a condition referred to as *patent ductus arteriosus* (also called a *persistent ductus arteriosus*) (Figure 3-4 ●). Septal defects (a hole in the wall between the atria or the ventricles) can also result in increased pulmonary blood flow. With *atrial septal defect*, a hole between the atria allows the commixing of blood (Figure 3-5 ●). With a *ventricular septal defect*, a hole between the two ventricles allows commixing of blood (Figure 3-6 ●). The increase in pulmonary blood flow that results from either type of septal defect can lead to congestive heart failure.

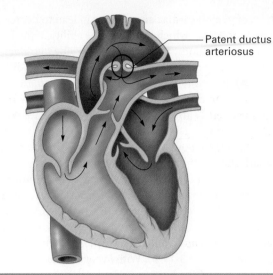

Patent ductus arteriosus

● **Figure 3-4**   Patent ductus arteriosus (PDA).

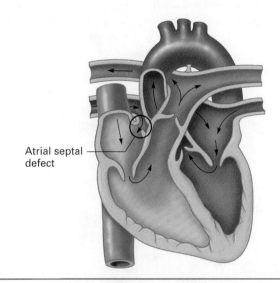

Atrial septal defect

● **Figure 3-5**   Atrial septal defect (ASD).

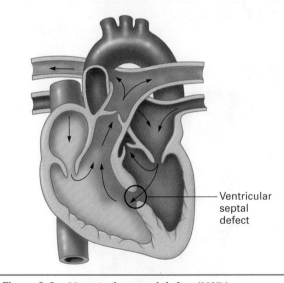

Ventricular septal defect

● **Figure 3-6**   Ventricular septal defect (VSD).

Other congenital cardiac anomalies can lead to decreased pulmonary blood flow, which decreases the ability of the lungs to oxygenate the blood. These defects include *tetralogy of Fallot*, which is a combination of four congenital conditions (Figure 3-7 ●). In addition, a condition called *transposition of the great vessels* can occur, whereby the normal outflow tracts of the right and left ventricles are switched (Figure 3-8 ●).

Finally, some congenital cardiac anomalies can result in obstruction of blood flow. Causes of blood flow obstruction include coarctation of the aorta, aortic or mitral stenosis/atresia, and hypoplastic left heart syndrome. With *coarctation of the aorta*, there is a narrowing in the arch of the aorta that obstructs blood flow (Figure 3-9 ●). Problems with either the mitral, pulmonary, or aortic valve can cause blood flow obstruction, a condition called *mitral stenosis, pulmonary stenosis* (Figure 3-10 ●), or *aortic stenosis* (Figure 3-11 ●). With *hypoplastic left heart syndrome,* the left side of the heart is underdeveloped, a condition that is usually fatal by 1 month of age if untreated.

There are some noncardiac congenital anomalies of note. For example, some children may be born with a defect in the dia-

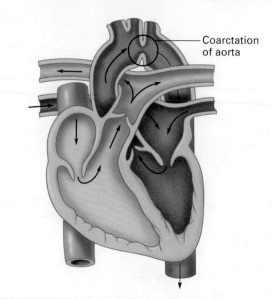

● **Figure 3-9**   Coarctation of the aorta.

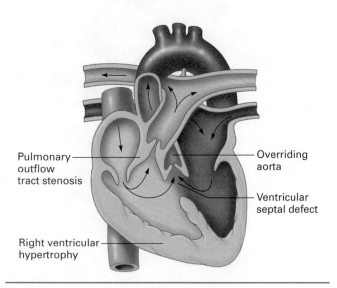

● **Figure 3-7**   Tetralogy of Fallot.

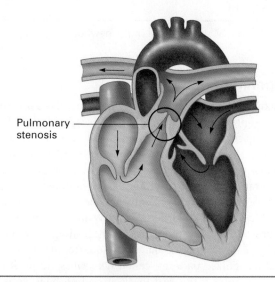

● **Figure 3-10**   Pulmonary stenosis.

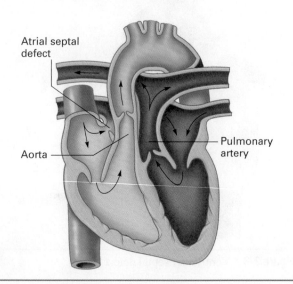

● **Figure 3-8**   Transposition of the great vessels.

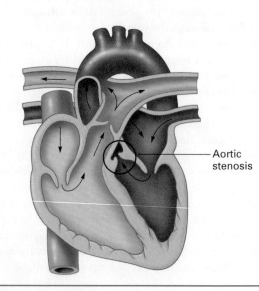

● **Figure 3-11**   Aortic stenosis.

phragm that allows some of the abdominal contents to enter the chest through the defect. This abnormality is referred to as a **diaphragmatic hernia**. If you suspect a diaphragmatic hernia, do not treat the infant with bag-valve-mask ventilation. If there is a diaphragmatic hernia, bag-valve-mask or other positive-pressure ventilation will cause stomach distention, which will cause the stomach to protrude into the chest cavity, thus decreasing ventilatory capacity. Instead, immediately intubate the infant. Diaphragmatic hernia will be discussed in more detail later in this chapter.

Some infants are born with a defect in the spinal cord. In some cases, the spinal cord and associated structures may be exposed. This abnormality is called a **meningomyelocele**. Infants born with a meningomyelocele should not be placed on the back. Instead, place them on the stomach or side and conduct resuscitation in this position, if possible. Cover the spinal defect with sterile gauze pads soaked in warm sterile saline and inserted in a plastic covering.

A newborn may exhibit a defect in the area of the umbilicus. In some cases, the abdominal contents will fill this defect, resulting in an **omphalocele**. If you encounter a newborn with an omphalocele, cover the defect with an occlusive plastic covering to decrease water and heat loss.

Because newborns are obligate nose breathers, **choanal atresia** can cause upper airway obstruction and respiratory distress. Choanal atresia is the most common birth defect involving the nose and is caused by the presence of a bony or membranous septum between the nasal cavity and the pharynx. Suspect this condition if you are unable to pass a catheter through either naris into the oropharynx. An oral airway will usually bypass the obstruction.

A fairly common congenital anomaly is cleft lip and cleft palate. During fetal development, the lip and palate come together in the middle, forming the oral cavity. Failure of the palate to completely close during fetal development can result in a defect known as **cleft palate**. Cleft palate may also be associated with failure of the upper lip to close. This condition, referred to as **cleft lip**, can make it difficult to obtain an adequate seal for effective mask ventilation. If a child with a cleft lip or cleft palate will require more than brief mechanical ventilation, you should place an endotracheal tube.

Pierre Robin syndrome is a congenital condition characterized by a small jaw and large tongue in conjunction with a cleft palate. In this condition, the tongue is likely to obstruct the upper airway. A nasal or oral airway usually bypasses the obstruction. If the obstruction cannot be bypassed with a simple airway, then intubation will be necessary, although intubation can be very difficult to carry out on newborns with this condition.

Assessment

Assess the newborn immediately after birth. (Ideally, if two paramedics are available, one paramedic attends the mother while the other attends the newborn.) Make a mental note of the time of birth and then quickly obtain vital signs. Remember that newborns are slippery and will require both hands to support the head and torso. Position yourself so you can work close to the surface where you have placed the infant.

The newborn's respiratory rate should average 40 to 60 breaths per minute. If respirations are not adequate or if the newborn is gasping, immediately start positive-pressure ventilation.

Expect a normal heart rate of 150 to 180 beats per minute at birth, slowing to 130 to 140 beats per minute thereafter. A pulse rate of less than 100 beats per minute indicates distress and requires emergency intervention.

Evaluate the skin color as well. Some cyanosis of the extremities is common immediately after birth. Unfortunately, cyanosis is a poor indicator of oxygen saturation in newborns. Pulse oximetry is a better indicator of oxygen saturation. It is important to remember that neonatal oxygen saturations do not reach normal levels until approximately 10 minutes after birth. They are initially in the 70 to 80 percent range (Table 3–2).[3] Supplemental oxygen should be provided only in cases in which oxygen saturation levels are lower than those detailed in Table 3–2. If needed, administer only enough oxygen to maintain the oxygen saturation levels as detailed.[4, 5]

The APGAR Score

As soon as possible, assign the newborn an **APGAR score** (Table 3–3). Ideally, try to do this at 1 and 5 minutes after birth. However, if the newborn is not breathing, *do not* withhold resuscitation in order to determine the APGAR score.

The APGAR scoring system helps distinguish between newborns who need only routine care and those who need greater assistance. The system also predicts long-term survival. An anesthesiologist named Dr. Virginia Apgar developed the system in 1952, and her name forms an acronym for its parameters.[6, 7] The parameters for APGAR scoring include:

- **A**ppearance
- **P**ulse rate
- **G**rimace
- **A**ctivity
- **R**espiratory effort

CONTENT REVIEW

▶ Normal Newborn Vital Signs

- Respirations: 30–60
- Heart rate: 100–180
- Blood pressure: 60–90 systolic
- Temperature: 36.7°C–37.8°C (98°F–100°F)

TABLE 3–2 | Targeted Predicted Oxygen Saturation (SpO$_2$) Levels after Birth

Time after Birth	Predicted SpO$_2$ Levels
1 minute	60–65%
2 minutes	65–70%
3 minutes	70–75%
4 minutes	75–80%
5 minutes	80–85%
10 minutes	85–95%

▶ APGAR

• **A**ppearance
• **P**ulse rate
• **G**rimace
• **A**ctivity
• **R**espiratory effort

A score of 0, 1, or 2 is given for each of these parameters. The minimum total score is 0 and the maximum is 10. A score of 7 to 10 indicates an active and vigorous newborn who requires only routine care. A score of 4 to 6 indicates a moderately distressed newborn who requires oxygenation and stimulation (Figure 3-12 ●). Severely distressed newborns—those with APGAR scores of less than 4—require immediate resuscitation. By determining the APGAR score at 1 and 5 minutes, you can determine whether intervention has caused a change in the newborn's status.

Treatment

Treatment starts prior to delivery. Begin care by preparing the environment and assembling the equipment needed for delivery and immediate care of the newborn. The initial care of a newborn follows the same priorities as care for all patients. Complete the primary assessment first. Correct any problems detected during the primary assessment before proceeding to the next step. The vast majority of term newborns—approximately 80 percent—require no resuscitation beyond suctioning of the airway if necessary, mild stimulation, and maintenance of body temperature by drying and warming with blankets.

Establishing the Airway

Airway management is one of the most critical steps in caring for the newborn. During delivery, fluid is forced out of the baby's lungs, into the oropharynx, and out through the nose and mouth. Fluid drainage occurs independently of gravity. Immediately following delivery, maintain the newborn at the same level as the mother's vagina, with the head approximately 15 degrees below the torso.

Bulb suctioning during delivery and following delivery was once a common practice. However, it has been found to be relatively ineffective and can actually cause neonatal bradycardia. It is no longer recommended. Thus, if the amniotic fluid is clear, suctioning (either bulb or otherwise) is indicated only in babies with an obstruction to spontaneous breathing or who require positive-pressure ventilation. If **meconium** is present, especially thick meconium, consider endotracheal intubation and endotracheal suctioning of nonvigorous neonates. (Meconium staining will be discussed in more detail in several later sections of this chapter.)

Drying and tactile stimulation usually produce enough stimulation to initiate respirations in most newborns. If the newborn does not cry immediately, stimulate him by flicking the soles of his feet or gently rubbing his back (Figure 3-13 ●). *Do not* spank or vigorously rub a newborn baby.

Preventing Heat Loss

Heat loss can be a life-threatening condition in newborns. Cold infants quickly become distressed infants. Heat loss occurs through evaporation, convection, conduction, and radiation. Most heat loss in newborns results from evaporation. The newborn comes into the world wet, and the amniotic fluid quickly evaporates. Immediately after birth, the newborn's core temperature can drop 1°C (1.8°F) or more from his birth temperature of 38°C (100.4°F).

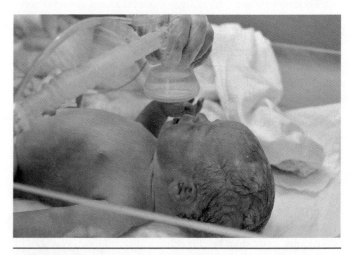

● **Figure 3-12** Administer supplemental oxygen if central cyanosis is present.

Sign	0	1	2	Score	
				1 min	5 min
Appearance (skin color)	Blue, pale	Body pink, extremities blue	Completely pink		
Pulse Rate (heart rate)	Absent	Below 100	Above 100		
Grimace (irritability)	No response	Grimace	Cries		
Activity (muscle tone)	Limp	Some flexion of extremities	Active motion		
Respiratory Effort	Absent	Slow and irregular	Strong cry		
			TOTAL SCORE =		

TABLE 3–3 | The APGAR Score

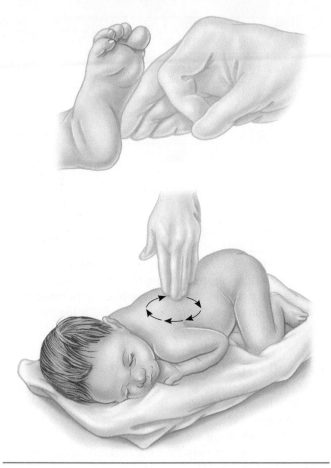

● **Figure 3-13** Stimulate the newborn as required.

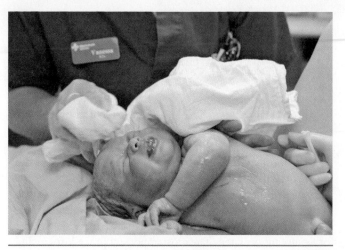

● **Figure 3-14** Dry the infant to prevent loss of evaporative heat.

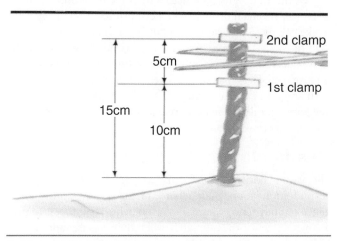

● **Figure 3-15** Clamping and cutting the cord.

Loss of heat can also occur through convection, depending on the temperature of the room and the movement of the air around the newborn. The newborn can lose additional heat through contact with surrounding surfaces (convection) or by radiating heat to colder objects nearby.

To prevent heat loss, take these steps:

● Dry the newborn immediately to prevent evaporative cooling (Figure 3-14 ●).

● Maintain the ambient temperature—the temperature in the delivery room or ambulance—at a *minimum* of 23°C to 24°C (74°F–76°F).

● Close all windows and doors.

● Discard the towel used to dry the newborn and swaddle the infant in a warm, dry receiving blanket or other suitable material. Cover the head.

● In colder areas, place well-insulated water bottles or rubber gloves filled with warm water (40°C [104°F]) around the newborn to help maintain a warm body temperature. To avoid burns, do not place these items against the skin. Be sure the newborn is wrapped in a blanket and place the water bottle or rubber glove against the blanket.

Cutting the Umbilical Cord

After you have stabilized the newborn's airway and minimized heat loss, clamp and cut the umbilical cord. You can prevent over- and undertransfusion of blood by maintaining the baby

at the same level as the mother's vagina, as previously described. Do not "milk" or strip the umbilical cord, as this increases blood viscosity, or **polycythemia**, and can lead to maternal–fetal transfusion. Polycythemia can cause cardiopulmonary problems. It can also contribute to excessive red blood cell destruction, which may in turn lead to **hyperbilirubinemia**—an increased level of bilirubin in the blood, which causes jaundice.

Apply the umbilical clamps within 30 to 45 seconds after birth. Place the first clamp approximately 10 cm (4 inches) from the newborn. Place the second clamp about 5 cm (2 inches) farther away than the first. Then cut the cord between the two clamps (Figure 3-15 ●). After the cord is cut, inspect it periodically to make sure there is no additional bleeding.

THE DISTRESSED NEWBORN

The distressed newborn can be either full term or premature. (See the Prematurity section later in this chapter.) The presence of fetal meconium at birth indicates that fetal distress has occurred at some point during pregnancy. If the newborn is simply meconium stained, then distress may have occurred at a remote time. If you see *particulate* meconium, however, distress may have occurred recently and the newborn should be managed accordingly.

CONTENT REVIEW

▶ Newborn Assessment Parameters

• Respiratory effort
• Heart rate
• Color
• APGAR score

Aspiration of meconium can cause significant respiratory problems. (More will be said about this topic in the Meconium-Stained Amniotic Fluid section later.) Be sure to report the presence of meconium to the medical direction physician.

The most common problem experienced by newborns during the first minutes of life is ventilation. For this reason, resuscitation usually consists of ventilation and, if needed, oxygenation. Except in special situations, the use of IV fluids, drugs, or cardiac equipment is usually not indicated. (See Inverted Pyramid for Resuscitation later.) The most important procedures include suctioning, drying, and stimulating the distressed newborn.

Of the vital signs, fetal heart rate is the most important indicator of neonatal distress. The newborn has a relatively fixed stroke volume. Thus, cardiac output depends more on heart rate than on stroke volume. Bradycardia, as caused by hypoxia, results in decreased cardiac output and, ultimately, poor perfusion. A pulse rate of less than 60 beats per minute in a distressed newborn should be treated with chest compressions. In distressed newborns, monitor the heart rate manually. Do not depend on external electronic monitors.

Resuscitation

The vast majority of newborns do not require resuscitation beyond stimulation, maintenance of the airway, and maintenance of body temperature. Unfortunately, it is difficult to predict which newborns ultimately will require resuscitation. Each EMS unit, therefore, should carry a neonatal resuscitation kit that contains the following items:

• Neonatal bag-valve-mask unit
• Bulb syringe
• **DeLee suction trap**
• Meconium aspirator
• Laryngoscope with size 0 and 1 blades
• Uncuffed endotracheal tubes (2.5, 3.0, 3.5, 4.0) with appropriate suction catheters
• Endotracheal tube stylet
• Tape or device to secure endotracheal tube
• Laryngeal mask airway
• Umbilical catheter and 10-mL syringe
• Three-way stopcock
• 20-mL syringe and 8-French (Fr.) feeding tube for gastric suction
• Glucometer
• Assorted syringes and needles
• Towels (sterile)
• Medications:
    ○ Epinephrine 1:10,000 and 1:1,000
    ○ Volume expander (lactated Ringer's solution or saline)

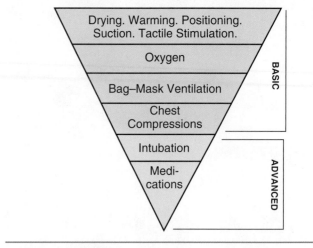

● **Figure 3-16**   The inverted pyramid of neonatal resuscitation showing approximate relative frequencies of neonatal care and resuscitative efforts. Note that a majority of infants respond to the simple measures noted at the top, wide part of the pyramid.

Inverted Pyramid for Resuscitation

Resuscitation of the newborn follows an inverted pyramid (Figure 3-16 ●). As this pyramid indicates, most distressed newborns respond to relatively simple maneuvers. Few require CPR or advanced life support measures.

The following are steps for the initial care of the newborn (also see Procedure 3–1).

Step 1: Drying, Warming, Positioning, Suctioning, and Tactile Stimulation   Resuscitation begins with drying, warming, positioning, and stimulating the newborn. Immediately upon delivery, minimize heat loss by drying the newborn. Next, place the newborn in a warm, dry blanket. Make sure the environment is warm and free of drafts.

After you have dried the newborn, place the infant on his back with his head slightly below his body and his neck slightly extended (Figure 3-17 ●). This facilitates drainage of secretions and fluids from the lungs. Place a small blanket, folded to a 2-cm (3/4-inch) thickness, under the newborn's shoulders to help maintain this position.

If the amniotic fluid is clear, suctioning is not required. If meconium is present, and the infant is vigorous (strong respiratory efforts, good muscle tone, and heart rate >100 per minute), tracheal intubation and suctioning is not recommended. If the infant is not vigorous, endotracheal intubation and suctioning should be immediately carried out (Procedure 3–2).

After carrying out the preceding procedures, assess the newborn as noted here:

Newborn Assessment Parameters

● *Respiratory effort.* The rate and depth of the newborn's breathing should increase immediately with tactile stimulation. If the respiratory response is adequate, evaluate the heart rate next. If the respiratory rate is inadequate, begin positive-pressure ventilation (see Step 2).

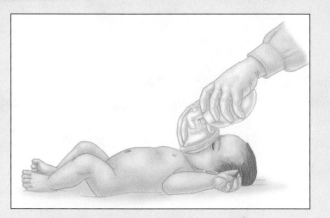

3-1a ● Ventilate for 15–30 seconds.

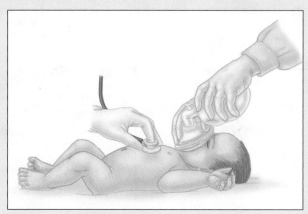

3-1b ● Evaluate heart rate.

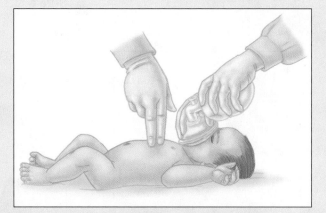

3-1c ● Initiate chest compressions if heart rate is less than 60.

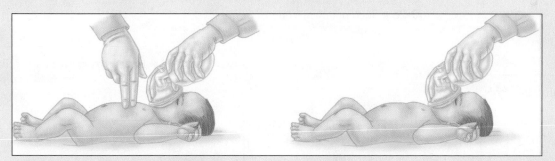

3-1d ● Evaluate heart rate: below 60—continue chest compressions; 60 or above—discontinue chest compressions.

● *Heart rate.* As noted earlier, heart rate is critical in the newborn. Check the heart rate by listening to the apical area of the heart with a stethoscope, feeling the pulse by lightly grasping the umbilical cord, or feeling either the brachial or femoral pulse. If the heart rate is greater than 100 and spontaneous respirations are present, continue the assessment. If the heart rate is less than 100,

immediately begin positive-pressure ventilation (see Step 2).

● *Color.* A newborn may be cyanotic despite a heart rate greater than 100 and spontaneous respirations. If you note central cyanosis, or cyanosis of the chest and abdomen, in a newborn with adequate ventilation and a pulse rate greater than 100, assess oxygen saturation and

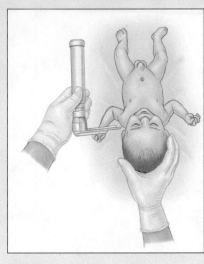

3-2a ● Position the infant.

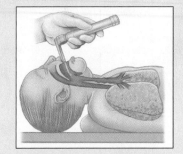

3-2b ● Insert the laryngoscope.

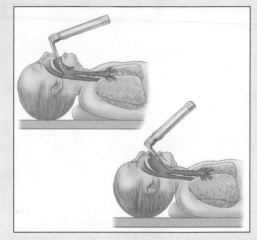

3-2c ● Elevate the epiglottis by lifting.

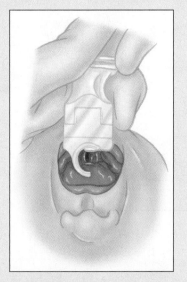

3-2d ● Visualize the cords.

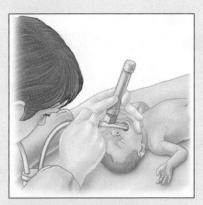

3-2e ● Suction any meconium present.

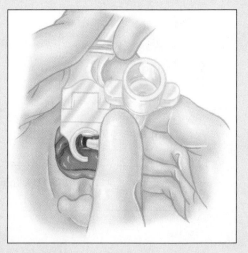

3-2f ● Insert a fresh tube for ventilation.

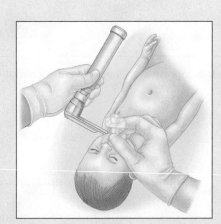

3-2g ● Remove the laryngoscope.

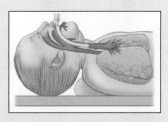

3-2h ● Check proper tube placement.

CORRECT

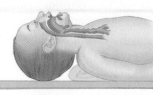

Neck slightly extended

Care should be taken to prevent hyperextension or underextension of the neck since either may decrease air entry.

INCORRECT

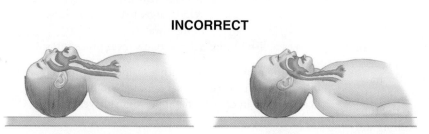

Neck hyperextended   Neck underextended

administer supplemental oxygen as needed to maintain appropriate oxygen saturation, as detailed in Table 3–2 (see Step 3). Newborns with peripheral cyanosis do not usually need supplemental oxygen *unless* the cyanosis is prolonged.

- *APGAR score.* Unless resuscitation is required, obtain 1- and 5-minute APGAR scores.

Step 2: Ventilation   Begin positive-pressure ventilation if *any* of the following conditions is present:

- Heart rate less than 100 beats per minute
- Apnea
- SpO_2 less than expected for post-birth values (Table 3–2)
- Persistence of central cyanosis

A ventilatory rate of 40 to 60 breaths per minute is usually adequate. A bag-valve-mask unit is the device of choice (Figure 3-18 ●). A self-inflating bag of an appropriate size (450 mL is optimal) should be used. Many self-inflating bags have a pressure-limiting pop-off valve that is preset at 30 to 45 cmH_2O. However, because the initial pressures required to ventilate a newborn may be as high as 40 to 60 cmH_2O, you may have to depress the pop-off valve to deactivate it and ensure adequate ventilation. If prolonged ventilation is required, you may have to disable the pop-off valve.

Face masks in various sizes must be available. The most effective ones are designed to fit the contours of the newborn's face and have a low dead space volume (less than 5 mL). When a mask is correctly sized and positioned, it covers the newborn's nose and mouth, but not the eyes.

Endotracheal intubation of a newborn should be carried out in the following situations:

- Chest compressions are performed.
- The patient cannot be ventilated with a mask.

● **Figure 3-17**   Positioning the newborn to open the airway.

- Tracheal suctioning is required (such as in cases of thick meconium).
- Prolonged ventilation will be required.
- A diaphragmatic hernia is suspected.
- Inadequate respiratory effort is found.

Because of the narrowness of the neonatal airway at the level of the cricoid cartilage, always use an *uncuffed* endotracheal tube. (Review Table 3–4 regarding tube size.) After inserting the tube, ensure proper placement by noting symmetrical chest wall motion and equal breath sounds. (Review Procedure 3–2.) Capnography should be used to ensure and monitor endotracheal tube placement.

Intubation has several effects in the newborn. First, it bypasses **glottic function**. Second, it eliminates **PEEP**—the physiologic positive end-expiratory pressure created during normal coughing and crying. To maintain adequate functional residual capacity, a PEEP of 2 to 4 cmH_2O should be provided when mechanical ventilation is initiated by adding a magnetic-disk PEEP valve to the bag-valve outlet.

Gastric distention, caused by a leak around an uncuffed endotracheal tube, may compromise ventilation of a newborn. This can be minimized by using a properly sized endotracheal tube. If significant gastric distention is present, a **nasogastric tube** or **orogastric tube** should be inserted (through the nose or mouth, respectively, then through the esophagus into the stomach) as soon as the airway is controlled. The endotracheal tube should be placed before the gastric tube is placed to avoid misplacing the gastric tube into the trachea.

Make sure the newborn is well ventilated before attempting to insert a gastric tube. To determine the depth of insertion, measure a nasogastric tube from the tip of the nose,

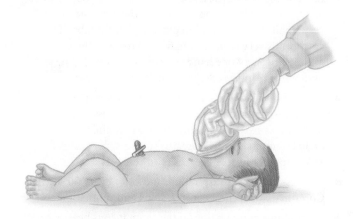

● **Figure 3-18**   Use of a bag-valve-mask unit to provide positive-pressure ventilation. Maintain a good mask seal and use just enough force to raise the infant's chest. Ventilate at a rate of 60 per minute for 30 seconds, then reassess.

TABLE 3–4 | Guidelines for Tracheal Tube Sizes and Depth of Insertion in the Newborn

Tube Size (mm ID)	Depth of Insertion from Upper Lip (cm)	Weight (g)	Gestation (wk)
2.5	6.5–7	<1000	<28
3.0	7–8	1000–2000	28–34
3.5	8–9	2000–3000	34–38
3.5–4.0	>9	>3000	>38

around the ear, to below the xiphoid process. Measure an orogastric tube from the lips to below the xiphoid process. Lubricate the end of the tube and pass it gently along the nasal floor or the mouth and into the esophagus. Confirm that the tube is in the stomach by injecting 10 mL of air into the tube and auscultating a bubbling sound, or sound of rushing air, over the epigastrium.

Step 3: Supplemental Oxygen   If central cyanosis is present or if SpO_2 levels are less than expected (see Table 3–2), administer only enough supplemental oxygen to maintain the SpO_2 within the normal range. Avoid both hypoxia and hyperoxia. Hyperoxia has been associated with numerous adverse outcomes in neonates and should be avoided to the same degree we avoid hypoxia. Generally speaking, supplemental oxygen will usually be provided in conjunction with mechanical ventilation. If possible, the oxygen should be warmed and humidified. Continue oxygen administration until the newborn's color has improved or the SpO_2 is maintained at target levels.[8]

Step 4: Chest Compressions   Initiate chest compressions if the heart rate is less than 60 beats per minute.[9] Perform chest compressions by following these steps:

- Encircle the newborn's chest, placing both of your thumbs on the lower third of the sternum. If the newborn is very small, you may need to overlap your thumbs. If the newborn is very large, you may need to place the ring and middle fingers of one hand just below the nipple line and perform two-finger compression (Figure 3-19 ●).

- Compress the lower half of the sternum at a rate of 100 times per minute. Accompany compressions with positive-pressure ventilation. Maintain a ratio of 30 compressions to 2 breaths (one rescuer) or 15 compressions to 2 breaths (two rescuers).

- Reassess heart rate, respiration, and color every 30 seconds. Coordinate with chest compressions and ventilation.

- Discontinue compressions if the spontaneous heart rate exceeds 80 per minute.

Step 5: Medications and Fluids   Most cardiopulmonary arrests in newborns result from hypoxia. Because of this, initial therapy consists of ventilation and oxygenation. However, when these measures fail, fluids and medications should be administered. They may also be necessary in cases of persistent bradycardia, hypovolemia, respiratory depression secondary to narcotics, and metabolic acidosis.

Vascular access for the administration of fluids and drugs can be managed most readily by using the umbilical vein. The umbilical cord contains three vessels—two arteries and one vein. The vein is larger than the arteries and has a thinner wall (Figure 3-20 ●).

To establish venous access, follow these procedures:

- Trim the umbilical cord with a scalpel blade to 1 cm above the abdomen. Be sure to save enough of the umbilical cord stump in case neonatal personnel have to place additional lines.

- Insert a 5-Fr. umbilical catheter into the umbilical vein. Connect the catheter to a three-way stopcock and fill it with saline.

- Insert the catheter until the tip is just below the skin and you note the free flow of blood. (If the catheter is inserted too far, it may become wedged against the liver, and it will not function.)

- After the catheter is in place, secure it with umbilical tape.

If an umbilical vein catheter cannot be placed, some medications can be given via the endotracheal tube. Other options for vascular access are peripheral vein cannulation and intraosseous cannulation. Fluid therapy should consist of 10 mL/kg of saline or lactated Ringer's solution given by syringe as a slow IV push.

Maternal Narcotic Use

Maternal abuse of narcotics—either illegal or prescribed—can complicate field deliveries. Maternal narcotic use has been shown to produce low-birth-weight infants. Such infants may demonstrate withdrawal symptoms—tremors, startles, and decreased alertness. They also face a serious risk of respiratory depression at birth. Although formerly used, the narcotic antagonist naloxone (Narcan) is not indicated in neonatal resuscitation. As with other newborns, continue all resuscitative measures until the newborn is resuscitated or until the emergency staff assumes care.

Neonatal Transport

Healthy newborns should be allowed to begin the bonding process with the mother as soon as possible. Distressed newborns, however, must be positioned on their side to prevent aspiration and must be rapidly transported.

In addition to field deliveries, paramedics are frequently called on to transport a high-risk newborn from a facility

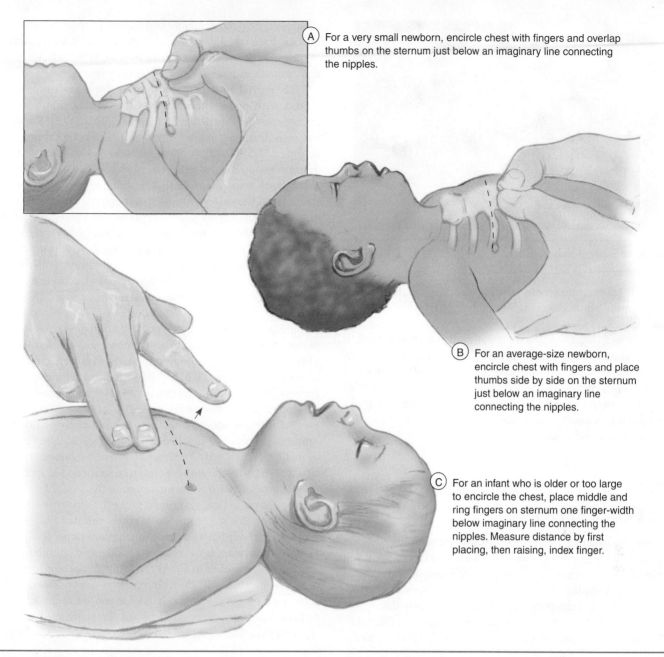

(A) For a very small newborn, encircle chest with fingers and overlap thumbs on the sternum just below an imaginary line connecting the nipples.

(B) For an average-size newborn, encircle chest with fingers and place thumbs side by side on the sternum just below an imaginary line connecting the nipples.

(C) For an infant who is older or too large to encircle the chest, place middle and ring fingers on sternum one finger-width below imaginary line connecting the nipples. Measure distance by first placing, then raising, index finger.

● **Figure 3-19** Position fingers for chest compressions according to the size of the infant.

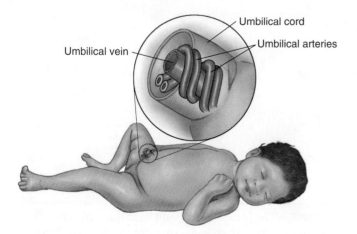

Umbilical cord

Umbilical arteries

Umbilical vein

where stabilization has occurred to a neonatal intensive care unit (NICU). The trip may be across the street or across the state. Usually a pediatric nurse, respiratory therapist, and, often, a physician accompany the newborn. During transport, a paramedic crew will help maintain a newborn's body temperature, control oxygen administration, and maintain ventilatory support. Often, a transport **isolette** with its own heat, light, and oxygen source is available (Figure 3-21 ●).

● **Figure 3-20** The umbilical cord contains two arteries and one vein. The umbilical vein can be accessed for vascular administration of fluids and drugs. The vein is larger than the arteries and has a thinner wall.

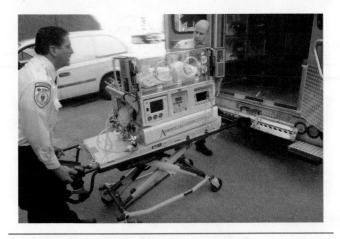

● **Figure 3-21**   Modern neonatal transport. (© *Mark C. Ide*)

In such cases, intravenous medications are usually infused through the umbilical vein. The umbilical artery is catheterized as well.

If a self-contained isolette is not available for transport, it is important to keep the ambulance warm. Wrap the newborn in several blankets, keep the head covered, and place hot-water bottles containing water heated to no more than 40°C (104°F) near, but not touching, the newborn. Do not use chemical packs to keep the newborn warm. These can generate excessive heat and may burn the infant.

SPECIFIC NEONATAL SITUATIONS

Rapid assessment and treatment of a distressed newborn are the keys to the infant's survival. The following information will help you to formulate treatment plans for specific emergencies involving newborns. Remember that, unless otherwise directed, you will need to transport these infants to a facility that is able to handle high-risk neonates. A reference card should be available in the ambulance and in the dispatch office that tracks the availability of neonatal unit beds. Whenever possible, keep the parents advised of what is happening and the reason for any treatments being given to the infant. However, do not discuss "chances of survival" with the family or caregivers.

Meconium-Stained Amniotic Fluid

Meconium-stained amniotic fluid occurs in approximately 10 to 15 percent of deliveries, mostly in post-term or in small-for-gestational-age (SGA) newborns. The mortality rate for meconium-stained infants is considerably higher than the mortality rate for non-meconium-stained infants, and meconium aspiration accounts for a significant proportion of neonatal deaths.

Fetal distress and hypoxia can cause the passage of meconium into the amniotic fluid. Meconium is a dark green substance found in the digestive tract of full-term newborns. It arises from secretions of the various digestive glands and amniotic fluid. Either *in utero*, or more often with the first breath, thick meconium is aspirated into the lungs, resulting in small-airway obstruction and aspiration pneumonia. This may produce respiratory distress within the first hours, or even minutes, of life as evidenced by tachypnea, retraction, grunting, and cyanosis in severely affected newborns.

The partial obstruction of some airways may lead to pneumothorax. A pneumothorax may occur in an infant, cause no distress, and require no active treatment. However, if the infant has significant respiratory distress, the pneumothorax must be evacuated. If tension pneumothorax has occurred, needle decompression may be required.

Infants born through thin meconium may not require treatment if they are vigorous (strong respiratory efforts, good muscle tone, and heart rate >100 per minute), but nonvigorous infants born through thick, particulate (pea-soup) meconium-stained fluid should be intubated immediately, prior to the first ventilation (Figure 3-22 ●).[10] Aspiration of meconium by a newborn can result in either partial or complete airway obstruction. Complete airway obstruction causes atelectasis (collapsed or airless lungs). In addition, some aspects of fetal blood flow resume a right-to-left shunt of blood across the foramen ovale (the opening between the atria of the fetal heart). This results from increased pulmonary pressures. Incomplete obstruction can act as a ball-valve in the smaller airways, thus preventing exhalation. The newborn is also at increased risk of developing a pneumothorax.

Before stimulating the infant to breathe, apply suction with a meconium aspirator attached to an endotracheal tube. Connect to suction at 100 cmH₂O or less to remove meconium from the airway. Withdraw the endotracheal tube as suction is applied.

Repeat intubation and suction until the meconium clears, usually not more than two times. Once the airway is clear and the infant is able to breathe on his own, ventilate and provide supplemental oxygen as needed to maintain target SpO₂ levels for age. If the infant is found to be hypotensive, consider a fluid challenge. Remember to warm the infant to prevent hypothermia. The parents will probably question the treatment being performed on the infant. Explain what you are doing and why, without discussing chances of survival. Stress the need for rapid transport to a facility able to handle high-risk infants.

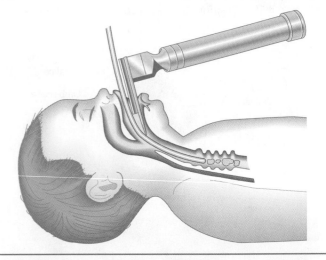

● **Figure 3-22**   Intubate the infant born through particulate, thick meconium immediately—prior to the first ventilation.

Apnea

Apnea is a common finding in preterm infants, infants weighing less than 1,500 grams (3 pounds, 5 ounces), infants exposed to drugs, or infants born after prolonged or difficult labor and delivery. Typically, the infant fails to breathe spontaneously after stimulation, or the infant experiences respiratory pauses of more than 20 seconds.

Although apnea is usually the result of hypoxia or hypothermia, there may be other causative factors. These include:

- Narcotic or central nervous depressants
- Weakness of the respiratory muscles
- Sepsis
- Metabolic disorders
- Central nervous system disorders

Begin management of apnea with tactile stimulation. Flick the soles of the infant's feet or gently rub his back. If necessary, ventilate using a bag-valve-mask unit with the pop-off valve disabled, as explained earlier. If the infant still does not breathe on his own, or if he has a heart rate of less than 60 with adequate ventilation and chest compressions, perform tracheal intubation with direct visualization. Gain circulatory access, and monitor the heart rate continuously. Generally, neonatal naloxone is no longer recommended.[11]

Early and aggressive treatment of apnea usually results in a good outcome. Throughout treatment, keep the infant warm to prevent hypothermia. Also explain to parents the procedures and the need for rapid transport.

Diaphragmatic Hernia

Diaphragmatic hernias rarely occur. They are seen in approximately 1 out of every 2,200 live births. When they do appear, the **herniation** takes place most often in the posterolateral segments of the diaphragm, and most commonly (90 percent) on the left side. The defect is caused by the failure of the pleuroperitoneal canal (foramen of Bochdalek) to close completely. The survival rate for infants who require mechanical ventilation in the first 18 to 24 hours is approximately 50 percent. However, if there is no respiratory distress in the first 24 hours of life, the survival rate approaches 100 percent.

Protrusion of abdominal viscera through the hernia into the thoracic cavity occurs in varying degrees. In severe cases, the stomach and a large part of the intestines and the spleen, liver, and kidneys displace the lungs and heart to the opposite side. The lung on the affected side is compressed, causing diminished total lung volume. In at least one-third of patients, pulmonary hypertension is present. With a patent ductus arteriosus, severe right-to-left shunting may occur, further aggravating tissue hypoxia.

Assessment findings may include:

- Little to severe distress present from birth
- Dyspnea and cyanosis unresponsive to ventilations
- Small, flat (scaphoid) abdomen
- Bowel sounds in the chest
- Heart sounds displaced to the right

As soon as you suspect a diaphragmatic hernia, position the infant with his head and thorax higher than the abdomen and feet (Figure 3-23 ●). This will help facilitate the downward displacement of the abdominal organs. Place a nasogastric or orogastric tube and apply low, intermittent suctioning. This will decrease the entrapment of air and fluid within the herniated viscera and will reduce the degree of ventilatory compromise. *Do not* use bag-valve-mask ventilation, which can worsen this condition by causing gastric distention. If necessary, cautiously administer positive-pressure ventilation through an endotracheal tube.

This condition usually requires surgical repair. Explain the possible need for surgery to parents, assuring them that their newborn child will be transported quickly to the facility best able to handle this procedure.

Bradycardia

Bradycardia in the newborn is most commonly caused by hypoxia. However, it may also be caused by several other factors, including increased intracranial pressure, hypothyroidism, or acidosis.

In cases of hypoxia, the infant experiences minimal risk if the hypoxia is corrected quickly. In providing treatment,

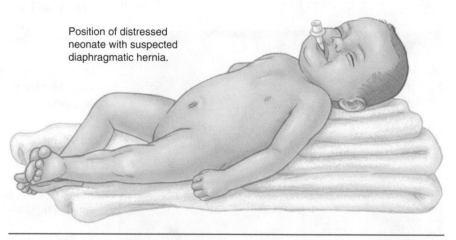

Position of distressed neonate with suspected diaphragmatic hernia.

● **Figure 3-23**   If a diaphragmatic hernia is suspected, position the infant with its head and thorax higher than the abdomen and feet to facilitate downward displacement of abdominal organs.

follow the procedures in the inverted pyramid, as discussed earlier. Check for secretions in the airway, check tongue and soft-tissue positioning, and check for possible foreign body obstruction. Resist the inclination to treat the bradycardia with pharmacological measures alone. Although epinephrine may be necessary, in all likelihood you will be able to correct the problem with ventilation and supplemental oxygen (if needed). Throughout treatment, keep the newborn warm and transport to the nearest facility.

Prematurity

A premature newborn is an infant born prior to 37 weeks of gestation or with weight ranging from 0.6 to 2.2 kg (1 pound, 5 ounces to 4 pounds, 13 ounces). Healthy premature infants weighing more than 1,700 grams (3 pounds, 12 ounces) have a survivability and outcome approximately equal to that of full-term infants. The mortality rate decreases weekly as the gestational age surpasses the age of fetal viability. With the technology currently available, fetal viability is considered to be 23 to 24 weeks of gestation.

Premature newborns are at greater risk of respiratory suppression, head or brain injury caused by hypoxemia, changes in blood pressure, intraventricular hemorrhage, and fluctuations in serum osmolarity. They are also more susceptible to hypothermia than full-term newborns. Reasons premature newborns lose heat more readily include the following:

- The premature newborn has a relatively large body surface area and comparatively small weight.
- The premature newborn has not sufficiently developed the various control mechanisms needed to regulate body temperature.
- The premature newborn has smaller subcutaneous stores of insulating fat.
- Newborns cannot shiver and must maintain body temperature through other mechanisms.

The degree of immaturity determines the physical characteristics of a premature newborn (Figure 3-24 ●). Premature newborns often appear to have a larger head relative to body

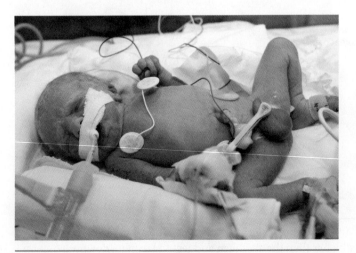

● **Figure 3-24** The premature newborn.

size. They may have large trunks and short extremities, transparent skin, and few wrinkles.

Prematurity should not be a factor in short-term treatment. Resuscitation should be attempted if there is any sign of life, and the measures of resuscitation should be the same as those for newborns of normal weight and maturity. Maintain a patent airway and avoid potential aspiration of gastric contents. Medical direction may advise administration of epinephrine. Throughout treatment, maintain the newborn's body temperature and transport to a facility with special services for low-birth-weight newborns.

Respiratory Distress/Cyanosis

Prematurity is the single most common factor causing respiratory distress and cyanosis in the newborn. The problem occurs most frequently in infants weighing less than 1,200 grams (2 pounds, 10 ounces) and who are born at less than 30 weeks' gestation. Premature infants have an immature central respiratory control center and are easily affected by environmental or metabolic changes. Multiple gestations or prenatal maternal complications may also increase the risk of respiratory distress and cyanosis.

The severely ill newborn with respiratory distress and cyanosis presents a difficult diagnostic challenge. Contributing factors include lung or heart disease, central nervous system disorders, meconium aspiration, metabolic problems, obstruction of the nasal passages, shock and sepsis, diaphragmatic hernia, and more. Assessment findings include:

- Tachypnea
- Paradoxical breathing
- Intercostal retractions
- Nasal flaring
- Expiratory grunt

Follow the inverted pyramid of treatment (Figure 3-16), paying particular attention to airway and ventilation. Suction as needed and provide high-concentration oxygen. Ventilate, as needed, with a bag-valve-mask unit. If prolonged ventilation will be required, consider placing an endotracheal tube. Perform chest compressions, if indicated. Sodium bicarbonate may be helpful for prolonged resuscitation. Consider dextrose ($D_{10}W$ or $D_{25}W$) solution if the newborn is hypoglycemic. Maintain body temperature and transport. Be sure to keep the parents informed and provide needed psychological support.

Hypovolemia

Hypovolemia is the leading cause of shock in newborns. It may result from dehydration, hemorrhage, or third-spacing of fluids. Dehydration is by far the most common cause. Signs of hypovolemia include:

- Pale color
- Cool skin
- Diminished peripheral pulses

- Delayed capillary refill, despite normal ambient temperature
- Mental status changes
- Diminished urination (oliguria) as evidenced by dark urine or dry diaper

When you observe these signs, administer a fluid bolus and assess the infant's response. If signs of shock continue, administer a second bolus. Additional boluses should be infused as indicated by repeated assessments. A hypovolemic infant may often need 40 to 60 mL/kg of fluid during the first hour of resuscitation.

Fluid bolus resuscitation consists of 10 mL/kg of an isotonic crystalloid solution, such as Ringer's lactate or normal saline. Administer the bolus over 5 to 10 minutes as soon as intravascular or intraosseous access is obtained. Do not use solutions containing dextrose, because they can produce hypokalemia or worsen ischemic brain injury. Avoid giving volume expanders too rapidly, as rapid infusion of large volumes of fluid has been associated with brain (intraventricular) hemorrhage.

Seizures

Although seizures occur in a very small percentage of all newborns, they usually indicate a serious underlying abnormality and represent a medical emergency. Prolonged and frequent multiple seizures may result in metabolic changes and cardiopulmonary difficulties.

Neonatal seizures differ from seizures in a child or an adult, because generalized tonic-clonic convulsions normally do not occur during the first month of life. Seizures in neonates include these types:

- *Subtle seizures.* These seizures consist of chewing motions, excessive salivation, blinking, sucking, swimming movements of the arms, pedaling movements of the legs, apnea, and changes in color.
- *Tonic seizures.* These seizures are characterized by rigid posturing of the extremities and trunk. They are sometimes associated with fixed deviation of the eyes. They occur more commonly in premature infants, especially those with an intraventricular hemorrhage.
- *Focal clonic seizures.* These seizures consist of rhythmic twitching of muscle groups, particularly in the extremities and face. They may occur in both full-term and premature infants.
- *Multifocal seizures.* These seizures are similar to focal clonic seizures, except that multiple muscle groups are involved. Clonic activity randomly migrates. These seizures occur primarily in full-term newborns.
- *Myoclonic seizures.* These seizures involve brief focal or generalized jerks of the extremities or parts of the body that tend to involve distal muscle groups. They may occur singly or in a series of repetitive jerks.

Causes of neonatal seizures include sepsis, fever, hypoglycemia, hypoxic-ischemic encephalopathy, metabolic disturbances, meningitis, developmental abnormalities, or drug withdrawal. Assessment findings include a decreased level of consciousness and seizure activities such as those just described. Treatment focuses on airway management and oxygen saturation. With medical direction, consider administration of an anticonvulsant. You might also administer a benzodiazepine (usually lorazepam) for status epilepticus or dextrose ($D_{10}W$ or $D_{25}W$) for hypoglycemia. As with all distressed newborns, maintain body temperature and transport rapidly.

Fever

Average normal temperature in a newborn is 37.5°C (99.5°F). A rectal temperature of 38.0°C (100.4°F) or higher is considered fever. Neonates do not develop fever as readily as older children. Thus, any fever in a neonate requires extensive evaluation because it may be caused by life-threatening conditions such as pneumonia, sepsis, or meningitis. Fever may be the only sign of meningitis in a neonate. Because of their immature development, neonates do not develop the classic symptoms such as a stiff neck. Thus, any neonate with a fever should be considered to have meningitis or sepsis until proven otherwise.

In assessing a neonate with fever, remember that infants have a limited ability to control their body temperature. As a result, fever can be a serious problem. Assessment findings will probably include the following:

- Mental status changes (irritability/somnolence)
- Decreased feeding
- Skin warm to the touch
- Rashes or *petechiae* (small, purplish, hemorrhagic spots on the skin)

Term infants may produce beads of sweat on their brow but not on the rest of their body. Premature infants will have no visible sweat at all.

Treatment of a neonate with fever will, for the most part, be limited to ensuring a patent airway and adequate ventilation. Do not use cold packs, which may drop the temperature too quickly and may also cause seizures. If the newborn becomes bradycardic, provide chest compressions. In the prehospital setting, administration of an antipyretic agent to a neonate is of questionable benefit and should be avoided. Select the appropriate treatment facility and explain the need for transport to the parents or caregivers.

Hypothermia

As previously noted, hypothermia presents a common and life-threatening condition for newborns. Adults sometimes fail to realize that a newborn may die because of exposure to temperatures that adults find comfortable. The increased surface-to-volume relationship in newborns makes them extremely sensitive to environmental temperatures, especially right after delivery when they are wet. As a result, it is important to control the four methods of heat loss: evaporation, conduction, convection, and radiation.

In treating hypothermia—a body temperature below 35°C (95°F)—keep in mind that it can also be an indicator of sepsis in the newborn. Regardless of the cause, the increased metabolic demands created by hypothermia can produce a variety of related conditions including metabolic acidosis, pulmonary hypertension, and hypoxemia.

In assessing hypothermic newborns, remember that they do not shiver. Instead, expect these findings:

- Pale color
- Skin cool to the touch, particularly in the extremities
- **Acrocyanosis**
- Respiratory distress
- Possible apnea
- Bradycardia
- Central cyanosis
- Initial irritability
- Lethargy in later stages

Management focuses on ensuring adequate ventilations and oxygenation. Chest compressions may be performed, if necessary. With medical direction, you might administer warm fluids through an IV fluid heater. Do not microwave fluids, because great variations in fluid temperature can result. Dextrose ($D_{10}W$ or $D_{25}W$) may also be given if the newborn is hypoglycemic. Above all, the newborn must be kept warm. Set the ambulance temperature at 24°C to 26°C (75.2°F–78.8°F). Also remember to warm your hands before touching the newborn. Select the appropriate receiving facility and transport rapidly.

Hypoglycemia

Newborns are the only age group that can develop severe hypoglycemia and not have diabetes mellitus. Hypoglycemia may be caused by inadequate glucose intake or increased glucose utilization. Stress and other factors can also cause the blood sugar to fall, sometimes to a critical level.

Hypoglycemia is more common in premature or small-for-gestational-age (SGA) infants, the smaller twin, and newborns of a diabetic mother, because these infants often have decreased glycogen stores. Hypoglycemia can also develop as a result of increased glucose utilization. Causes include respiratory illnesses, hypothermia, toxemia, CNS hemorrhage, asphyxia, meningitis, and sepsis. In an older infant, hypoglycemia may be caused by an inadequate glucose intake or increased utilization of glucose. Infants receiving glucose infusions can develop hypoglycemia if the infusion is suddenly stopped.

Infants with hypoglycemia may be asymptomatic or they may exhibit symptoms such as apnea, color changes, respiratory distress, lethargy, seizures, acidosis, and poor myocardial contractility.

Persistent hypoglycemia can have catastrophic effects on the brain. The normal newborn's glycogen stores are sufficient to meet glucose requirements for only 8 to 12 hours. This time frame is diminished in infants with decreased glycogen stores or the presence of other problems in which glucose utilization increases. As a result, you should determine the blood glucose level on all sick infants. A blood glucose screening test of less than 45 mg/dL indicates hypoglycemia.

In response to hypoglycemia, the newborn's body will release counterregulatory hormones such as glucagon, epinephrine,

cortisol, and growth hormone. These hormones help raise the blood glucose level by mobilizing glucose stores. In fact, this hormone response may cause transient symptoms of hyperglycemia that can last for several hours. However, when the infant's glucose stores are depleted, the glucose level will again fall.

In assessing hypoglycemic newborns, expect these findings:

- Twitching or seizures
- Limpness
- Lethargy
- Eye rolling
- High-pitched cry
- Apnea
- Irregular respirations
- Possible cyanosis

Treatment begins with management of the airway and ventilations. Ensure adequate oxygenation. Perform chest compressions, if indicated. With medical direction, administer dextrose ($D_{10}W$ or $D_{25}W$). Maintain a normal body temperature in the newborn and transport to the appropriate facility.

Vomiting

Vomiting in a neonate may result from a variety of causes and rarely presents as an isolated symptom. Vomiting (a forceful ejection of stomach contents) is uncommon during the first weeks of life and may be confused with regurgitation (a simple backflow of stomach contents into the mouth, or "spitting up"). Vomiting in the neonate usually occurs because of an anatomic abnormality such as a tracheoesophageal fistula or upper gastrointestinal obstruction. More often, it may be a symptom of a serious disorder, such as increased intracranial pressure or an infection. Vomitus containing dark blood often signals a life-threatening illness. Keep in mind, however, that vomiting of mucus, which may occasionally be blood streaked, in the first few hours after birth is not uncommon.

Assessment findings may include a distended stomach, signs of infection, increased intracranial pressure, or drug withdrawal. Because vomitus can be aspirated, management considerations focus on ensuring a patent airway. If you detect respiratory difficulties or obstruction of the airway, suction or clear vomitus from the airway and ensure adequate oxygenation. Fluid administration may be needed to prevent dehydration. Also remember that, as with older patients, **vagal stimulation** may cause bradycardia in the neonate.

After you have protected the airway, place the infant on his side and transport to an appropriate facility. As with all other situations involving distressed neonates, advise parents or caregivers of the steps taken and why.

Diarrhea

Diarrhea in a neonate can cause severe dehydration and electrolyte imbalances. Although diarrhea may be harder to assess in neonates than in other patients, consider five to six stools per day as normal, especially in breast-fed infants.

Causes of diarrhea in a neonate include:

- Bacterial or viral infection
- Gastroenteritis
- Lactose intolerance
- **Phototherapy**
- **Neonatal abstinence syndrome (NAS)**
- **Thyrotoxicosis**
- Cystic fibrosis

In treating neonates with diarrhea, remember to take Standard Precautions, just as you would do in any situation involving body fluids. Expect to find loose stools, decreased urinary output, and other signs of dehydration, such as prolonged capillary refill time, cool extremities, and listlessness or lethargy. It is often difficult for the parents to estimate the number of stools. In such cases, it might be better to inquire about the number of diapers the baby is using.

Management consists of maintenance of airway and ventilations, adequate oxygenation, and chest compressions, if indicated. With medical direction, you might also consider fluid therapy. Explain all treatments to parents or caregivers, and transport the neonate to a facility able to handle high-risk infants.

Common Birth Injuries

A **birth injury** occurs in an estimated 2 to 7 of every 1,000 live births in the United States. About 5 to 8 of every 100,000 infants die of birth trauma and 25 of every 100,000 die of anoxic injuries. Such injuries account for 2 to 3 percent of infant deaths. Risk factors for birth injury include:

- Prematurity
- Postmaturity
- Cephalopelvic disproportion
- Prolonged labor
- Breech presentation
- Explosive delivery
- Shoulder dystocia
- Diabetic mother

Birth injuries take various forms. Cranial injuries may include molding of the head and overriding of the parietal bones, erythema (reddening of the skin), abrasions, ecchymosis (black-and-blue discoloration) and subcutaneous fat necrosis, subconjunctival and retinal hemorrhage, subperiosteal hemorrhage, and fracture of the skull. Intracranial hemorrhage may result from trauma or asphyxia. Often the infant will develop a large scalp hematoma during the birth process. This injury, called *caput succedaneum*, will usually resolve over a week's time. Damage to the spine and spinal cord may occur as a result of strong traction exerted when the spine is hyperextended or there is a lateral pull. Other birth injuries include peripheral nerve injury, injury to the liver, rupture of the spleen, adrenal hemorrhage, fractures of the clavicle or extremities, and, of course, hypoxia/ischemia.

Assessment findings may include:

- Diffuse, sometimes ecchymotic, edematous swelling of soft tissues around the scalp
- Paralysis below the level of the spinal cord injury
- Paralysis of the upper arm with or without paralysis of the forearm
- Diaphragmatic paralysis
- Movement on only one side of the face when crying
- Inability to move the arm freely on the side of the fractured clavicle
- Lack of spontaneous movement of the affected extremity
- Hypoxia
- Shock

Management of a newborn with birth injuries usually centers on protection of the airway, provision of adequate ventilation and oxygen, and, if needed, chest compressions. With medical direction, you may administer medications or take other nonpharmacological steps to support the specific injury. Newborns with birth injuries usually require treatment at specialized facilities. As in the management of other neonatal emergencies, provide professional and compassionate communication to parents or caregivers.

Cardiac Resuscitation, Postresuscitation, and Stabilization

The incidence of neonatal cardiac arrest is related primarily to hypoxia. As explained previously, the outcome will be poor unless you immediately initiate appropriate interventions. As

CULTURAL CONSIDERATIONS

When Parents Request Baptism

Occasionally, prehospital childbirth may result in the delivery of a stillborn infant. The reasons for the infant's demise may be obvious or the infant may appear otherwise normal. Some Christian families may request that the infant be baptized as soon as possible after birth. In fact, in some faiths, failure to baptize the infant might "deny a child the priceless grace of becoming a child of God." Infant baptism is primarily a practice of the Roman Catholic Church, although similar faiths (Episcopalian, Anglican) also often practice the rite. If you are asked to baptize an infant, remember that, despite your own personal religious beliefs, this is very important to the parents and they have put a great deal of trust in you. According to the Catechism of the Catholic Church, dip your finger into a bowl of water and make a sign of the cross on the infant's forehead. Then say, "I baptize you in the name of the Father and of the Son and of the Holy Spirit. Amen." Even if you are not baptized, in an emergency you may baptize an infant if that is the parents' wish, provided you act in the spirit of church teaching. Most parents will appreciate the act. Sometimes, even in this era of sophisticated medical technology, there is little we can do other than provide support to the survivors.

CONTENT REVIEW

► Causes of Neonatal Cardiac Arrest

- Primary or secondary apnea
- Bradycardia
- Persistent fetal circulation
- Pulmonary hypertension

you might expect, cases involving cardiac arrest have an increased chance of brain and organ damage. Risk factors for cardiac arrest in newborns include:

- Bradycardia
- Intrauterine asphyxia

- Congenital malformations
- Intrapartum hypoxemia

Cardiac arrest can be caused by primary or secondary apnea, bradycardia, persistent fetal circulation, or pulmonary hypertension. Assessment findings may include peripheral cyanosis, inadequate respiratory effort, and ineffective or absent heart rate.

In managing neonatal cardiac arrest, follow the inverted pyramid for resuscitation (Figure 3-16). Administer drugs or fluids according to medical direction. Maintain normal body temperature while you transport the distressed newborn to the appropriate facility. This situation will require delicate handling of the parents or caregivers. Explain what is being done for the infant, without discussing the possibilities of survival.

- Prematurity
- Drugs administered to or taken by the mother
- Congenital neuromuscular diseases

SUMMARY

After a woman gives birth, you must care for two patients—the mother and her newborn child. The newborn has several special needs, the most important of which are protection of the airway and support of ventilations. The most important aspects of newborn care, aside from airway and ventilation, are preventing heat loss and warming the newborn, who must be kept warm at all times.

If assessment reveals a distressed newborn, you should initiate ventilatory support, stimulation, and, if required, CPR. Keep in mind that it is not uncommon for the newborn to require a little oxygen and even ventilatory support following birth. Generally, oxygen therapy and ventilatory support will dramatically improve the majority of poorly presenting infants. Remember to start simply (blow-by oxygen) and progress to the more invasive procedures (CPR) when the newborn presents with a low APGAR score. When possible, newborns born away from a facility should be transported to a facility with an NICU.

YOU MAKE THE CALL

You are called to assist a BLS unit with a difficult delivery. When you arrive at the scene, the EMTs report that the patient is a 35-year-old woman who is two weeks past full term. Her amniotic sac has just ruptured, and thick meconium staining is observed. The infant is crowning. Just after your arrival at the scene, the mother begins to scream that the baby is coming.

1. Should you stimulate this baby to breathe as soon as it is delivered? Why or why not?

2. What is the major danger associated with this type of problem?

3. Once you have stabilized this infant, where should he be transported?

See Suggested Responses at the back of this book.

REVIEW QUESTIONS

1. About 80 percent of newborns weighing less than _____ grams at birth require resuscitation.
   a. 1,500
   b. 2,000
   c. 2,500
   d. 2,800

2. Factors that stimulate the baby's first breath include all of the following *except* _____.
   a. hypoxia
   b. hyperthermia
   c. mild acidosis
   d. initiation of stretch reflexes in the lungs

3. Most fetal development occurs during the _____ trimester of pregnancy.
   a. last
   b. third
   c. first
   d. second

4. The newborn's respiratory rate should average _____ breaths per minute and the heart rate should fall within the range of _____ beats per minute.
   a. 20–30, 90–110
   b. 25–35, 100–110
   c. 30–40, 110–120
   d. 40–60, 130–140

5. The maximum APGAR score is _____.
   a. 6   c. 8
   b. 7   d. 10

6. Most heat loss in newborns results from _____.
   a. radiation
   b. convection
   c. conduction
   d. evaporation

7. In a newborn, _____ refers to an excess of red blood cells and may reflect hypovolemia or prolonged intrauterine hypoxia.
   a. choanal atresia
   b. polycythemia
   c. omphalocele
   d. Pierre Robin syndrome

8. When caring for a newborn, suctioning should last no longer than _____ seconds.
   a. 5   c. 15
   b. 10   d. 20

9. In the newborn, vascular access for the administration of fluids and drugs can most readily be managed by using the _____ vein.
   a. cephalic   c. umbilical
   b. brachial   d. saphenous

10. A premature newborn is an infant born prior to _____ weeks of gestation or with weight ranging from 0.6 to 2.2 kg.
   a. 40   c. 38
   b. 39   d. 37

See Answers to Review Questions at the back of this book.

REFERENCES

1. Perlman, J. M. and R. Risser. "Cardiopulmonary Resuscitation in the Delivery Room: Associated Clinical Events." *Arch Pediatr Adolesc Med* 149 (1995): 20–25.

2. Barber, C. A. and M. H. Wyckoff. "Use and Efficacy of Endotracheal versus Intravenous Epinephrine during Neonatal Cardiopulmonary Resuscitation in the Delivery Room." *Pediatrics* 118 (2006): 1028–1034.

3. Toth, B., A. Becker, and B. Seelbach-Gobel. "Oxygen Saturation in Healthy Newborn Infants Immediately after Birth Measured by Pulse Oximetry." *Arch Gynecol Obstet* 266 (2002): 105–107.

4. Davis, P. G., A. Tan, C. P. O'Donnell, and A. Schulze. "Resuscitation of Newborn Infants with 100% Oxygen or Air: A Systematic Review and Meta-Analysis." *Lancet* 364 (2004): 1329–1333.

5. Rabi, Y., D. Rabi, and W. Yee. "Room Air Resuscitation of the Depressed Newborn: A Systematic Review and Meta-Analysis." *Resuscitation* 72 (2007): 353–363.

6. Apgar, V. "A Proposal for a New Method of Evaluation of the Newborn Infant." *Anesth Analg* 32 (1953): 260–267.

7. Mieczyslaw, F. and M. Wood. "The APGAR Score has Survived the Test of Time." *Anesthesiology* 102 (2005): 855–857.

8. Kattwinkel, J., J. M. Perlman, K. Aziz, et al. "Part 15: Neonatal Resuscitation: 2010 American Heart Association Guidelines for Cardiopulmonary Resuscitation and Emergency Cardiovascular Care." *Circulation* 122 (2010): S909–S919.

9. Berg, M. D., S. M. Schexnayder, L. Chameides, et al. "Part 13: Pediatric Basic Life Support: 2010 American Heart Association Guidelines for Cardiopulmonary Resuscitation and Emergency Cardiovascular Care." *Circulation* 122 (2010): S862–S875.

10. Roggensack, A., A. L. Jeffries, D. Farine, et al. "Management of Meconium at Birth." *J Obstet Gynaecol Can* 31 (2009): 355–357.

11. Raghuveer, T. S. and A. J. Cox. "Neonatal Resuscitation: An Update." *Am Family Physician* 83 (2011): 911–918.

FURTHER READING

American Heart Association. *2010 American Heart Association Guidelines for CPR and ECC.* Dallas: American Heart Association, 2010.

American Heart Association and American Academy of Pediatrics. *PALS Provider Manual.* 6th ed. Dallas: American Heart Association, 2011.

Braner, D., J. Kattwinkel, S. Denson, and S. Niermeyer, eds. *Neonatal Resuscitation.* 5th ed. Elk Grove Village, IL: American Academy of Pediatrics, 2011.

DeBoer, J. L. *Emergency Newborn Care: The First Minutes of Life.* Chicago: ACM Publications, 2004.

Kleigman, R. M., et al. *Nelson Textbook of Pediatrics.* 19th ed. Philadelphia: W. B. Saunders, 2011.

Tintinalli, J. E., J. Stapczynski, O. John Ma, D. Cline, and R. Cydulka. *Emergency Medicine: A Comprehensive Study Guide.* 7th ed. New York: McGraw-Hill, 2010.

Pediatrics

Bryan Bledsoe, DO, FACEP, FAAEM, EMT-P

STANDARD
Special Patient Populations (Pediatrics)

COMPETENCY
Integrates assessment findings with principles of epidemiology and pathophysiology and knowledge of psychosocial needs to formulate a field impression and implement a comprehensive treatment/disposition plan for patients with special needs.

OBJECTIVES

Terminal Performance Objective
After reading this chapter, you should be able to integrate patient assessment findings, patient history, and knowledge of anatomy, physiology, pathophysiology, and basic and advanced life support interventions to recognize and manage emergencies in pediatric patients.

Enabling Objectives
To accomplish the terminal performance objective, you should be able to:

1. Define key terms introduced in this chapter.

2. Describe the roles of paramedics in pediatric illness and injury prevention and in the management of ill and injured children.

3. Formulate a plan for becoming and remaining proficient in assessing and managing pediatric patients.

4. Relate the developmental, anatomic, and physiologic differences of children of various ages to adaptations in communication, assessment, and management of pediatric patients.

5. Consider the psychosocial needs of the parents or caregivers of a pediatric patient.

6. Use a process of clinical reasoning to guide and interpret the patient assessment and management process for pediatric patients.

7. Adapt the scene size-up, primary assessment, patient history, secondary assessment, and use of monitoring technology to meet the needs of pediatric patients.

8. Recognize specific problems in pediatric patients, including infection, respiratory emergencies, hypoperfusion, cardiac emergencies, neurologic emergencies, gastrointestinal problems, diabetic emergencies, poisoning and toxicologic emergencies, trauma, drowning, and burns.

9. Relate the pathophysiology of specific pediatric problems to the priorities of patient assessment and management.

10. Adapt equipment and techniques of management to meet the needs of pediatric patients in positioning and immobilization, airway management, ventilation, oxygenation, vascular access, fluid and medication administration, and cardiac arrest management.

11. Recognize indications of abuse or neglect of a pediatric patient.

12. Describe special considerations in management and documentation of situations involving SIDS, ALTE, abuse, and neglect.

13. Work with caregivers to troubleshoot home care equipment for special needs pediatric patients and intervene as needed.

14. Apply the JumpSTART triage method to multiple-casualty incidents involving children.

15. Communicate relevant patient information orally and in writing when transferring care of the pediatric patient to hospital personnel.

KEY TERMS

asthma, p. 110

bacterial tracheitis, p. 109

bend fractures, p. 126

bronchiolitis, p. 111

buckle fractures, p. 126

cardiogenic shock, p. 113

central IV line, p. 131

congenital, p. 114

croup, p. 107

diabetic ketoacidosis, p. 119

distributive shock, p. 113

Emergency Medical Services for Children (EMSC), p. 72

epiglottitis, p. 108

febrile seizures, p. 117

foreign body airway obstruction (FBAO), p. 75

greenstick fractures, p. 126

growth plate, p. 79

hyperglycemia, p. 119

hypoglycemia, p. 118

hypovolemic shock, p. 113

noncardiogenic shock, p. 113

shunt, p. 131

status epilepticus, p. 116

stoma, p. 130

sudden infant death syndrome, p. 127

tracheostomy, p. 130

CASE STUDY

Three tones sound on the paramedic radios in the ED. A message crackles: "LA Fifty-Four, I need you to be in-service." The crew of LA 54 transfers care of the patient in Bed 6 to the hospital staff. Within 60 seconds, they depart the hospital parking lot. En route to the emergency, they review information provided by the dispatcher. They will be treating a 5-month-old girl who is described as "not breathing" by the father.

The response time is 4 minutes. On arrival, the parents lead the paramedics into the patient's bedroom. The little girl is lying in a crib. Immediately, paramedics note that she has pale, cool, clammy skin. Her anterior fontanelle is noticeably sunken. The respiratory rate and quality are 20 and shallow. Upon mild painful stimuli, the infant cries vigorously, increasing her tidal rate and volume. However, no tears appear. After taking Standard Precautions, the paramedics check the diaper and find that it is dry. "She hasn't kept any food down for three days," explains the mother. "She hasn't wet her diaper in hours."

The crew administers supplemental oxygen via a nonrebreather mask. The infant responds to the mask by crying, but she makes no effort to remove it. Capillary refill is borderline (2.5 seconds). The paramedics prepare to transport the infant to the ED, informing the parents of all the steps that will be taken to help their daughter.

En route to the hospital, the crew establishes an IV and administers a fluid bolus of 20 mL/kg of normal saline. By the time they pull up to the ambulance ramp at the ED, the patient's color and respiratory rate have improved greatly. Capillary refill time and pulse rate move toward normal limits. The ED staff evaluates the patient and admits her for 24-hour observation and IV fluid therapy. She returns home the following day. The paramedics later learn that she had contracted a viral gastroenteritis that was going around her day care center. Within 48 hours she was back to her usual playful self.

INTRODUCTION

The ill or injured child presents special concerns for prehospital personnel. Current research indicates that more than 20,000 pediatric deaths occur each year in the United States. The leading causes of death are age specific. They include motor vehicle collisions, burns, drownings, suicides, and homicides. These alarming facts become even more troublesome when experts theorize that many of them could have been prevented by early intervention. Tragedies involving children—neonates to adolescents—account for some of the most stressful incidents that you will encounter in EMS practice.[1]

Treatment of pediatric patients presents a number of challenges for the paramedic. Children, especially young ones, often cannot describe what is bothering them or what has happened to them. In addition to the child patient, you must deal with the parents or caregivers. Finally, a child's size often makes routine procedures more difficult. Keep in mind that children are not simply small adults. They have special considerations and needs. This chapter will present the topic of pediatric emergencies as it applies to advanced prehospital care.

ROLE OF PARAMEDICS IN PEDIATRIC CARE

When considering the reduction of pediatric morbidity and mortality, your role as a paramedic centers around two key concepts. First, you must realize that pediatric injuries have become a major health concern. Second, you should remember that children are at a higher risk of injury than adults and that they are more likely to be adversely affected by the injuries that they suffer.

Numerous factors account for the high pediatric injury rates. Some factors, such as geography and weather, cannot be altered. However, other factors, particularly dangers within the home and community, can be eliminated or minimized. As health care professionals, we must all get involved in identifying and implementing methods and mechanisms that prevent injuries to infants and children. Those of us who deliver prehospital care must do more than simply enter the picture after an injury has taken place.

In addition to treating pediatric injuries, paramedics are often responsible for treating the ill child. Many aspects of disease and disease processes are unique to children. It is important that the paramedic be familiar with these, because early intervention is often the key to reduced morbidity and mortality.

Continuing Education and Training

Your role in improving the health care offered to pediatric patients begins with your own training. Because you will encounter pediatric patients less frequently than adult patients, you have a professional responsibility to maintain and improve on your pediatric knowledge, particularly your clinical skills.[2] Continuing education programs include:

- Pediatric Advanced Life Support (PALS)
- Pediatric Education for Paramedic Professionals (PEPP)

- Advanced Pediatric Life Support (APLS)
- Prehospital Pediatric Care (PPC)

In addition to these programs, you can also attend regional conferences and seminars designed to increase your knowledge of pediatric care. These are often conducted by regional children's hospitals. You can further enhance your clinical skills by spending time in pediatric emergency departments, pediatric hospitals, or pediatric departments in local hospitals. You might also visit the offices of pediatricians or talk with pediatric nurse practitioners—registered nurses who provide primary health care to children.

Improved Health Care and Injury Prevention

Funding for a significant amount of prehospital pediatric education comes largely from a program known as **Emergency Medical Services for Children (EMSC)**.[3] This federally funded program falls under the management of the Maternal and Child Health Bureau, an agency of the U.S. Department of Health and Human Services. The EMSC was formed for the express purpose of improving the health of pediatric patients who suffer potentially life-threatening illnesses or injuries. This nationally coordinated effort has identified a number of pediatric health care concerns, including:

- Community education
- Data collection
- Quality improvement
- Injury prevention
- Access
- Prehospital care
- Emergency care
- Definitive care
- Finance
- Rehabilitation
- A systems approach to pediatric care
- Ongoing health care from birth to young adulthood

As a paramedic, you can take part in this national effort by actively participating in programs that promote injury prevention. Let's face it—as prehospital care providers, we see the consequences of pediatric trauma all too often. You can help reduce the rate of injury by taking advantage of opportunities to share "teaching points" in your daily life, both personally and professionally. Take part in, or offer to organize, school or community programs in injury prevention or health care (Figure 4-1 ●). Engage student interest in the EMS profession by volunteering to speak at "career days," emphasizing those aspects of your job that relate to young people. Use nonurgent ambulance calls as a chance to educate family members or caregivers on the importance of "childproofing" a home or neighborhood. Work with appropriate agencies in initiating or conducting safety inspections, block watches, and more.

Increased effort has been made to identify the severity and nature of prehospital pediatric emergencies. Many regions now

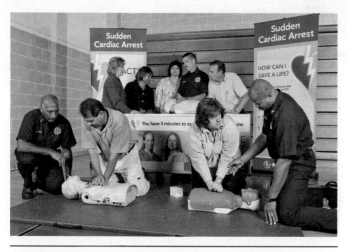

● **Figure 4-1**   It is important to organize or participate in programs that educate the public about injury prevention and health care.

have both pediatric and trauma registries. These, in addition to standard epidemiological research conducted by local health departments, are dependent on quality prehospital documentation. If your area is participating in a registry program or research study, be sure to obtain and record all required data. Information gained from these registries will help identify the need for more or specialized resources.

Advanced Life Support Skills in Pediatrics

Several recent research studies have shown that up to 85 percent of children treated by EMS personnel need nothing more than basic life support skills.[4] These include such things as bandaging and splinting, oxygen administration, and similar fundamental skills. In addition, only a limited percentage of EMS transports involve children. Thus, it is fairly rare that a paramedic will be called on to perform an advanced life support (ALS) skill such as intubation, IV access, or drug administration in a child. Because these skills are used infrequently in EMS, it is difficult for paramedics to remain proficient in them. For this reason, several large EMS systems have abandoned the practice of pediatric endotracheal intubation in favor of simple bag-valve-mask (BVM) ventilation. Likewise, some systems have opted for less aggressive pediatric prehospital care.

Regardless of how your system operates, it is important to remember that the less frequently a skill is used, the more frequently it should be practiced. Certain ALS skills can be lifesaving when properly applied. Thus, it is incumbent on each paramedic to realize that pediatric ALS skills will be needed infrequently. When they are needed, however, they must be applied competently.

GENERAL APPROACH TO PEDIATRIC EMERGENCIES

The approach to the pediatric patient varies with the age of the patient and with the problem being treated. Foremost in approaching any pediatric emergency is consideration of the patient's

emotional and physiologic development. Care also involves the family members or caregivers responsible for the child. They will demand information, express fears, and, ultimately, give or refuse consent for treatment and/or transport.

CONTENT REVIEW

▶ Top Causes of Pediatric Deaths

• Motor vehicle crashes
• Burns
• Drownings
• Suicides
• Homicides

Communication and Psychological Support

Treatment of an infant, child, or teenager begins with communication and psychological support. Interaction with pediatric patients and related adults continues throughout assessment and management. When obtaining the medical history of the pediatric patient, you should gather information as quickly and as accurately as possible. The parents and caregivers are often the primary source of information, especially in the case of infants. However, as children become older, they can also be a good source of information. Older children, for example, can often give accurate descriptions of symptoms or other details.

Treat pediatric patients with respect, allowing them to express opinions and ask questions. Your listening skills will play an important role in alleviating the fears of child patients. You can even communicate a calm and caring attitude to infants, who respond to touch and voice just like any other human being.

Responding to Patient Needs

As previously mentioned, a child's response to an emergency will vary, depending on the age and emotional maturity of the child. The child's most common response to illness or injury is fear. Common fears of children include:

● Fear of being separated from the parents or caregivers
● Fear of being removed from a family place, such as home, and never returning
● Fear of being hurt
● Fear of being mutilated or disfigured
● Fear of the unknown

These fears may be intensified if the child detects fear or anxiety from the parents or caregivers. The general chaos and panic that often surround pediatric emergency situations may further distress the child.

Remember that children have the right to know what is being done to them. You should be as honest as possible with them. If a procedure such as an IV needlestick will hurt, tell them so—but tell them immediately before performing a procedure. Do not say that a procedure will be painful and then take 5 minutes to prepare the equipment, allowing time for the child's anticipation of pain to build.

Always use language that is appropriate for the age of the child. Medical and anatomic terms that we routinely use may be completely foreign to children. Telling a child that you are going to "apply a cervical collar" means nothing. Instead, tell the child: "I'm going to put this collar around your neck to keep it from moving." "Try to hold your head still." "Tell me if it is too tight." Communication such as this will involve children in their own care and reduce their feelings of helplessness.

Responding to Parents or Caregivers

As you might expect, the reactions of parents or caregivers to a pediatric emergency will vary. Initial reactions might include shock, grief, denial, anger, guilt, fear, or complete loss of control. Their behavior may change during the course of the emergency. Communication is the key. Preferably only one paramedic will speak with adults at the scene. This will reduce any chance of providing conflicting information and allow a second paramedic to focus on the child. If parents or caregivers sense your confidence and professionalism, they will regain control and trust your suggestions for care. As with the child, most parents and caregivers feel overwhelmed by fear. They often express their fears in questions such as the following:

"Is my child going to die?"
"Did my child suffer brain damage?"
"Is my child going to be all right?"
"What are you doing to my child?"
"Will my child be able to walk?"

It may be difficult to answer these questions in the prehospital setting. However, the following actions may help allay parents' fears:

- Tell them your name and qualifications.
- Acknowledge their fears and concerns.
- Reassure them that it is all right to feel the way they do.
- Redirect their energies toward helping you care for the child.
- Remain calm and appear in control of the emergency.
- Keep the parents or caregivers informed as to what you are doing.
- Don't "talk down" to them.
- Assure parents or caregivers that everything possible is being done for their child.

If conditions permit, you should allow one of the parents or caregivers to remain with the child at all times. Some family members may be extremely emotional in emergency situations. The child will react more positively to a family member who appears calm and reassuring. If a parent or caregiver is "out of control," have another person take him or her away from the immediate area to settle down. Maintain a reasonable level of suspicion if a child shows a pattern of injuries, some old and some new. In such cases, the parent or caregiver may try to cover up what may be an abusive situation. They may also try to block examination and treatment. (Potential abuse or neglect will be discussed in more detail later in this chapter.)

GROWTH AND DEVELOPMENT

Children progress through developmental stages on their way to adulthood. You should tailor your approach to the developmental level of your pediatric patient, as discussed in the following segments.

Newborns (First Hours after Birth)

Although the terms *newborn* and *neonate* are often used interchangeably, *newborn* refers to a baby in the first hours of extrauterine life. The term *neonate* describes infants from birth to one month of age. The method most frequently used to assess newborns is the APGAR scoring system, which was described in Chapter 3. Resuscitation of the newborn generally follows the inverted pyramid described in Chapter 3 and the guidelines established in the Neonatal Advanced Life Support (NALS) curriculum.

Neonates (Birth to One Month)

The neonate, as just noted and as described in Chapter 3, is an infant up to one month of age. This is a major stage of development. Soon after birth, the neonate typically loses up to 10 percent of his birth weight as he adjusts to extrauterine life. This lost weight, however, is ordinarily recovered within ten days. Gestational age affects early growth. Children born at term (40 weeks) should follow accepted developmental guidelines. Infants born prematurely will not be as developed, either neurologically or physically, as their term counterparts.

The neonatal stage of development centers on reflexes. The neonate's personality also begins to form. The infant is close to the mother and may stare at faces and smile. The mother, and occasionally the father, can comfort and quiet the child. Common illnesses in this age group include jaundice, vomiting, and respiratory distress. Serious illnesses, such as meningitis, are difficult to distinguish from minor illnesses in neonates. Often, fever is the only sign, although the majority of neonates with fever have minor illnesses (96 to 97 percent). The few who are seriously ill can be easily missed. For this reason, any fever in a neonate requires extensive evaluation.

The approach to this age group should include several factors. First, the child should always be kept warm. Observe skin color, tone, and respiratory activity. The absence of tears when crying may indicate dehydration. The lungs should be auscultated early during the exam, while the infant is quiet. You might find it helpful to have the child suck on a pacifier during the examination. Allowing the infant to remain in a parent's or caregiver's lap may help keep the child calm. Obviously, the history must be obtained from the parents or caregivers. However, it is also important to observe the child.

Infants (Ages One to Five Months)

Infants should have doubled their birth weight by five to six months of age. They should be able to follow the movements of others with their eyes. Muscle control develops in a cephalocaudal progression. This means, literally, that development of muscular control begins at the head (cephalo) and moves toward the tail (caudal). Muscular control also spreads from the trunk toward the extremities during this period. The infant's personality at this stage still centers closely on the parents or caregivers. The history must be obtained from these individuals, with close attention to possible illnesses and accidents, including sudden infant death syndrome (SIDS), vomiting, dehydration, meningitis, child abuse, and household accidents.

Concentrate on keeping these patients warm and comfortable. Allow the infant to remain in the parent's or caregiver's lap. A pacifier or bottle can be used to help keep the baby quiet during the examination.

Infants (Ages Six Months to One Year)

Infants in this age group may stand or even walk with assistance. They are quite active and enjoy exploring the world with their mouths. In this stage of development, the risk of **foreign body airway obstruction (FBAO)** becomes a serious concern.

Infants six months and older have more fully formed personalities and express themselves more readily. They have considerable anxiety toward strangers. They do not like lying on their backs. Children in this age group tend to cling to the mother, although the father "will do" in many cases. Common illnesses and accidents include febrile seizures, vomiting, diarrhea, dehydration, bronchiolitis, car crashes, croup, child abuse, poisonings, falls, airway obstructions, and meningitis.

These children should be examined while sitting in the lap of the parent or caregiver (Figure 4-2 ●). The exam should progress in a toe-to-head order, because starting at the face may upset the child. If time and conditions permit, allow the child to become familiar with you before beginning the examination.

Toddlers (Ages One to Three Years)

Great strides occur in gross motor development during this stage. Children tend to run underneath or stand on almost everything. They seem to always be on the move. As they grow older, toddlers become braver and more curious or stubborn.

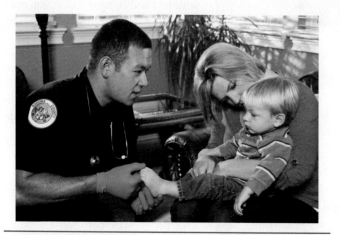

● **Figure 4-2** Infants and young children should be allowed to remain in their mother's arms.

They begin to stray away from the parents or caregivers more frequently. These remain the only people who can comfort them quickly, however, and most children will cling to a parent or caregiver if frightened.

At ages one to three years, language development begins. Often children can understand better than they can speak. Therefore, the majority of the medical history will still come from the parents or caregivers. Remember, however, that you can ask toddlers simple and specific questions.

Accidents of all types are the leading cause of injury deaths in pediatric patients ages 1 to 15 years. Common accidents in this age group include motor vehicle collisions, homicides, burn injuries, drownings, and pedestrian collisions. Common illnesses and injuries in the toddler age group include vomiting, diarrhea, febrile seizures, poisonings, falls, child abuse, croup, and meningitis. Keep in mind that FBAO is still a high risk for toddlers.

Be cautious when treating toddlers. Approach toddlers slowly and try to gain their confidence. Conduct the exam in a toe-to-head order. The child may be difficult to examine and may resist being touched. Speak quietly and use only simple words. Avoid asking questions that allow the child to say "no." If the situation permits, allow toddlers to hold transitional objects such as a favorite blanket or toy. Be sure to tell the child if something will hurt. If at all possible, avoid procedures on the dominant arm/hand, which the child will try to pull away.

Preschoolers (Ages Three to Five Years)

Children in this age group show a tremendous increase in fine and gross motor development. Language skills increase greatly. Children in this age group know how to talk. However, if frightened, they often refuse to speak, especially to strangers. They often have vivid imaginations and may see monsters as part of their world. Preschoolers may have tempers and will express them. During this stage of development, children fear mutilation and may feel threatened by treatment. Avoid frightening or misleading comments.

Preschoolers often run to a particular parent or caregiver, depending on the occasion. They stick up for the people they love and are openly affectionate. They still seek support and comfort from within the home.

When evaluating children in this age group, question the child first, keeping in mind that imagination may interfere with the facts. The child often has a distorted sense of time; thus, you must rely on the parents or caregivers to fill in the gaps. Common illnesses and injuries in this age group include croup, asthma, poisonings, auto collisions, burns, child abuse, ingestion of foreign bodies, drownings, epiglottitis, febrile seizures, and meningitis.

Treatment of preschoolers requires tact. Avoid baby talk. If time and situation permit, give the child health care choices. Often the use of a doll or stuffed animal will assist in the examination. Allow the child to hold a piece of equipment, such as a stethoscope, and to use it. Let the child sit on your lap. Start the examination with the chest and evaluate the head last. Avoid misleading comments. Do not trick or lie to the child and always explain what you are going to do.

School-Age Children (Ages 6 to 12 Years)

Children in this age group are active and carefree. Growth spurts sometimes lead to clumsiness. The personality continues to develop. School-age children are protective and proud of their parents or caregivers and seek their attention. They value peers, but also need home support.

When examining school-age children, give them the responsibility of providing the history. However, remember that children may be reluctant to provide information if they sustained an injury while doing something forbidden. The parents or caregivers can fill in the pertinent details. When assessing children in this age group, it is important to respect their modesty. Be honest and tell the child what is wrong. A small toy may help to calm the child (Figures 4-3 ● and 4-4 ●). Common illnesses and injuries for this age group include drownings, auto collisions, bicycle accidents, falls, fractures, sports injuries, child abuse, and burns.

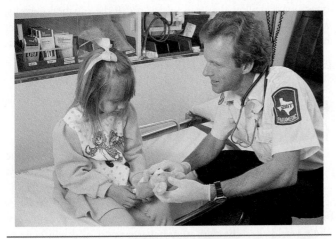

● **Figure 4-3** A small toy may calm a child in the six- to ten-year age range.

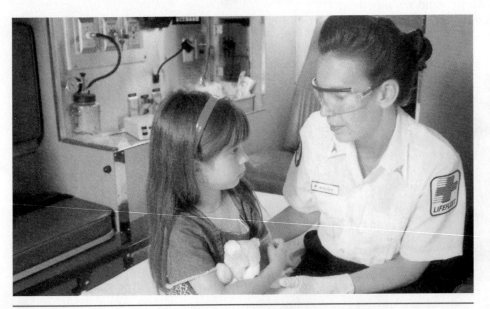

● **Figure 4-4** The approach to the pediatric patient should be gentle and slow.

Adolescents (Ages 13 to 18 Years)

Adolescence covers the period from the end of childhood to the start of adulthood (age 18). It begins with puberty, roughly age 13 for male children and age 11 for female children. (For this reason, adolescence is often defined as including ages 11 to 18, rather than 13 to 18.) Puberty is highly child specific and can begin at various ages. A female child, for example, may experience her first menstrual period as early as age 7 or 8.

Adolescents vary significantly in their development. Those over age 15 are physically nearer to adults in terms of their vital signs, but emotionally they may still be children. Regardless of physical maturity, remember that teenagers as a group are "body conscious." They worry about their physical image more than any other pediatric age group. You should tactfully address their stated concerns about body integrity or disfigurement. The slightest possibility of a lasting scar may be a tremendous issue to the adolescent patient.

Although patients in this age group are not yet legally adults, most consider themselves to be grown up. They take offense at the use of the word "child." They have a strong desire to be liked by their peers and to be included. Relationships with parents and caregivers may at times be strained as the adolescent demands greater independence. They value the opinions of other adolescents. Generally, these patients make good historians. Do not be surprised, however, if their perception of events differs from that of their parents or caregivers.

Common illnesses and injuries in this age group include mononucleosis, asthma, auto collisions, sports injuries, drug and alcohol problems, suicide gestures, and sexual abuse. Remember that pregnancy is also possible in female adolescents. When assessing teenagers, remember that their vital signs will approach those of adults. In gathering a history, be factual and address the patient's questions. It may be wise to interview the patient away from the parents or caregivers. Listen to what the teenager is saying, as well as what he is *not* saying. If you suspect substance abuse or endangerment of the patient or others, approach the subject with tact and compassion. If you must perform a detailed physical exam, respect the teenager's sense of privacy. If the patient exhibits modesty or bodily shame, have a paramedic of the same sex as the teenager conduct the examination, if possible. Regardless of the situation, provide psychological support and reassurance.

ANATOMY AND PHYSIOLOGY

The differences between the anatomy and physiology of infants and children and those of adults form

TABLE 4–1 | Anatomic and Physiologic Characteristics of Infants and Children

Differences in Infants and Children as Compared with Adults	Potential Effects That May Affect Assessment and Care
Tongue proportionately larger	More likely to block airway
Smaller airway structures	More easily blocked
Abundant secretions	Can block the airway
Deciduous (baby) teeth	Easily dislodged; can block the airway
Flat nose and face	Difficult to obtain good face mask seal
Head heavier relative to body and less-developed neck structures and muscles	Head may be propelled more forcefully than body, producing a higher incidence of head injury in trauma
Fontanelle and open sutures (soft spots) palpable on top of young infant's head	Bulging fontanelle can be a sign of increased intracranial pressure (but may be normal if infant is crying); shrunken fontanelle may indicate dehydration
Thinner, softer brain tissue	Susceptible to serious brain injury
Head larger in proportion to body	Tips forward when supine; possible flexion of neck, which makes neutral alignment of airway difficult
Shorter, narrower, more elastic (flexible) trachea	Can close off trachea with hyperextension of neck
Short neck	Difficult to stabilize or immobilize
Abdominal breathers	Difficult to evaluate breathing
Faster respiratory rate	Muscles easily fatigue, causing respiratory distress
Newborns breathe primarily through the nose (obligate nose breathers)	May not automatically open mouth to breathe if nose is blocked; airway more easily blocked
Larger body surface relative to body mass	Prone to hypothermia
Softer bones	More flexible, less easily fractured; traumatic forces may be transmitted to internal organs, causing injury without fracturing the ribs; lungs easily damaged with trauma
Spleen and liver more exposed	Organ injury likely with significant force to abdomen

the basis for the differences in the emergency medical care offered to the two groups (Table 4–1). As previously mentioned, children are not simply small adults. They possess bodies well suited to growth. As a rule, they have healthier organs, a greater ability to compensate for most illnesses, and softer, more flexible tissues. Because you will probably have infrequent contact with pediatric patients, you need to regularly review the physical characteristics that distinguish them from the adult patients that you encounter more often (Figure 4-5 ●).

Head

The pediatric patient's head is proportionately larger than an adult's and the occipital region is significantly larger. In comparison to their head size, most pediatric patients have small faces and flat noses, which makes it difficult to obtain a good face–mask seal.

With infants, pay special attention to the fontanelles—areas of the skull that have not yet fused. The fontanelles allow for compression of the head during childbirth and for rapid growth of the brain during early life. The posterior fontanelle generally closes by 4 months of age. The anterior fontanelle diminishes after 6 months of age and usually closes between 9 and 18 months.

During assessment, always inspect the anterior fontanelle. Normally, it should be level with the surface of the skull or slightly sunken. It also may pulsate. With increased intracranial pressure, as with meningitis or head trauma, the fontanelle may become tight and bulging, thus causing the pulsations to diminish or disappear. In the presence of dehydration, the anterior fontanelle often falls below the level of the skull and appears sunken.

The heavy head relative to body size places an infant or child at risk of blunt head trauma. In accidents, the head may be propelled more forcefully than the body, resulting in a higher

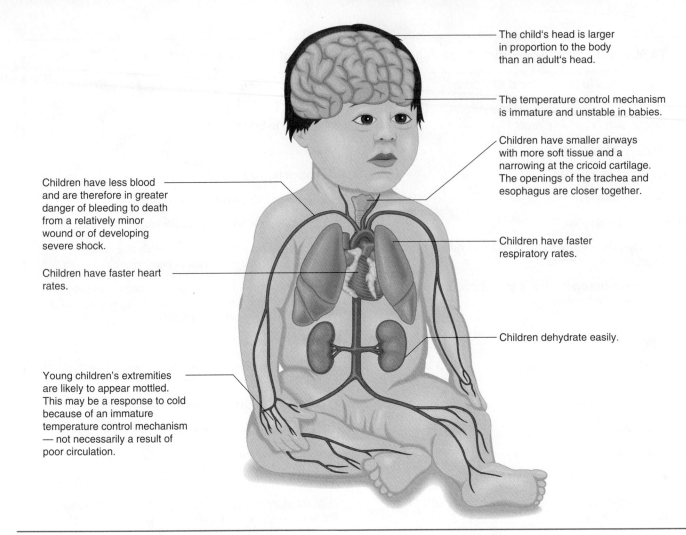

The child's head is larger in proportion to the body than an adult's head.

The temperature control mechanism is immature and unstable in babies.

Children have smaller airways with more soft tissue and a narrowing at the cricoid cartilage. The openings of the trachea and esophagus are closer together.

Children have less blood and are therefore in greater danger of bleeding to death from a relatively minor wound or of developing severe shock.

Children have faster heart rates.

Children have faster respiratory rates.

Children dehydrate easily.

Young children's extremities are likely to appear mottled. This may be a response to cold because of an immature temperature control mechanism — not necessarily a result of poor circulation.

● **Figure 4-5**   Anatomic and physiologic considerations in the infant and child.

incidence of brain injury. Head size also affects the airway positioning techniques you should use in treating pediatric patients. In general, follow these guidelines:

● In treating seriously injured patients less than three years of age, place a thin layer of padding under their back to obtain a neutral position. This will prevent

the head from tipping forward when supine, causing flexion of the neck (Figure 4-6 ●).

● In treating medically ill children over three years of age, place a folded sheet or towel under the occiput to obtain a sniffing position (neck flexed slightly forward, head extended slightly backward to align pharynx and trachea).

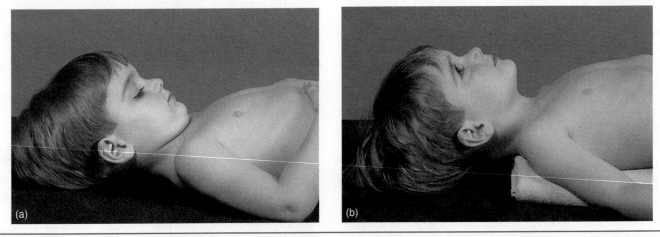

(a)

(b)

● **Figure 4-6**   (a) In the supine position, an infant's or child's larger head tips forward, causing airway obstruction. (b) Placing padding under the patient's back and shoulders will bring the airway to a neutral or slightly extended position.

Airway

In managing the airway of an infant or child, keep in mind these anatomic and physiologic considerations:

- Pediatric patients have narrower airways than adults at all levels, and these are more easily blocked by secretions or obstructions.
- Infants are obligate nose breathers. If their noses are blocked by secretions, for example, they may not automatically "know" to open their mouths to breathe.
- The tongue takes up more space proportionately in a child's mouth than in an adult's and can more easily obstruct breathing in an unconscious patient.
- The trachea is softer and more flexible in a child than in an adult and can collapse if the neck and head are hyperextended.
- A child's larynx is higher (C3–C4) than an adult's and extends into the pharynx.
- In young children, the cricoid ring is the narrowest part of the airway.
- Infants have an omega-shaped (horseshoe-shaped) epiglottis that extends at a 45-degree angle into the airway. Because epiglottic folds in pediatric patients have softer cartilage than in adults, they can be more floppy, especially in infants.

Take these anatomic and physiologic differences into account by following these general procedures: Always keep the nares clear in infants less than six months of age. Do not overextend the neck, which may collapse the trachea. Open the airway gently to avoid soft-tissue injury. Because any device placed in the infant's or child's airway further narrows the passage's diameter and may result in localized swelling, consider use of an oral or a nasal airway only after other manual maneuvers have failed to keep the airway open. (More information on pediatric airway management is provided later in this chapter.)

Chest and Lungs

In evaluating the chest and lungs of an infant or child, remember that tissues and muscles are more immature than in adults. Chest muscles tire easily, and lung tissues are more fragile. The soft, pliable ribs offer less protection to organs. Expect the ribs to be positioned horizontally and the mediastinum to be more mobile.

Take into account the following anatomic and physiologic considerations when assessing the chest and lungs of a pediatric patient:

- Infants and children are diaphragmatic breathers.
- Pediatric patients, especially young infants, are prone to gastric distention.
- Although rib fractures occur less frequently in children, they are not uncommon in cases of child abuse.
- Because of the softness of a child's ribs, greater energy can be transmitted to underlying organs following trauma. As a result, significant internal injury can be present without external signs.
- Pulmonary contusions are more common in pediatric patients who have been subjected to major trauma.
- An infant's or child's lungs are more prone than an adult's to pneumothorax following barotrauma.
- The mediastinum of a child or infant will shift more with tension pneumothorax than in an adult.
- Thin chest walls in infants and children allow for easily transmitted breath sounds. This may result in perception of breath sounds from elsewhere in the chest, which may cause you to miss a pneumothorax or misplaced intubation.

Abdomen

The liver and spleen, both very vascular organs, are proportionately larger in the pediatric patient than in the adult patient. Abdominal organs lie closer together. Because of the immature abdominal muscles in an infant or child, expect to find more frequent damage to the liver and spleen and more multiple organ injuries than in an adult.

Extremities

Until pediatric patients reach adolescence, they have softer and more porous bones than adults. Therefore, you should treat "sprains" and "strains" as fractures and immobilize them accordingly.

During early stages of development, injuries to the **growth plate** may also disrupt bone growth. Keep this in mind when inserting an intraosseous needle, which could mistakenly pierce the plate. (Intraosseous infusion will be discussed later in this chapter.)

Skin and Body Surface Area

The pediatric patient's skin and body surface area (BSA) have three distinguishing features. First, the skin of an infant or child is thinner than that of an adult. Second, infants and children generally have less subcutaneous fat. Finally, they have a larger BSA-to-weight ratio.

As a result of these features, children risk greater injury than adults do from extremes in temperature or thermal exposure. They lose fluids and heat more quickly than adults and have a greater likelihood of dehydration and hypothermia. They also burn more easily and deeply than adults, explaining why burns account for one of the leading causes of death among pediatric trauma patients.

Respiratory System

Although infants and children have a tidal volume proportionately similar to that of adolescents and adults, they require double the metabolic oxygen. They also have proportionately smaller oxygen reserves. The combination of increased oxygen requirements and decreased oxygen reserves makes infants and children especially susceptible to hypoxia.

Cardiovascular System

Cardiac output is rate dependent in infants and small children. They possess vigorous, but limited, cardiovascular reserves. Although infants and children have a circulating blood volume proportionately larger than that of adults, their absolute blood volume is smaller. As a result, they can maintain blood pressure longer than an adult but still be at risk of shock (hypoperfusion). In assessing a pediatric patient for shock, keep in mind the following points:

- A smaller absolute volume of fluid/blood loss is needed to cause shock in infants and children.

- A larger proportional volume of fluid/blood loss is needed to cause shock in these same patients.

- As with all categories of patients, hypotension is a late sign of shock. In pediatric patients, it is an ominous sign of imminent cardiopulmonary arrest.

- A child may be in shock despite a normal blood pressure.

- Shock assessment in children and infants is based on clinical signs of tissue perfusion. (See the later discussion of circulation assessment.)

- Suspect shock if tachycardia is present.

- Monitor the pediatric patient carefully for the development of hypotension.

Once again, remember that children are not small adults. Bleeding that would not be dangerous in an adult may be a serious and life-threatening condition in an infant or child. Shock can develop in the small child who has a laceration to the scalp (with its many blood vessels) or in the 3-year-old who loses as little as a cup of blood. (Management of shock in pediatric patients will be discussed in detail later in the chapter.)

Nervous System

The nervous system develops continually throughout childhood. Even so, the neural tissue remains more fragile than in adults. The skull and spinal column, which are softer and more pliable than in adults, offer less protection of the brain and spinal cord. Therefore, greater force can be transmitted to a child's neural tissue with more devastating consequences. These injuries can occur without injury to the skull or to the spinal column. (Treatment of head and neck trauma is discussed later in the chapter.)

Metabolic Differences

You may have noticed the repeated emphasis on the need to keep neonatal and pediatric patients warm during treatment and transport. The emphasis on warming techniques is based on the following metabolic considerations:

- Infants and children have a limited store of glycogen and glucose.

- Pediatric patients are prone to hypothermia because of their greater BSA-to-weight ratio.

- Significant volume loss can result from vomiting and diarrhea.

- Newborns and neonates lack the ability to shiver.

To prevent heat loss, always cover the patient's head and maintain adequate temperature controls in the ambulance. Ensure that the ambulance is always stocked with an adequate supply of blankets and, if you live in a cold area, hot-water bottles.

GENERAL APPROACH TO PEDIATRIC ASSESSMENT

Priorities in the management of the pediatric patient, as with all patients, are established on a threat-to-life basis. If life-threatening problems are not present, you will complete each of the general steps discussed in the following sections.

Basic Considerations

Many of the components of the primary assessment can be done during a visual examination of the scene. (This is sometimes called the "assessment from the doorway," during which you quickly note signs of an ill child, such as lethargy.) Whenever possible, involve the parent or caregiver in efforts to calm or comfort the child. Depending on the situation, you may decide to allow the parent or caregiver to remain with the child during treatment and transport. As mentioned previously, the developmental stage of the patient and the coping skills of the parents or guardians will be key factors in making this decision.

When interacting with parents or other responsible adults, keep in mind the communication techniques suggested earlier. Pay attention to the way in which parents or caregivers interact with the child. Are the interactions appropriate to the emergency? Are family members concerned? Are they angry? Are they overly emotional or entirely indifferent?

From the time of dispatch, you will continually acquire information relative to the patient's condition. As with all patients, personal safety must be your first priority. In treating pediatric patients, follow the same guidelines in approaching the scene as you would with any other patient. Observe for potentially hazardous situations and make sure you take appropriate Standard Precautions. Remember that infants and young children are at especially high risk of an infectious process.

Scene Size-Up

On arrival, conduct a quick scene size-up. Dispatch information received en route, as well as your own observations, can provide critical indicators of scene safety. Be aware of the increased anxiety and stress in any situation involving an infant or child. Try to set aside thoughts of your own children and adopt the professional, systematic approach to assessment necessary for scene safety and effective patient management. If you find yourself getting angry or upset, temporarily turn over care to another paramedic until you compose yourself.

As you survey the scene, look for clues to the mechanism of injury (MOI) or the nature of the illness (NOI). These clues will help guide your assessment and determine appropriate interventions. Note the presence of dangerous substances (e.g., medicine bottles, household chemicals, or poisonous plants) that the child may have ingested. Spot environmental hazards

When Is a Child No Longer a Child?

A difficult question EMS providers face is this: Legally, when is a child no longer a child? The answer varies from state to state. Children, as a rule, are considered to have reached the age of majority on their eighteenth birthday. At this point, the law allows them to make decisions for themselves, sign contracts, join the military, and provide consent for medical care. In addition, a married person—even if younger than 18 years of age—generally is considered to be able to provide consent, especially for any children he or she might have.

Some children under the age of 18 live independent of their parents. Although the laws pertaining to this vary somewhat, the true emancipated minor is one who has appealed to a court to be declared emancipated and granted the ability to make decisions for himself, including providing consent for medical care. Again, the laws vary from state to state. Know the laws of the state or states where you work.

When confronted with a minor seeking medical care, you must contact the parents, if possible, and obtain consent. The refusal of care by a minor is a particular problem. If the parents cannot be contacted, it is usually safest to transport the minor and have the emergency department staff or law enforcement try to locate the parents and obtain consent for treatment or a refusal-of-care declaration. Similarly, when confronted by a minor who claims to be emancipated but who cannot provide the documentation, it might be better to err on the side of transport. In any of these situations, involve your supervisor and law enforcement in the decision-making process.

such as unprotected stairwells, kerosene heaters, and so on. Identify possible causes of trauma, especially in motor vehicle collisions. Remain alert for evidence of child abuse, particularly in cases in which the injury and history do not coincide. As already mentioned, pay attention to the way parents or caregivers respond to the child and the way the child responds to them.

Keep the child in mind while conducting your scene size-up. Pace your approach to give the child time to adjust to your presence. Speak in a soft voice, using simple words. As soon as you reach the child, position yourself at eye level with the patient and make every effort to win his trust. If the child bonds more readily with one member of the team than another, allow that person to remain with the child and, if possible, allow him to conduct most of the secondary assessment.

Primary Assessment

The patient's condition determines the course of your primary assessment. An active and alert child will allow for a more comfortable approach, with more time spent on communication with the child and appropriate adults. A critically ill or injured child, however, may require quick intervention and rapid transport. Your choice of action depends on your general impression of the patient. (For a summary of the primary assessment of a pediatric patient, see Figure 4-7 ●.)

General Impression

The major points in forming your general impression are outlined in an assessment tool called the *pediatric assessment triangle* (PAT, included in Figure 4-7). Many experts recommend this assessment tool as a way of quickly evaluating the level of severity and the need for immediate intervention.[5, 6] It is a rapid "eyes-open, hands-on" approach that allows you to detect a life-threatening situation without the use of a stethoscope, blood pressure cuff, pulse oximeter, or other medical device. The triangle's three components are:

- *Appearance*—focuses on the child's mental status and muscle tone
- *Breathing*—directs attention to respiratory rate and respiratory effort
- *Circulation*—uses skin signs and color as well as capillary refill as indicators of the patient's circulatory status

Vital Functions

After quickly applying the pediatric assessment triangle to form a general impression, you will evaluate vital functions—mental status (level of consciousness) and the ABCs—as they apply to infants and children. Although assessment steps are basically the same as for adults, certain modifications must be made to collect accurate data.

Level of Consciousness Employ the AVPU method (**A**lert, responds to **V**erbal stimuli, responds to **P**ainful stimuli, **U**nresponsive) to evaluate the pediatric patient's level of consciousness. Adjust the techniques for the child's age. With an infant, you may need to shout to elicit a response (perhaps crying) to verbal stimulus. An infant should withdraw from a noxious stimulus. *Never shake an infant or child.*

Airway Assess the airway using the techniques shown in Figures 4-8 ● through 4-11 ●. If at any point the patient shows little or no movement of air, intervene immediately. Keep this fact in mind: *Airway and respiratory problems are the most common cause of cardiac arrest in infants and young children.*

As you inspect the airway, ask yourself the following questions:

- Is the airway patent?
- Is the airway maintainable with head positioning, suctioning, or airway adjuncts?
- Is the airway *not* maintainable? If so, what action is required? (Airway management techniques are discussed later in this chapter.)

Breathing In assessing the breathing of a pediatric patient, recall the CPR certification courses in which you learned to "look, listen, and feel." *Look* at the patient's chest and abdomen for movement. *Listen* for breath sounds—both normal and abnormal. *Feel* for air movement at the patient's mouth.

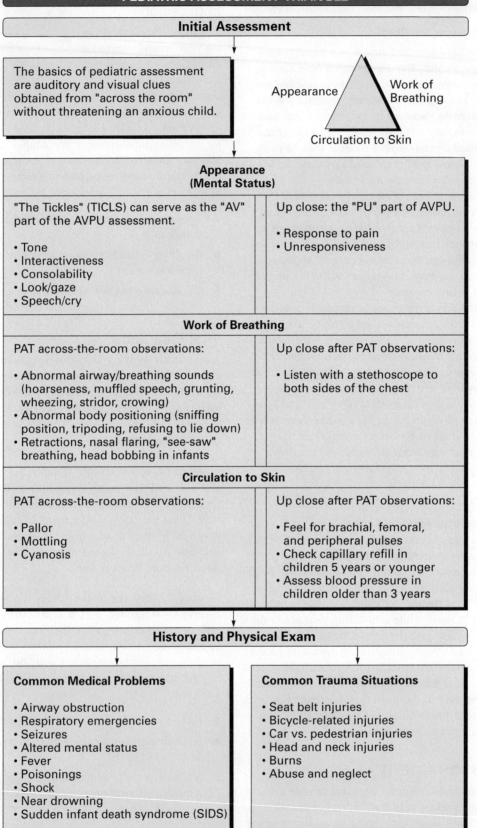

PEDIATRIC ASSESSMENT TRIANGLE

Initial Assessment

The basics of pediatric assessment are auditory and visual clues obtained from "across the room" without threatening an anxious child.

Appearance   Work of Breathing

Circulation to Skin

Appearance (Mental Status)

"The Tickles" (TICLS) can serve as the "AV" part of the AVPU assessment.

• Tone
• Interactiveness
• Consolability
• Look/gaze
• Speech/cry

Up close: the "PU" part of AVPU.

• Response to pain
• Unresponsiveness

Work of Breathing

PAT across-the-room observations:

• Abnormal airway/breathing sounds (hoarseness, muffled speech, grunting, wheezing, stridor, crowing)
• Abnormal body positioning (sniffing position, tripoding, refusing to lie down)
• Retractions, nasal flaring, "see-saw" breathing, head bobbing in infants

Up close after PAT observations:

• Listen with a stethoscope to both sides of the chest

Circulation to Skin

PAT across-the-room observations:

• Pallor
• Mottling
• Cyanosis

Up close after PAT observations:

• Feel for brachial, femoral, and peripheral pulses
• Check capillary refill in children 5 years or younger
• Assess blood pressure in children older than 3 years

History and Physical Exam

Common Medical Problems

• Airway obstruction
• Respiratory emergencies
• Seizures
• Altered mental status
• Fever
• Poisonings
• Shock
• Near drowning
• Sudden infant death syndrome (SIDS)

Common Trauma Situations

• Seat belt injuries
• Bicycle-related injuries
• Car vs. pedestrian injuries
• Head and neck injuries
• Burns
• Abuse and neglect

● **Figure 4-7**   The basic steps in pediatric assessment.

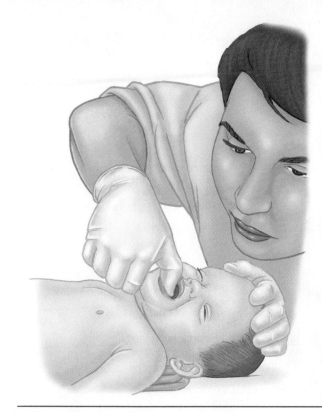

● **Figure 4-8** Opening the airway in a child.

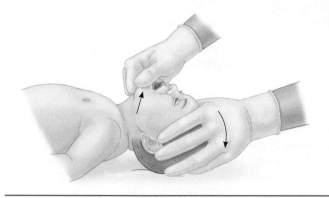

● **Figure 4-9** Head-tilt/chin-lift method.

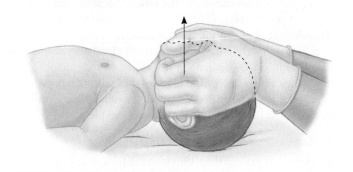

● **Figure 4-10** Jaw-thrust method.

Keep in mind that pediatric patients have small chests. For this reason, place the stethoscope near each of the armpits in order to minimize transmitted breath sounds. When considering the respiratory rate, remember that pain or fear can increase a child's

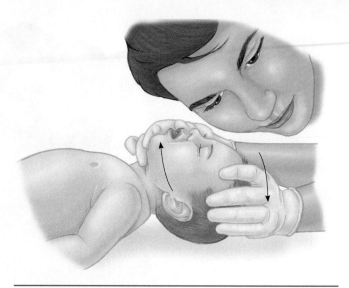

● **Figure 4-11** Assessing breathing.

respiratory efforts. Tachypnea, an abnormally rapid rate of breathing, may indicate fear, pain, inadequate oxygenation, or, in the case of neonates, exposure to cold.

If you suspect trauma, check the infant or child for life-threatening chest injuries. Keep in mind that even a minor injury to the chest can interfere with a child's breathing efforts. A chest injury can also interfere with your effort to provide adequate oxygenation or ventilation.

Your goal is to identify any evidence of compromised breathing (Figure 4-12 ●). Evaluation of breathing includes assessment of the following conditions:

● *Respiratory rate.* Tachypnea is often the first manifestation of respiratory distress in infants. Regardless of the cause, an infant breathing at a rapid rate will eventually tire. Keep in mind that a decreasing respiratory rate may be a result of tiring and is not necessarily a sign of improvement. A slow respiratory rate in an acutely ill infant or child is an ominous sign. (Normal respiratory rates are listed in Table 4–2.) In short, be alert for a respiratory rate that is *either* abnormally fast *or* abnormally slow.

● *Respiratory effort.* The quality of air entry can be assessed by observing for chest rise, breath sounds, stridor, or wheezing. An increased respiratory effort in the infant or child is also evidenced by nasal flaring and the use of accessory respiratory muscles. (Signs of respiratory effort are listed in Table 4–3.)

● *Color.* Cyanosis is a fairly late sign of respiratory failure and is most frequently seen in the mucous membranes of the mouth and the nail beds. Cyanosis of the extremities alone is more likely due to circulatory failure (shock) than to respiratory failure.

Circulation   As mentioned earlier, you should assess a pediatric patient's circulation by first checking the child's color. Keep in mind that the pediatric patient tends to become hypothermic; therefore, you should check the capillary refill time in an area of central circulation, such as the sternum or forehead. (Capillary refill time, as discussed later in this chapter, is considered

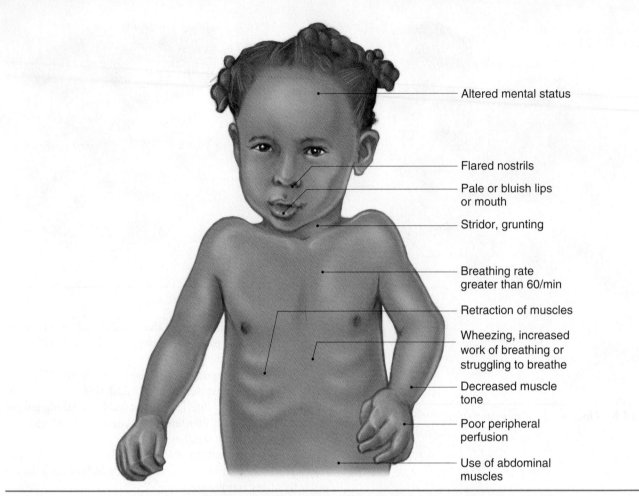

Altered mental status

Flared nostrils

Pale or bluish lips or mouth

Stridor, grunting

Breathing rate greater than 60/min

Retraction of muscles

Wheezing, increased work of breathing or struggling to breathe

Decreased muscle tone

Poor peripheral perfusion

Use of abdominal muscles

● **Figure 4-12** Signs of respiratory distress. Notice the conditions that can be determined by quick observation.

reliable as a sign of perfusion, primarily in children less than six years of age.) In general, evaluate the following conditions when assessing circulation during the primary assessment:

● **Heart rate.** As previously mentioned, infants develop sinus tachycardia in response to stress. Thus, any tachycardia in an infant or child requires further evaluation to determine the cause. Bradycardia in a distressed infant or child may indicate hypoxia and is an ominous sign of impending cardiac arrest. (Normal heart rates are listed in Table 4–2.)

● **Peripheral circulation.** The presence of peripheral pulses is a good indicator of the adequacy of end-organ perfusion. Loss of central pulses is an ominous sign.

● **End-organ perfusion.** End-organ perfusion is most evident in the skin, kidneys, and brain. Decreased perfusion of the skin is an early sign of shock. A capillary refill time of greater than 2 seconds is indicative of low cardiac output. Impairment of brain perfusion is usually evidenced by a change in mental status. The child may become confused or lethargic. Seizures may occur. Failure of the child to recognize the parents' faces is often an ominous sign. Urine output directly relates to kidney perfusion. Normal urine output is 1 to 2 mL/kg/hr. Urine flow of less than 1 mL/kg/hr is an indicator of poor renal perfusion.

Remember that evaluation of mental status and ABCs during the primary assessment is rapid and not detailed because it is aimed at discovering and correcting immediate life threats. More thorough measurements will be performed during the secondary assessment.

Anticipating Cardiopulmonary Arrest

Your primary assessment and the repeated assessments that follow help you to recognize and prevent cardiopulmonary arrest. At each stage of evaluating vital functions, ask yourself this question: "Does this child have pulmonary or circulatory failure that may lead to cardiopulmonary arrest?" Early recognition of the physiologically unstable child is one of the main goals of pediatric advanced life support (PALS). Conditions that place a pediatric patient at risk of cardiopulmonary arrest include:

● Respiratory rate greater than 60

● Heart rate greater than 180 or less than 80 (under five years of age)

● Heart rate greater than 180 or less than 60 (over five years of age)

● Respiratory distress

● Trauma

● Burns

TABLE 4–2 | Normal Vital Signs: Infants and Children*

Normal Pulse Rates (Beats per Minute, at Rest)

Newborn (0–1 month)	100–180
Infant (1–12 months)	100–160
Toddler (1–3 years)	80–110
Preschooler (3–5 years)	70–110
School age (6–10 years)	65–110
Early adolescence (11–14 years)	60–90

Normal Respiratory Rates (Breaths per Minute, at Rest)

Newborn (0–1 month)	30–60
Infant (1–12 months)	30–60
Toddler (1–3 years)	24–40
Preschooler (3–5 years)	22–34
School age (6–10 years)	18–30
Early adolescence (11–14 years)	12–26

Normal Blood Pressure Ranges (mmHg, at Rest)

	Systolic Approx. 90 + 2 × Age	Diastolic Approx. 2/3 Systolic
Preschooler (3–5 years)	Average 98 (78–116)	Average 65
School age (6–10 years)	Average 105 (80–122)	Average 69
Early adolescence (11–14 years)	Average 114 (88–140)	Average 76

*Adolescents ages 15 to 18 approach the vital signs of adults.

Note: *A high pulse in an infant or child is not as great a concern as a low pulse. A low pulse may indicate imminent cardiac arrest. Blood pressure is usually not taken in a child under three years of age. In cases of blood loss or shock, a child's blood pressure will remain within normal limits until near the end, then fall swiftly.*

TABLE 4–3 | Signs of Increased Respiratory Effort

Retraction	Visible sinking of the skin and soft tissues of the chest around and below the ribs and above the collarbone
Nasal flaring	Widening of the nostrils; seen primarily on inspiration
Head bobbing	Observed when the head lifts and tilts back as the child inhales and then moves forward as the child exhales
Grunting	Sound heard when an infant attempts to keep the alveoli open by building back pressure during expiration
Wheezing	Passage of air over mucous secretions or airway constrictions in the bronchi; heard more commonly on expiration; a low- or high-pitched sound
Gurgling	Coarse, abnormal bubbling sound heard in the airway during inspiration or expiration; may indicate an open chest wound
Stridor	Abnormal, musical, high-pitched sound, more commonly heard on inspiration

result of progressive deterioration in respiratory and cardiac function. Therefore, you need to determine whether the patient's condition is deteriorating or improving. Any decompensation or change in the patient's status will prompt you to perform basic or advanced life support measures, as detailed in American Heart Association guidelines and system protocols.

Transport Priority

Based on your primary assessment, you will assign the patient one of the following transport priorities:

- *Urgent.* Proceed with the rapid secondary assessment, if trauma is suspected, then transport immediately with further assessment and treatment performed en route.

- *Nonurgent.* Complete the secondary assessment at the scene, then transport.

To help determine transport priority, some EMS systems use a trauma score that is modified for pediatric patients, which includes the elements of the Glasgow Coma Scale, also modified for pediatric patients (Table 4–4). These scores can help predict patient outcome and help in the decision on whether rapid transport to a trauma center is required. If used in your EMS system, your medical director and/or system protocols will determine what numerical score mandates rapid transport.

- Cyanosis
- Altered level of consciousness
- Seizures
- Fever with petechiae (small purple spots resulting from skin hemorrhages)

Evaluate the patient for these conditions throughout assessment and transport. Cardiopulmonary arrest in infants and children is usually not a sudden event. Instead, it is the end

TABLE 4–4 | Pediatric Trauma Score and Glasgow Coma Scale Score

Pediatric Trauma Score

Score	+2	+1	−1
Weight	>44 lb (>20 kg)	22–44 lb (10–20 kg)	<22 lb (<10 kg)
Airway	Normal	Oral or nasal airway	Intubated, tracheostomy, invasive airway
Blood Pressure	Pulse at wrist >90 mmHg	Carotid or femoral pulse palpable, 50–90 mmHg	No palpable pulse or <50 mmHg
Level of Consciousness	Completely awake	Obtunded or any loss of consciousness	Comatose
Open Wound	None	Minor	Major or penetrating
Fractures	None	Closed fracture	Open or multiple fractures

Pediatric Glasgow Coma Scale

		>1 Year	<1 Year	
Eye Opening	4	Spontaneous	Spontaneous	
	3	To verbal command	To shout	
	2	To pain	To pain	
	1	No response	No response	

		>1 Year	<1 Year	
Best Motor Response	6	Obeys		
	5	Localizes pain	Localizes pain	
	4	Flexion-withdrawal	Flexion-withdrawal	
	3	Flexion-abnormal (decorticate rigidity)	Flexion-abnormal (decorticate rigidity)	
	2	Extension (decerebrate rigidity)	Extension (decerebrate rigidity)	
	1	No response	No response	

		>5 Years	2–5 Years	0–23 Months
Best Verbal Response	5	Oriented and converses	Appropriate words and phrases	Smiles, coos, cries appropriately
	4	Disoriented and converses	Inappropriate words	Cries
	3	Inappropriate words	Cries and/or screams	Inappropriate crying and/or screaming
	2	Incomprehensible sounds	Grunts	Grunts
	1	No response	No response	No response

Transitional Phase

The way in which the pediatric patient is transferred to EMS care depends entirely on the seriousness of the patient's condition. A transitional phase is intended for the conscious, nonacutely ill child. This phase of assessment allows the infant or child to become familiar with you and the equipment that you will be using. When dealing with the unconscious or acutely ill patient, however, you will skip this phase and proceed directly to the treatment and transport phases of assessment. In essence, you assign the patient an "urgent" status.

Secondary Assessment

After you have prioritized patient care at the end of the primary assessment, you will perform the secondary assessment, including a history and a physical exam. If the patient has a medical illness, the history will precede the physical exam. If the patient is suffering from trauma, the physical exam will take precedence. If partners are working together, the history and physical exam may be performed simultaneously. (For a summary of conditions that may be found during the focused history and physical exam, review Figure 4-7.)

History

Whenever a patient is identified as a priority patient, the focused history will occur en route to the hospital, after essential treatments or interventions for life-threatening conditions have been performed.

To obtain a history for a pediatric patient, you will probably need to involve a family member or caregiver. Remember, however, that school-age children and adolescents like to take part in their own care. As previously mentioned, you can elicit valuable information from even very young patients. As a general precaution, question older adolescent patients in private, especially about issues such as sexual activity, pregnancy, or illicit drug and alcohol use. If you question adolescents about these subjects in the presence of an adult, they will probably be more reticent for fear of later repercussions.

As with any patient, you will use the history to uncover additional pertinent injuries or medical conditions. The history should center on the chief complaint and past medical history.

To evaluate the nature of the chief complaint, determine each of the following:

- Nature of the illness/injury
- Length of time the patient has been sick/injured
- Presence of fever
- Effects of the illness/injury on patient behavior
- Bowel/urine habits
- Presence of vomiting/diarrhea
- Frequency of urination

The past medical history identifies chronic illnesses, use of medications, and allergies. Be sure to inquire whether the infant or child is currently under a doctor's care. If so, obtain the name of the physician and present it at the receiving hospital. In the case of trauma patients, reconsider the mechanism of injury and the results of your on-scene physical examination (which, as noted earlier, will precede the history in the case of trauma).

Physical Exam

Focused Exam Carry out the physical exam after all life-threatening conditions have been identified and addressed. If there is a significant mechanism of injury or if the patient is unresponsive, perform a complete rapid trauma assessment or rapid medical assessment. Use the toe-to-head approach with the younger child (or begin with the chest and examine the head last) and the head-to-toe approach in the older child. If the injury is minor or if the ill patient is responsive, perform a physical exam that is focused on the affected areas and systems.

Perform the physical exam as described in Volume 3. Depending on the particular situation, some or all of the following assessment techniques may be appropriate to include in the exam:

- *Pupils.* Inspect the patient's pupils for equality and reaction to light.
- *Capillary refill.* As noted earlier, this technique is valuable for pediatric patients less than six years of age. Blanch the nail bed, base of the thumb, or sole of one of the feet. Remember that normal capillary refill is 2 seconds or less. Recall that this technique is less reliable in cold environments.
- *Hydration.* Note skin turgor, presence of tears and saliva, and, with infants, the condition of the fontanelles.
- *Pulse oximetry.* Use this electronic device on injured or ill infants and children. Readings will give you immediate information regarding peripheral oxygen saturation and allow you to follow trends in the patient's pulse rate and oxygenation status. Keep in mind, however, that hypothermia or shock can affect readings.

Glasgow Coma Scale In cases of trauma, you may need to apply the Glasgow Coma Scale (GCS), a scoring system for monitoring the neurologic status of patients with possible head injuries. The GCS assigns scores based on verbal responses, motor functions, and eye movements.

In using the GCS with pediatric patients, you will have to make certain modifications; the younger the patient, the more adjustments you will need to make. Verbal responses, for example, will not be possible for neonates and infants. However, motor function may be assessed in very young children by observing voluntary movement. Infants under four months of age should have a grasp reflex when an object is placed on the palmar surface of their hand. The grasp should be immediate. Children over three years of age will follow directions, when encouraged. Sensory function can be observed by the withdrawal reaction from "tickling" the patient. (Review Table 4–4 for a modified GCS for pediatric patients.)

After you score the GCS for the patient, prioritize the patient according to severity. Guidelines are:

- *Mild*—GCS 13 to 15
- *Moderate*—GCS 9 to 12
- *Severe*—GCS less than or equal to 8

Vital Signs Remember that poorly taken vital signs are of less value than no vital signs at all. The following guidelines will help you obtain accurate pediatric readings. (Review Table 4–2 for normal pediatric vital signs.)

- Take vital signs with the patient in as close to a resting state as possible. If necessary, allow the child to calm down before attempting vital signs. Vital signs in the field should include pulse, respiration, blood pressure, and temperature.

- Obtain blood pressure with an appropriate-sized cuff. The cuff should be two-thirds the width of the upper arm. The pulse pressure (the difference between the systolic and diastolic blood pressure) narrows as shock develops. *Note that hypotension is a late and often sudden sign of cardiovascular decompensation.* Even mild hypotension

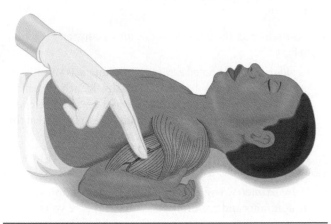

● **Figure 4-13a**   Taking the brachial pulse.

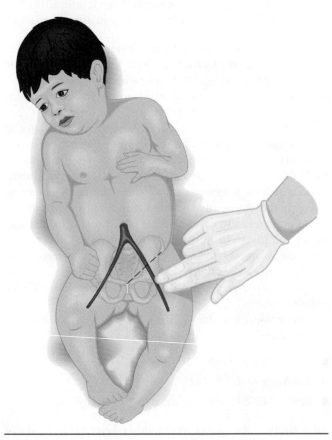

● **Figure 4-13b**   Taking the femoral pulse.

should be taken seriously and treated quickly and vigorously, because cardiopulmonary arrest is probably imminent.

- Feel for peripheral, brachial, or femoral pulses (Figures 4-13a ● and b ●). There is often a significant variation in pulse rate in children owing to varied respirations. Therefore, it is important to monitor the pulse for at least 30 seconds, with one full minute being preferable.

- It is generally not possible to weigh the child. However, if medications are required, make a good estimate of the child's weight. Often the parents or caregivers can provide a fairly reliable weight from a recent visit to the doctor. Table 4–5 lists the average weights by age for pediatric patients. (Remember, these are only averages.)

- Observe the child's respiratory rate before beginning the examination. After the examination is started, the child will often begin to cry. It will then be impossible to determine the respiratory rate. For an estimate of the upper limit of respiratory rate, subtract the child's age from 40. It is also important to identify the respiratory pattern, as well as retractions, nasal flaring, or paradoxical chest movement.

- Measure temperature early in the patient encounter and repeat toward the end. IV fluid and exposure to the environment can cause a drop in core temperature.

TABLE 4–5	Pediatric Weights and Pound–Kilogram Conversion		
Age	**Weight (lb)**	**Weight (kg)**
Birth	7	3.5
3 Months	10	5
6 Months	15	7
9 Months	18	8
1 Year	22	10
2 Years	26	12
3 Years	33	15
4 Years	37	17
5 Years	40	18
6 Years	44	20
7 Years	50	23
8 Years	56	25
9 Years	60	28
10 Years	70	33
11 Years	75	35
12 Years	85	40
13 Years	98	44

- Continue to observe the child for level of consciousness. The level of consciousness and activity during treatment may vary widely.

Noninvasive Monitoring Modern noninvasive monitoring devices all have their applications in pediatric emergency care (Figure 4-14 ●). These may include the pulse oximeter, capnography, automated blood pressure devices, self-registering thermometers, and ECGs.

To promote the goal of early recognition of cardiopulmonary arrest, every seriously ill or injured child should receive continuous pulse oximetry. This will provide you with essential information regarding the patient's heart rate and peripheral O_2 saturation. It will also help you monitor the effects of any medications administered. Hyperoxia can be harmful. Thus, pulse oximetry can be used to guide supplemental oxygen therapy. The goal is to maintain a SpO_2 of 94 percent or greater.

Capnography, also called end-tidal carbon dioxide monitoring ($PETCO_2$), is useful in pediatrics (Figure 4-15 ●). It provides

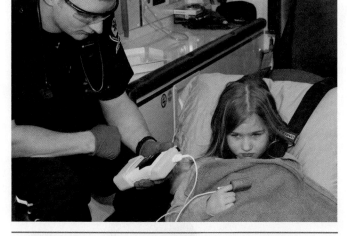

● **Figure 4-14**   If available, noninvasive monitoring, including pulse oximetry and temperature measurement, should be used in prehospital pediatric care.

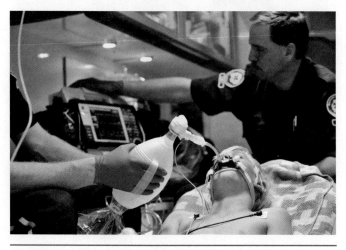

● **Figure 4-15**   Capnography is an effective tool for evaluation and monitoring of pediatric patients.

essential information about ventilation and can also provide diagnostic information. If the $PETCO_2$ is consistently greater than 10 to 15 mmHg, focus efforts on improving ventilation and ensuring that the patient does not receive excessive ventilation (hyperventilation).[7, 8]

An ECG and automated blood pressure/pulse monitor should also be considered. However, these devices may frighten the child. Before applying any monitoring device, explain what you are going to do. Demonstrate the display or lights. If the monitoring device makes noise, allow the child to hear the noise before you apply it. Reassure the child that the device will not hurt him.

Reassessment

Because a pediatric patient's condition can rapidly change for the better or the worse, it is necessary to repeat relevant portions of the assessment. You should continually monitor the patient's respiratory effort, skin color, mental status, temperature, and pulse oximetry. Retake vital signs and compare them with baseline vitals. In general, reassess stable patients every 15 minutes, critical patients every 5 minutes.

GENERAL MANAGEMENT OF PEDIATRIC PATIENTS

The same ABCs that guide the management of adult patients apply to pediatric patients: Your top priorities in treating an infant or child are airway, breathing, and circulation. However, because of the special anatomic and physiologic considerations that influence the management of pediatric patients, you need to practice these skills on an ongoing and regular basis.

Basic Airway Management

In treating the pediatric patient, basic life support (BLS) should be applied according to current standards and protocols. BLS should include maintenance of the airway, artificial ventilation, and, if required, chest compressions (Table 4–6). As with all patients, your priority is to ensure an open airway. The following modifications of BLS airway skills will ensure that you take into account the clinical implications of the pediatric airway.

Manual Positioning

Allow the pediatric patient to assume a position of comfort, if possible. When placing the patient in a supine position, avoid hyperextension of the neck. As previously mentioned, infants and small children risk collapsed tracheas from hyperextension of the neck. For trauma patients less than three years old, place support under the upper torso or shoulders. For supine medical patients three years old and older, provide occipital elevation.

Foreign Body Airway Obstruction

Before administering treatment, determine whether an airway obstruction is mild or severe. Infants or children with a mild

TABLE 4–6 | Summary of BLS Maneuvers in Infants and Children

Target of Maneuver	Infant (<1 Year)	Child (1 Year–Puberty)
Airway		
Open airway	Head-tilt/chin-lift (unless trauma present)	Head-tilt/chin-lift (unless trauma present)
	Jaw thrust	Jaw thrust
Clear foreign body obstruction	Back blows/chest thrusts	Abdominal thrusts
Breathing		
Initial	2 breaths that make the chest rise	2 breaths that make the chest rise
Subsequent	1 breath every 3 seconds (12–20/minute)	1 breath every 3 seconds (12–20/minute)
Circulation		
Pulse check	Brachial/femoral	Carotid
Compression area	Lower third of sternum	Lower third of sternum
Compression width	2 or 3 fingers	Heel of one hand
Depth	Approximately ⅓ to ½ AP diameter of chest	Approximately ⅓ to ½ AP diameter of chest
Rate	At least 100/minute	100/minute
Compression-to-ventilation ratio	30:2 (1 rescuer); 15:2 (2 rescuers)	30:2 (1 rescuer); 15:2 (2 rescuers)

airway obstruction will have a cough, hoarse voice or cry, stridor, or some other evidence that at least some air is passing through the airway. Avoid any maneuvers that will turn a mild obstruction into a severe obstruction. Instead, place the patient in a position of comfort and transport immediately.

In the case of severe airway obstruction, take one of the following age-specific maneuvers:

- *Children.* For children older than one year of age, perform a series of abdominal thrusts until the item is expelled or the victim becomes unresponsive (Figure 4-16 ●). If the victim becomes unresponsive, start CPR.

- *Infants.* For an infant, deliver a series of five back blows followed by five chest thrusts (abdominal thrusts are not recommended for infants). Inspect the infant's mouth on completion of each series (Procedure 4–1). If the infant becomes unresponsive, begin CPR.

As you recall from the basic CPR courses, never check a pediatric patient's mouth with blind finger sweeps.

Suctioning

Apply suctioning whenever you detect heavy secretions in the nose or mouth of a pediatric patient, especially if the patient has a diminished level of consciousness. You can use a bulb syringe, flexible suction catheter, or rigid-tip suction catheter, depending on the patient's age or size (Figure 4-17 ●). Make sure that flexible catheters are correctly sized (Table 4–7).

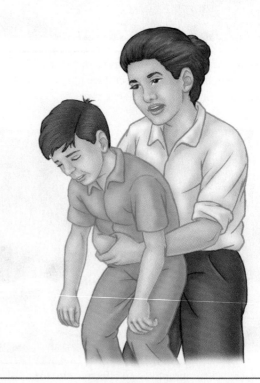

● **Figure 4-16** Delivering abdominal thrusts to a child.

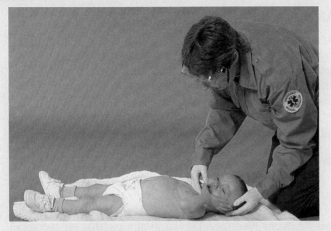

4-1a ● Recognize and assess for choking. Look for breathing difficulty, ineffective cough, and lack of a strong cry.

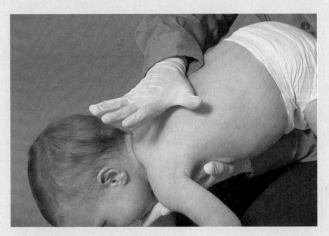

4-1b ● Give up to five back blows.

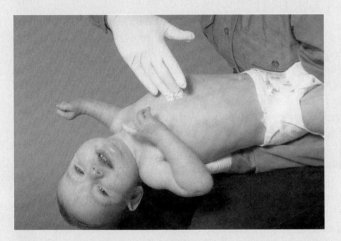

4-1c ● Then administer five chest thrusts.

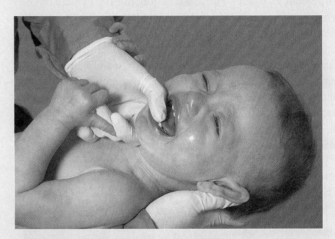

4-1d ● If the infant becomes unresponsive, begin CPR.

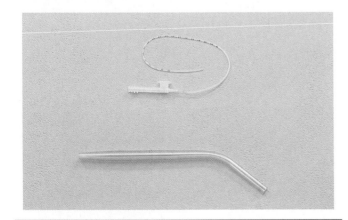

● **Figure 4-17** Pediatric-size suction catheters. Top: soft suction catheter. Bottom: rigid or hard suction catheter.

TABLE 4–7 | Suction Catheter Sizes for Infants and Children	
Age	Suction Catheter Size (French)
Up to 1 year	8
1 to 6 years	8–10
7 to 15 years	10–12
16 years	12

Although pediatric suctioning techniques vary very little from adult suctioning techniques, keep the following modifications in mind:

- Decrease suction pressure to less than 100 mmHg in infants.
- Avoid excessive suctioning time (suction less than 10 seconds) in order to decrease the possibility of hypoxia.
- Avoid stimulation of the vagus nerve, which may produce bradycardia. As a general rule, suction no deeper than you can see and for no more than 10 seconds per attempt.
- Frequently check the patient's pulse. If bradycardia occurs, stop suctioning immediately and oxygenate.

Oxygenation

Adequate oxygenation is the hallmark of pediatric patient management, but excess oxygen can be harmful. When possible, use pulse oximetry to guide supplemental oxygen administration. The goal is to provide just enough oxygen to maintain a SpO_2 of 94 percent or greater. For resuscitation, use 100 percent oxygen when possible (except in newborns). Methods of oxygen delivery include "blow-by" techniques (especially for neonates) and pediatric-sized nonrebreather masks. Although nonrebreather masks provide the highest concentration of supplemental oxygen, children may resist their use. Try to overcome their fear by demonstrating the use of the mask on yourself (Figure 4-18 ●). Better yet, enlist the support of a parent or caregiver and ask him or her to demonstrate the mask. As an alternative, you might place the mask over the face of a stuffed animal.

If the child refuses to accept the nonrebreather mask, resort to high-concentration blow-by oxygen. Some units place oxygen tubing through the bottom of a colorful paper cup and use it to deliver the blow-by supplemental oxygen. Children often find a familiar object less frightening than complicated medical equipment.

Airway Adjuncts

As a general rule, use airway adjuncts in pediatric patients only if prolonged artificial ventilations are required. There are two reasons for this. First, infants and children often improve quickly through the administration of 100 percent oxygen. Second, airway adjuncts may create greater complications in children than in adults. Pediatric patients risk soft-tissue damage, vomiting, and stimulation of the vagus nerve.

Oropharyngeal Airways Oropharyngeal airways should be used only in pediatric patients who lack a gag reflex. (Patients with a gag reflex risk vomiting and bradycardia.) Size the airway by measuring from the corner of the mouth to the front of the earlobe. Remember, oropharyngeal airways that are too small can obstruct breathing; ones that are too large can both block the airway and cause trauma. (For general sizing suggestions, see Table 4–8.)

In placing an oropharyngeal airway, use a tongue blade to depress the tongue and jaw (Figure 4-19 ●). If you detect a gag reflex, continue to maintain an open airway with a manual (head-tilt/chin-lift) maneuver and consider the use of a nasal airway. Remember that with a pediatric patient, the oral airway is inserted with the tip pointing toward the tongue and pharynx. For a comparison with insertion in the adult patient, see Figures 4-20a ● and b ●.

Nasopharyngeal Airways Use nasopharyngeal airways for those children who possess a gag reflex and who require prolonged artificial ventilations. *Do not* use them on any child with midface or head trauma. You might mistakenly pass the airway through a fracture into the sinuses or the brain.

Size the pediatric nasal airway in the same fashion as for adult patients. Pay particular attention to determining

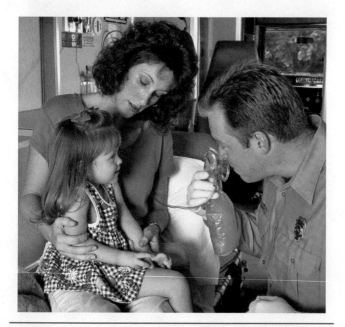

● **Figure 4-18** To overcome the child's fear of the nonrebreather mask, try it on yourself or have the parent try it on before attempting to place it on the child.

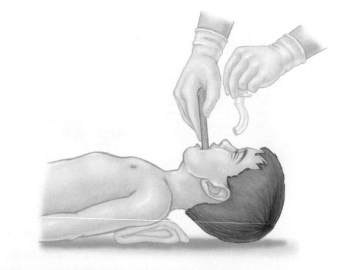

● **Figure 4-19** Inserting an oropharyngeal airway in a child with the use of a tongue blade.

TABLE 4–8 | Airway Management: Pediatric Equipment Guidelines

Equipment	Premature (1–2.5 kg; 2.2–5.5 lb*)	Neonate (2.5–4 kg; 5.5–8.8 lb)	6 Months (6–8 kg; 13.2–17.6 lb)	1–4 Years (10–14 kg; 22–30.8 lb)	5 Years (16–18 kg; 35.2–39.6 lb)	5–10 Years (24–30 kg; 52.8–66 lb)
Airway	Infant	Infant/small	Small	Small	Medium	Medium/large
Oral	(00)	(0)	(1)	(2)	(3)	(4.5)
Breathing						
O₂ ventilation mask	Premature	Newborn	Infant/child	Child	Child	Small adult
Bag-valve device	Infant	Infant	Child	Child	Child	Child/adult
Endotracheal tube	2.5–3.0 (uncuffed)	3.0–3.5 (uncuffed)	3.5–4.0	4.0–4.5	5.0–5.5	5.5–6.5
Suction/stylet (French)	6–8/6	8/6	8–10/6	10/6	14/14	14/14
Laryngoscope blade	0 (straight)	1 (straight)	1 (straight)	1–2 (straight)	2 (straight or curved)	2–3 (straight or curved)
Circulation						
Blood pressure cuff	Newborn	Newborn	Infant	Child	Child	Child/adult
Orogastric Tube (French)	5	5–8	8	10	10–12	14–18
Chest Tube (French)	10–14	12–18	14–20	14–24	20–32	28–38

Weights are the 50th percentile for the given age range.

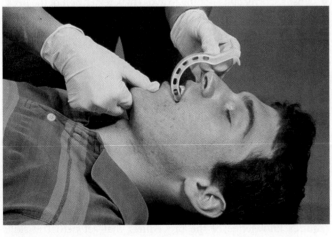

(a)   (b)

● **Figure 4-20**   (a) In an adult, the airway is inserted with the tip pointing to the roof of the mouth, then rotated into position. (b) In an infant or small child, the airway is inserted with the tip pointing toward the tongue and pharynx, in the same position it will be in after insertion.

proper airway diameter and length. A nasopharyngeal airway that is too short may not maintain an open airway. One that is too long may obstruct the airway. A small-diameter nasopharyngeal airway may be easily obstructed by secretions, thus requiring frequent suctioning. Use the outside diameter of the patient's little finger as a rough measure of airway diameter. Nasopharyngeal airways come in a variety of sizes, but they are not readily available for infants less than one year old. Equipment required for insertion of a nasal airway includes:

- Appropriately sized soft, flexible latex tubing
- Water-based lubricant

When inserting the nasal airway, follow the same basic method as you would in an adult patient. It is important to remember that younger children often have enlarged adenoids (lymphatic tissues in the nasopharynx), which can be easily lacerated when inserting a nasopharyngeal airway. Because of this, always use care when inserting a nasopharyngeal airway in a younger child. Gentle rotation of the airway may help it slide past obstructions. If resistance is met, do not force the airway because significant bleeding can result.

Ventilation

Adequate tidal volume and ventilatory rate provide more than just a high oxygen saturation for your patient. Ventilation is a two-way physiologic street regarding maintenance of appropriate oxygen and carbon dioxide levels. However, you will achieve neither of these clinically important events without tailoring the ventilatory device and technique to your pediatric patient. Important points to remember include the following:

- Avoid excessive bag pressure and volume (hyperventilation). Ventilate at an age-appropriate rate, using only enough ventilation to make the chest rise.
- Use continuous waveform capnography to monitor and guide ventilation.
- Use a properly sized mask to ensure a good fit. In general, the mask should fit on the bridge of the nose and the cleft of the chin (Figure 4-21 ●).
- Obtain a chest rise with each breath.
- Allow adequate time for full chest recoil and exhalation.
- Assess bag-valve-mask (BVM) ventilation. (Provide 100 percent oxygen by using a reservoir attached to the BVM for resuscitation.)

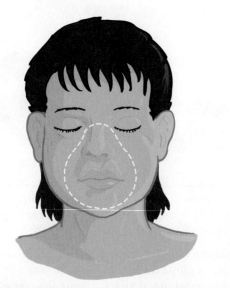

● **Figure 4-21** A mask used for a child should fit on the bridge of the nose and the cleft of the chin.

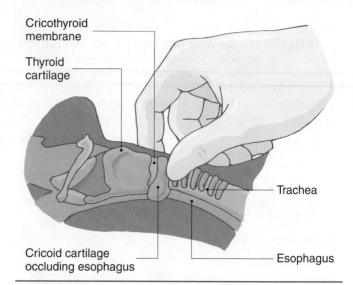

Cricothyroid membrane

Thyroid cartilage

Trachea

Cricoid cartilage occluding esophagus

Esophagus

● **Figure 4-22** In the Sellick maneuver, pressure is placed on the cricoid cartilage, compressing the esophagus. This reduces regurgitation and helps bring the vocal cords into view, which is useful if intubation is to be performed.

- Remember that flow-restricted, oxygen-powered ventilation devices are contraindicated in pediatric resuscitation.
- Do not use BVMs with pop-off valves unless they can be readily occluded, if necessary. (Ventilatory pressures required during pediatric CPR may exceed the limit of the pop-off valve.)
- Apply cricoid pressure to minimize gastric inflation and passive regurgitation in unresponsive children.[9] Avoid excessive cricoid pressure so as not to obstruct the trachea (Figure 4-22 ●).
- Ensure correct positioning to avoid hyperextension of the neck.

Advanced Airway and Ventilatory Management

As a paramedic, you will be expected to master the advanced life support (ALS) procedures that make you a leader in the EMS system. Your clinical skills will help save the lives of pediatric patients whose respiratory systems have failed so severely that BLS measures are insufficient. When signs of impending cardiopulmonary arrest have been identified (as discussed earlier), you may be called on to implement the following pediatric advanced life support (PALS) techniques, either in your own unit or in a transfer of care from a BLS unit. The success of these techniques requires knowledge of the procedures that set pediatric skills apart from the ALS skills used on adults. (Review the advanced airway skills for adults discussed in Volume 2, Chapter 5.)

Foreign Body Airway Obstruction

One advantage of being able to perform endotracheal intubation is that it gives you another treatment modality for children with foreign body airway obstructions. If a child's airway cannot be cleared by basic airway procedures, visualize the airway with the laryngoscope. Often, the obstructing foreign body can be seen. Once it is visualized, grasp the foreign body with Magill forceps and remove it. If you cannot remove the foreign body with Magill forceps, try to intubate around the obstruction. This often requires using an endotracheal tube smaller than you would normally choose. However, this will provide an adequate airway until the foreign body can be removed at the hospital. Finally, if the foreign body cannot be removed with Magill forceps and it is impossible to intubate around it, then you should consider placing a cricothyrotomy needle. This should only be done as a last resort. Be sure to follow local protocols regarding needle cricothyrotomy.

Needle Cricothyrotomy

Needle cricothyrotomy in children is the same as in adult patients (as discussed in Volume 2, Chapter 5). It is important to remember that the anatomic landmarks are smaller and more difficult to identify. For years it was taught that needle cricothyrotomy was contraindicated in children less than one year of age. However, current thinking is that the possible benefit (life) exceeds the risks (bleeding, local tissue damage). Remember, the only indication for cricothyrotomy is failure to obtain an airway by any other method.

Endotracheal Intubation

Endotracheal intubation allows direct visualization of the lower airway through the trachea, bypassing the entire upper airway. It is the most effective method of controlling a patient's airway, whether the patient is an adult or a child. However, endotracheal intubation is not without complications. It is an invasive technique with little room for error. A tube that is mistakenly sized or misplaced, especially in an apneic patient, can quickly lead to hypoxia and death.

Pediatric endotracheal intubation has come under increasing scrutiny in EMS. Several studies have questioned the effectiveness of prehospital pediatric endotracheal intubation.[10] Bag-mask ventilation can be as effective, and may be safer, than endotracheal tube ventilation for short periods during prehospital resuscitation.[11]

Anatomic and Physiologic Concerns   Although endotracheal intubation of a child and an adult follow the same basic procedures, the special features of the pediatric airway complicate placement of any orotracheal tube. In fact, variations in the airway size of children preclude the use of certain airways, including esophageal obturator airways (EOAs), pharyngeotracheal lumen airways (PtLs), and esophageal–tracheal combitubes (ETCs). Properly sized laryngeal mask airways (LMAs) may be used in children but do not protect the airway from aspiration. In using an endotracheal tube, keep in mind these points:

- In infants and small children, it is often more difficult to create a single clear visual plane from the mouth, through the pharynx, and into the glottis. A straight-blade laryngoscope is preferred, as it provides greater displacement of the tongue and better visualization of the relatively cephalad and anterior glottis. For larger children, a curved blade may sometimes be used. (Review Table 4–8.)

- Variations in the sizes of pediatric airways, coupled with the fact that the narrowest portion of the airway is at the level of the cricoid ring, make proper sizing of the endotracheal tube crucial. To determine correct size, apply any of the following methods:

  ○ Use a resuscitation tape, such as the Broselow™ tape, to estimate tube size based on height.

  ○ Estimate the correct tube size by using the diameter of the patient's little finger or the diameter of the nasal opening.

  ○ Calculate the correct tube size by using this simple numerical formula: (Patient's age in years + 16) ÷ 4 = Tube size.

- The depth of insertion can be estimated based on age (Table 4–9). However, the best method of determining depth is direct visualization. Because of the distance between the mouth and the trachea, a stylet is rarely needed to position the tube properly. When a stylet is used, select a malleable yet rigid style.

- Either cuffed or uncuffed endotracheal tubes can be used in children (but not in neonates). In certain conditions, a cuffed tube may be superior, but cuff pressure should be limited to 20 cmH$_2$O. If using a cuffed endotracheal tube, it may be necessary to select a tube that is 0.5 mm smaller than an uncuffed tube.

- Infants and small children may have greater vagal response than adults. Therefore, laryngoscopy and passage of an endotracheal tube are likely to cause a vagal response, dramatically slowing the child's heart rate and decreasing the cardiac output and blood pressure. As a result, pediatric intubations must be carried out swiftly, accurately, and with continuous monitoring.

Indications   The indications for endotracheal intubation in a pediatric patient are the same as those for an adult. They include:

- Need for prolonged artificial ventilations
- Inadequate ventilatory support with a BVM
- Cardiac or respiratory arrest
- Control of an airway in a patient without a cough or gag reflex
- Need to provide a route for drug administration
- Need to gain access to the airway for suctioning

TABLE 4–9 | Infant/Child Endotracheal Tubes	
Age of Patient	**Measurement of the Endotracheal Tube at the Teeth to the Midtrachea (cm)**
6 Months to 1 year	12
2 Years	14
4–6 Years	16
6–10 Years	18
10–12 Years	20

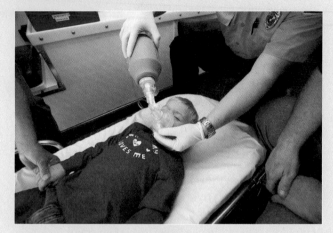

4-2a ● Hyperventilate the child.

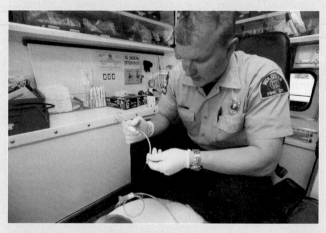

4-2b ● Prepare the equipment.

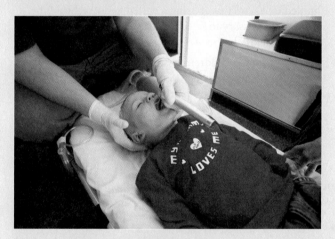

4-2c ● Insert the laryngoscope.

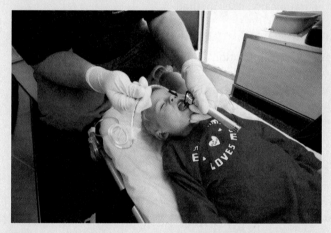

4-2d ● Visualize the child's larynx and insert the ETT.

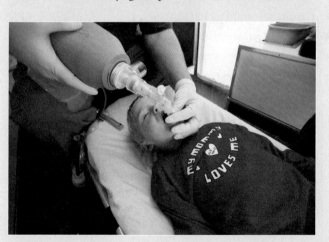

4-2e ● Ventilate, inflate the ETT cuff (if it is a cuffed tube), and auscultate.

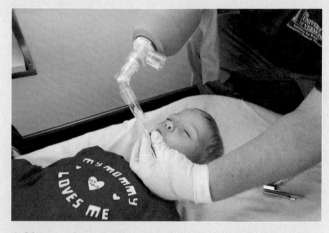

4-2f ● Confirm placement with an $ETCO_2$ detector or waveform capnography.

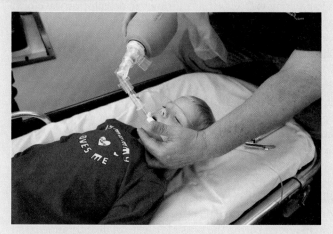

4-2g ● Secure the tube.

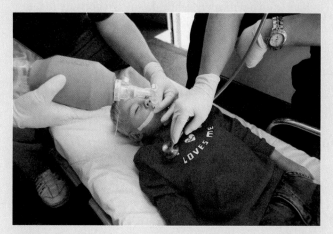

4-2h ● Reconfirm proper ETT placement.

Additionally, if local protocols allow it, endotracheal intubation may be used in a child who is suffering croup or epiglottitis with an increasingly compromised airway.

Techniques for Pediatric Intubation To perform endotracheal intubation on a pediatric patient, follow the basic steps shown in Procedure 4–2. Detailed steps are as follows:

1. While maintaining ventilatory support, ventilate the patient with 100 percent oxygen. If time allows, ventilate for a full 2 minutes.

2. Assemble and check your equipment. As stated earlier, a straight-blade laryngoscope is preferred. Assorted sizes of endotracheal tubes, both cuffed and uncuffed, should be stocked in the pediatric kit aboard your ambulance.

3. Place the patient's head and neck into an appropriate position. With a pediatric patient, the head should be maintained in a sniffing position.

4. Hold the laryngoscope in your left hand.

5. Insert your laryngoscope blade into the right side of the patient's mouth. With a sweeping action, displace the tongue to the left.

6. Move the blade slightly toward the midline, then advance it until the distal end is positioned at the base of the tongue (Figure 4-23 ●).

7. Look for the tip of the epiglottis, and place the laryngoscope blade into its proper position. Keep in mind that a child—particularly an infant—has a shorter airway and a higher glottis than an adult. Because of this, you will see the cords much sooner than you may expect.

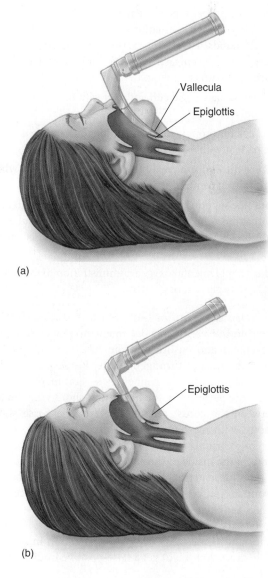

(a)

(b)

● **Figure 4-23** Placement of the laryngoscope: (a) MacIntosh (curved) blade and (b) Miller (straight) blade.

8. With your left wrist straight, use your shoulder and arm to lift the mandible and tongue at a 45-degree angle to the floor until the glottis is exposed. Use the little finger of your left hand to apply gentle downward pressure to the cricoid cartilage. This will permit easier visualization of the cords.

9. Grasp the endotracheal tube in your right hand. To pass the tube into your patient's mouth, it may be helpful to hold it so that its curve is in a horizontal plane (bevel sideways). Insert the tube through the right corner of the child's mouth.

10. Under direct observation, insert the endotracheal tube into the glottic opening and pass it through until its distal cuff disappears past the vocal cords—approximately 5 to 10 cm. As a tube is advanced, it should be rotated into the proper plane. In some cases, it will be difficult to advance an endotracheal tube at the level of the cricoid. *Do not* force the tube through this region, because it can cause laryngeal edema.

11. Hold the tube in place with your left hand. Attach an infant- or child-size bag-valve device to the 15/22-mm adapter and deliver several breaths.

12. Check for proper tube placement. Watch for chest rise and fall with each ventilation and listen for equal, bilateral breath sounds. There should also be an absence of sounds over the epigastrium with ventilations. Confirm placement with capnography.

13. If the tube has a distal cuff, inflate it with the recommended amount of air.

14. Recheck for proper placement of the tube and ventilate the patient with 100 percent oxygen.

15. Secure the endotracheal tube with umbilical tape while maintaining ventilatory support.

16. Continue supporting the tube manually while maintaining ventilations. Check periodically to ensure proper tube position. As with adults, allow no more than 30 seconds to pass without ventilating your patient.

17. Adjust supplemental oxygen administration to maintain a SpO_2 of 94 percent or greater.

Tube Placement Verification in the Pediatric Patient

You must *always* verify and document proper endotracheal tube placement and ensure that the tube remains properly situated in the trachea throughout care. Proper endotracheal tube placement can be determined by several methods. First, the paramedic performing the intubation should see the tube pass between the cords. Second, bilateral chest rise should be observed with mechanical ventilation, and breath sounds over the epigastrium should be absent. The presence of condensation on the inside of the endotracheal tube also suggests proper tube placement. Additionally, the lack of phonation (vocal sounds) indicates that the tube is properly placed into the trachea. Esophageal detector devices are sometimes used in prehospital care to confirm proper tube placement. However, it is important to use these devices with caution in pediatric patients because you might get a false-positive finding even if the tube is improperly placed. This is particularly true when uncuffed endotracheal tubes have been used. The preferred method of endotracheal tube verification is through the use of capnography with either a colorimetric detector or waveform capnography. (Esophageal detector devices and end-tidal carbon dioxide detection devices were discussed in Volume 2, Chapter 5.)

It is not uncommon for an endotracheal tube to become displaced during patient care, movement, or transport. Because of this, paramedics must be extremely vigilant about repeatedly or continuously monitoring proper endotracheal tube placement. Monitoring can be accomplished through repeated assessments or through the use of continuous waveform capnography. Continuous waveform capnography provides breath-to-breath verification of proper tube placement and will rapidly alert providers of a problem with ventilation or with endotracheal tube placement. The mnemonic DOPE will help in remembering the possible causes of deterioration in an intubated child:

- **D**isplacement of the endotracheal tube from the trachea
- **O**bstruction of the tube
- **P**neumothorax
- **E**quipment failure

Problems with endotracheal tube placement remain a major malpractice risk for EMS personnel. For this reason, it is essential that proper endotracheal tube placement is not only verified *but also documented* by at least three methods. Continuous waveform capnography is rapidly becoming a standard of care and, if properly used, becomes irrefutable evidence of proper endotracheal tube placement, not only immediately after tube insertion but also throughout patient care.

Rapid Sequence Intubation

Advanced airway management may sometimes be indicated in pediatric patients with a significant level of consciousness and the presence of a gag reflex. Examples may include a combative child with head trauma or an adolescent with a drug overdose. In such cases, clenched teeth and resistance may make intubation difficult or impossible. As a result, medical direction may authorize the use of "paralytics" to induce a state of neuromuscular compliance. All skeletal muscles, including the muscles of respiration, respond to these drugs, known as *neuromuscular blocking agents*. Following their administration, the patient will require mechanical ventilation.

An example of a commonly used neuromuscular blocker is succinylcholine (Anectine). Typically, it is administered at 1 to 2 mg/kg IV push. It acts in 60 to 90 seconds and lasts approximately 3 to 5 minutes. Remember that succinylcholine has no effect on consciousness or pain. Thus, a sedative agent must be used for all children except those who are unconscious. Commonly used drugs include midazolam (Versed), diazepam (Valium), thiopental, and fentanyl. A bite block should be placed to prevent the patient from biting the endotracheal tube. Medical direction may authorize sedation to minimize the emotional trauma to the patient or drugs such as pancuronium or vecuronium if longer paralysis is required.

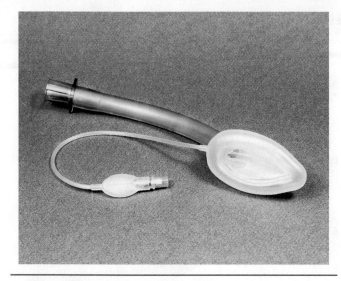

● **Figure 4-24** Pediatric laryngeal mask airway (LMA).

Extraglottic Airways

Endotracheal intubation has long been regarded as the "gold standard" for airway management. However, the use of alternative airways has become more common. This same trend is also occurring in pediatric airway management. The laryngeal mask airway (LMA) and the King LT-D are available in pediatric sizes and are now routinely used in several EMS systems for prehospital airway management.[12] The LMA is easy to insert and requires less education and practice than endotracheal intubation (Figure 4-24 ●).

Nasogastric Intubation

If gastric distention is present in a pediatric patient, you may consider placing a nasogastric (NG) tube. In infants and children, gastric distention may result from overly aggressive artificial ventilations or from air swallowing. Placement of an NG tube will allow you to decompress the stomach and proximal bowel of air. An NG tube can also be used to empty the stomach of blood or other substances. Indications for use of a nasogastric intubation include:

● Inability to achieve adequate tidal volumes during ventilation due to gastric distention

● Presence of gastric distention in an unresponsive patient

As with nasopharyngeal airways, an NG tube is contraindicated in pediatric patients who have sustained head or facial trauma. Because the NG tube might migrate into the cranial sinuses, consider the use of an orogastric tube instead. Other contraindications include possible soft-tissue damage in the nose and inducement of vomiting.

Equipment for placing an NG tube includes:

● Age-appropriate NG tubes
● 20-mL syringe
● Water-soluble lubricant
● Emesis basin
● Tape
● Suctioning equipment
● Stethoscope

In sizing the NG tube, keep in mind the following recommended guidelines:

● Newborn/infant: 8.0 French
● Toddler/preschooler: 10 French
● School-age children: 12 French
● Adolescents: 14–16 French

In determining the correct length, measure the tube from the tip of the nose, over the ear, to the tip of the xiphoid process. The steps in Procedure 4–3 can be followed for inserting the tube. Keep in mind, as you examine these steps, that many experts believe that an NG tube should be inserted only when an endotracheal tube is in place. This precaution will prevent misplacement of the tube into the trachea instead of the esophagus. Consult protocols in your area on the use of NG tubes.

Circulation

As mentioned earlier, the respiratory and cardiovascular systems are interdependent. In pediatrics, you are encouraged to look at the total child. You should assess the child by assessing the various body systems. For example, instead of simply checking a pulse, you should look for end-organ changes that indicate the effectiveness of respiratory and cardiovascular function. These include such things as mental status, skin color, skin temperature, urine output, and others.

Two problems lead to cardiopulmonary arrest in children: shock and respiratory failure. Both must be identified and corrected early. The following section will address assessment of the cardiovascular system. Particular emphasis is placed on venous access and fluid resuscitation, because these are essential skills for prehospital ALS personnel who treat pediatric patients.

Vascular Access

Intravenous techniques for children are basically the same as for adults (see Volume 2, Chapter 4). However, additional veins may be accessed in the infant. These include veins of the neck and scalp as well as those of the arms, hands, and feet. The external jugular vein, however, should be used only for life-threatening situations.

Intraosseous Infusion

The use of intraosseous (IO) infusion has become popular in treating pediatric patients (Figure 4-25a ●). This is especially true when large volumes of fluid must be administered, as occurs in hypovolemic shock, and when other means of venous access are unavailable. Certain medications can be administered intraosseously, including epinephrine, atropine, dopamine, lidocaine, sodium bicarbonate, and dobutamine. Indications for IO infusion include:

● Existence of shock or cardiac arrest
● An unresponsive patient
● Suspected sepsis
● Unsuccessful attempts at peripheral IV insertion

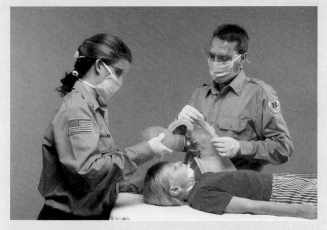

4-3a ● Oxygenate and continue to ventilate, if possible.

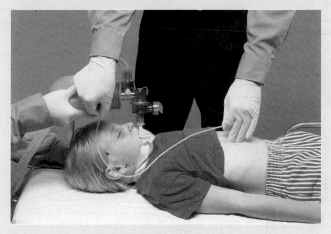

4-3b ● Measure the NG tube from the tip of the nose, over the ear, to the tip of the xiphoid process.

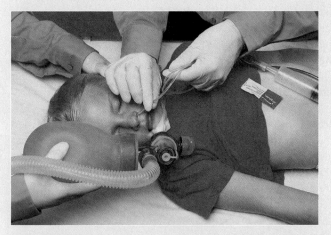

4-3c ● Lubricate the end of the tube. Then pass it gently downward along the nasal floor to the stomach.

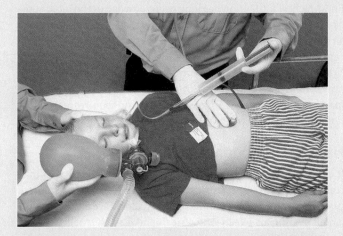

4-3d ● Auscultate over the epigastrium to confirm correct placement. Listen for bubbling while injecting 10–20 cc of air into the tube.

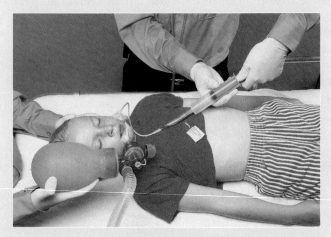

4-3e ● Use suction to aspirate stomach contents.

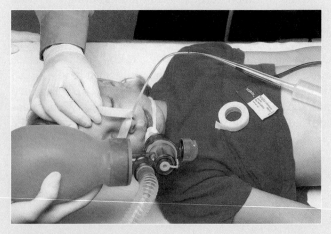

4-3f ● Secure the tube in place.

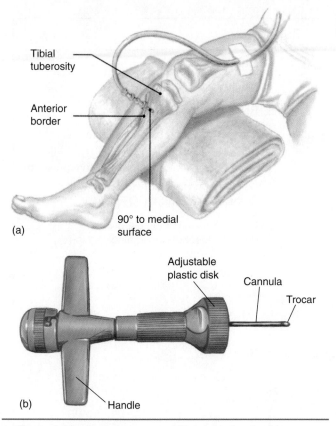

(a)

(b)

- **Figure 4-25** (a) Intraosseous administration in the pediatric patient. (b) An intraosseous needle.

The primary contraindications for IO infusion include:

- Presence of a fracture in the bone chosen for infusion
- Fracture of the pelvis or extremity fracture in the bone proximal to the chosen site

In performing IO perfusion, you can use a standard 16- or 18-gauge needle (either hypodermic or spinal). However, an intraosseous needle is preferred and is significantly better (Figure 4-25b ●). The anterior surface of the leg below the knee should be prepped with antiseptic solution. The needle is then inserted, in a twisting fashion, 1 to 3 cm below the tuberosity. Insertion should be slightly inferior in direction (to avoid the growth plate) and perpendicular to the skin (Figure 4-26 ●). Placement of the needle into the marrow cavity can be determined by noting a lack of resistance as the needle passes through the bony cortex. Other indications include the needle standing upright without support, the ability to aspirate bone marrow into a syringe, or free flow of the infusion without infiltration into the subcutaneous tissues. Several of the intraosseous devices, such as the EZ-IO® and the Bone Injection Gun (B.I.G.), are approved for usage in children. (See also the discussion of intraosseous infusion in Volume 2, Chapter 4.)

Fluid Therapy

The accurate dosing of fluids in children is crucial. Too much fluid can result in heart failure and pulmonary edema. Too little fluid can be ineffective. The primary dosage of fluid in hypovolemic shock should be 20 mL/kg of an isotonic solution

such as lactated Ringer's or normal saline as soon as IV access is obtained. After the infusion, the child should be reassessed. If perfusion is still diminished, then a second bolus of 20 mL/kg should be administered. A child with hypovolemic shock may require 40 to 60 mL/kg, whereas a child with septic shock may require at least 60 to 80 mL/kg. Fluid therapy should be guided by the child's clinical response.

Intravenous infusions in children should be closely monitored with frequent patient reassessment. Minidrip administration sets, flow limiters, or infusion pumps should be used routinely in pediatric cases.

Medications

Cardiopulmonary arrest in infants and children is almost always the result of a primary respiratory problem, such as drowning, choking, or smoke inhalation. The major aim in pediatric resuscitation is airway management and ventilation, as well as replacement of intravascular volume, if indicated. In certain cases, medications may be required. The objectives of medication therapy in pediatric patients include:

- Correction of hypoxemia
- Increased perfusion pressure during chest compressions
- Stimulation of spontaneous or more forceful cardiac contractions
- Acceleration of the heart rate
- Correction of metabolic acidosis
- Suppression of ventricular ectopy
- Maintenance of renal perfusion

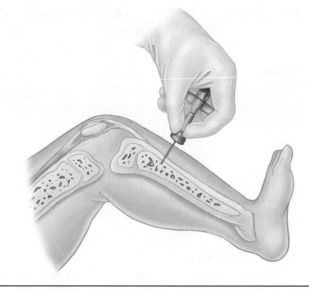

- **Figure 4-26** Correct needle placement for intraosseous administration. Note that the needle tip is in the marrow cavity.

TABLE 4–10 | Drugs Used in Pediatric Advanced Life Support*

Drug	Dose	Remarks
Adenosine	0.1–0.2 mg/kg Maximum strength dose 12 mg	Monitor ECG Rapid IV/IO bolus
Amiodarone	5 mg/kg IV/IO; repeat up to 15 mg/kg. Maximum: 300 mg	Monitor ECG and blood pressure Adjust administration rate to urgency (give more slowly when perfusing rhythm present) Use caution when administering with other drugs that prolong the QT interval.
Atropine Sulfate	0.02 mg/kg IV/IO 0.03 mg/kg ET† Repeat once if needed Minimum dose: 0.1 mg Maximum single dose: Child: 0.5 mg Adolescent: 1.0 mg	Higher doses may be used with organophosphate poisoning.
Calcium Chloride (10%)	20 mg/kg per dose IV/IO (0.2 mL/kg)	Give slowly.
Epinephrine	0.01 mg/kg (0.1 mL/kg 1:10,000) IV/IO 0.1 mg/kg (0.1 mL/kg 1:1,000) ET† Maximum dose: 1 mg IV/IO; 10 mg ET†	May repeat every 3–5 minutes.
Glucose	0.5–1.0 g/kg IV/IO	$D_{10}W$: 5–10 mL/kg $D_{25}W$: 2–4 mL/kg $D_{50}W$: 1–2 mL/kg
Magnesium Sulfate	20–50 mg/kg IV/IO over 10–20 minutes; faster in *torsades de pointes*. Maximum dose: 2 g	
Naloxone	<5 years or <20 kg: 0.1 mg/kg IV/IO/ET* >5 years or >20 kg: 2 mg IV/IO/ET*	Use lower doses to reverse respiratory depression associated with therapeutic opioid use (1–15 mcg/kg).
Procainamide	15 mg/kg IV/IO over 30–60 minutes Adult dose: 20 mg/min IV up to a total dose of 17 mg/kg	Monitor ECG and blood pressure. Use caution when administering with other drugs that prolong the QT interval.
Sodium Bicarbonate	1 mEq/kg per dose IV/IO slowly	After adequate ventilation.

*IV indicates intravenous route; IO, intraosseous route; ET, endotracheal route.
†Flush with 5 mL of normal saline and follow with five ventilations.

The dosages of medications must be modified for the pediatric patient. Tables 4–10 and 4–11 illustrate recommended pediatric drug dosages in advanced cardiac life support.

Electrical Therapy

You are less likely to use electrical therapy on pediatric patients than on adult patients, because ventricular fibrillation is much less common in children than adults. However, you should review and keep the following principles in mind for times when these emergencies arise:

- Administer an initial dosage of 2 to 4 joules per kilogram of body weight. (Keep in mind the estimated body weights in Table 4–5.)
- If this is unsuccessful, focus your attention on correcting hypoxia and acidosis.
- Transport to a pediatric critical care unit, if possible.

TABLE 4–11 | Preparation of Infusions

Drug	Preparation*	Dose
Epinephrine	0.6 × body weight (kg) equals milligrams added to diluent[†] to make 100 mL	Then 1 mL/hr delivers 0.1 mcg/kg per minute; titrate to effect
Dopamine/dobutamine	0.6 × body weight (kg) equals milligrams added to diluent[†] to make 100 mL	Then 1 mL/hr delivers 0.3 mcg/kg per minute; titrate to effect

*Standard concentration can be used to provide more dilute or more concentrated drug solution, but then individual dose must be calculated for each patient and each infusion rate:

$$\text{Infusion Rate (mL/h)} = \frac{\text{Weight (kg)} \times \text{Dose (mcg/kg/min)} \times 60 \text{ min/hr}}{\text{Concentration (mcg/mL)}}$$

[†]Diluent may be 5 percent dextrose in water, 5 percent dextrose in half-normal, normal saline, or Ringer's lactate.

C-Spine Immobilization

Spinal injuries in children are not as common as in adults. However, because of a child's disproportionately larger and heavier head, the cervical spine (C-spine) is vulnerable to injury. Any time an infant or child sustains a significant head injury, assume that a neck injury may also be present. Children can suffer a spinal cord injury with no noticeable damage to the vertebral column as seen on cervical spine X-rays, referred to as spinal cord injury without radiographic abnormality (SCIWORA). Thus, negative cervical spine X-rays do not necessarily ensure that a spinal cord injury does not exist. Because of this, children should remain immobilized until a spinal cord injury has been excluded by hospital personnel—typically through magnetic resonance imaging (MRI) and other imaging technologies. As previously noted, even a child secured in a car safety seat can suffer a neck injury if the head is propelled forward during a collision or sudden stop.

Always make sure that you use the appropriate-sized pediatric immobilization equipment. These supplies may include rigid cervical collars, towel or blanket rolls, foam head blocks, commercial pediatric immobilization devices, vest-type or short wooden backboards, and long boards with the appropriate padding. For pediatric patients found in car seats, you can also use the seat for immobilization (Procedure 4–4). The Kendrick extrication device (KED) can be quickly modified to immobilize a pediatric patient. Because of the significant variations in the size of children, you must be creative in devising a plan for pediatric immobilization.

In securing the pediatric patient to the backboard, use appropriate amounts of padding to secure infants, toddlers, and preschoolers in a supine, neutral position. Never use sandbags when immobilizing a pediatric patient's head. If you must tip the board to manage vomiting, the weight of the sandbag may worsen the head injury. For steps in applying a pediatric immobilization system, see Procedure 4–5.

Whenever you immobilize a pediatric patient, remember that many children, especially those under age 5, will protest or fight restraint. Try to minimize the emotional stress by having a parent or caretaker stand near or touch the child. Often the child will stop struggling when secured totally in an immobilization device. Ideally, a rescuer or family member should remain with the child at all times to reassure and calm the child, if possible.

Transport Guidelines

In managing a pediatric patient, never delay transport to perform a procedure that can be done en route to the hospital. After deciding on necessary interventions—first BLS, then ALS—determine the appropriate receiving facility. In reaching your decision, consider three factors:

- Time of transport
- Specialized facilities
- Specialized personnel

If you live in an area with specialized prehospital crews, such as critical care crews and neonatal nurses, their availability should weigh in your decision as well. Consider whether the patient would benefit from transfer by one of these crews. If so, request support. If not, determine the closest definitive care facility for the infant or child placed in your care. Continue to reassure the child to reduce the fear involved in transition of care from the family to the hospital (Figure 4-27 ●). Think of what you would do or say to calm your own child or the child of a close relative or friend.

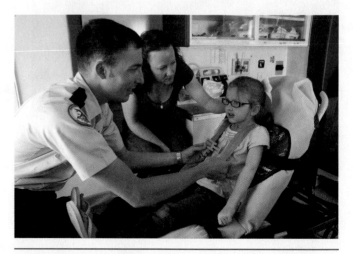

● **Figure 4-27** Emotional support of the infant or child continues during transport.

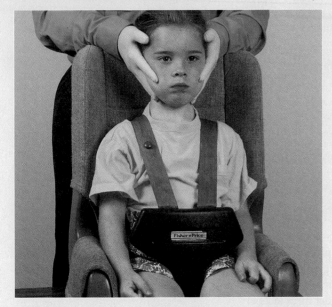

4-4a ● One paramedic stabilizes the car seat in an upright position and applies and maintains manual in-line stabilization to the child's head throughout the immobilization process.

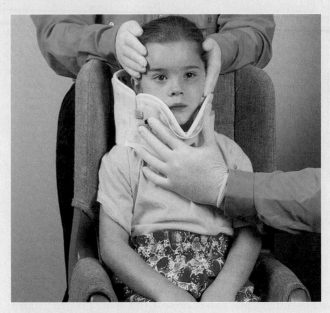

4-4b ● A second paramedic applies an appropriately sized cervical collar. If one is not available, improvise using a rolled hand towel.

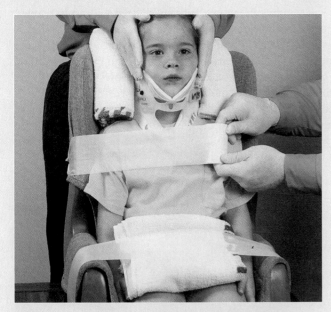

4-4c ● The second paramedic places a small blanket or towel on the child's lap, then uses straps or wide tape to secure the chest and pelvic areas to the seat.

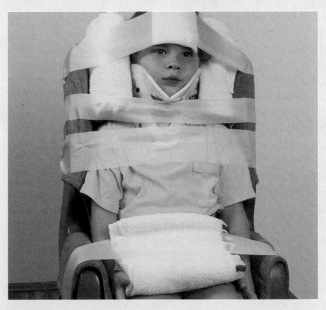

4-4d ● The second paramedic places towel rolls on both sides of the child's head to fill voids between the head and seat. The medic tapes the head into place, taping across the forehead and the collar, but avoiding taping over the chin, which would put pressure on the neck. The patient and seat can be carried to the ambulance and strapped to the stretcher, with the stretcher head raised.

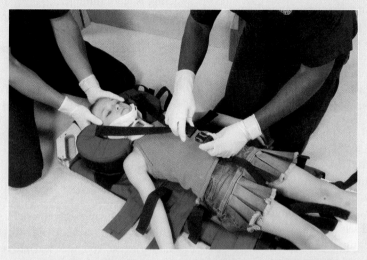

4-5a ● Position the patient on the immobilization system and adjust the color-coded straps to fit the child.

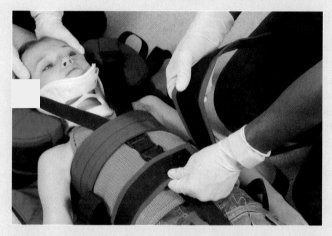

4-5b ● Attach the four-point safety system.

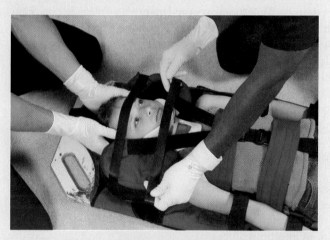

4-5c ● Fasten the adjustable head-support system.

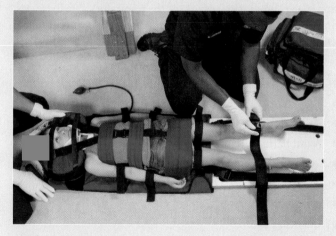

4-5d ● At this point, the patient is fully immobilized to the system.

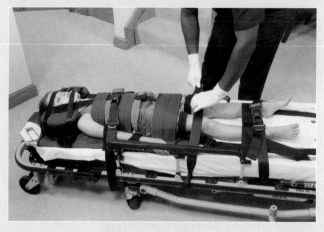

4-5e ● Move the immobilized patient onto the stretcher and fasten the loops at both ends to connect to the stretcher straps.

SPECIFIC MEDICAL EMERGENCIES

As you already realize from your earlier training and experience, a variety of pediatric medical problems can activate the EMS system. Although the majority of childhood medical emergencies involve the respiratory system, other body systems can be involved as well. To help you recognize and treat pediatric medical emergencies, the following sections cover some of the specific conditions you may encounter.

Infections

Childhood is a time of frequent illnesses because of the relative immaturity of the pediatric immune system. Infectious diseases may be caused by the infection or infestation of the body by an infectious agent such as a virus, bacterium, fungus, or parasite. Most infections are minor and self-limiting. Several infections, however, can be life threatening. These include meningitis, pneumonia, and septicemia, a systemic infection (usually bacterial) in the bloodstream.

The impact of an infection on physiologic processes depends on the type of infectious agent and the extent of the infection. Signs and symptoms also vary, depending on the type of infection and the time since exposure. Any of the following conditions may indicate the presence of an infection: fever, chills, tachycardia, cough, sore throat, nasal congestion, malaise, tachypnea, cool or clammy skin, petechiae, respiratory distress, poor appetite, vomiting, diarrhea, dehydration, hypoperfusion (especially with septicemia), purpura (purple blotches resulting from hemorrhages into the skin that do not disappear under pressure), seizures, severe headache, irritability, stiff neck, or bulging fontanelle (infants).

The management of infections depends on the body system or systems affected. Treatment of some of the most common and serious infections will be found in the sections that follow. As a general rule, you should adhere to these guidelines when treating an infectious illness:

- Take Standard Precautions because of the unknown cause of the infection.
- Become familiar with the common pediatric infections encountered in your area.
- If possible, try to determine which, if any, pediatric infections you have not been exposed to or vaccinated for. For example, if you did not have chickenpox (varicella) or measles (rubeola) as a child and were not vaccinated for them, then you should consider receiving vaccination for these illnesses. If you encounter a child suspected of having an infectious disease to which you may be susceptible, consider allowing another rescuer to be the primary person to care for the child.

Respiratory Emergencies

Respiratory emergencies constitute the most common reason EMS is summoned to care for a pediatric patient. Respiratory illnesses can cause respiratory compromise because of their effect on the alveolar/capillary interface. Some illnesses are quite minor, causing only mild symptoms, but others can be rapidly fatal. Your approach to the child with a respiratory emergency will depend on the severity of respiratory compromise. If the child is alert and talking, then you can take a more relaxed approach. However, if the child appears ill and exhibits marked respiratory difficulty, then you must immediately intervene to prevent respiratory arrest and possible cardiopulmonary arrest.

Severity of Respiratory Compromise

The severity of respiratory compromise can be quickly classified into the following categories:

- Respiratory distress
- Respiratory failure
- Respiratory arrest

Respiratory emergencies in pediatric patients may quickly progress from respiratory distress to respiratory failure to respiratory arrest. You must learn to recognize the phase your patient is in and take the appropriate interventions. Prompt recognition and treatment can literally mean the difference between life and death for an infant or child suffering from respiratory compromise.

Respiratory Distress The mildest form of respiratory impairment is classified as respiratory distress. The most noticeable finding is an increased work of breathing. One of the earliest indicators of respiratory distress is an increase in respiratory rate. Unfortunately, respiratory rate is one of the vital signs that is most often "estimated." As mentioned previously, it is essential to obtain an accurate respiratory rate in children. Ideally, the respiratory rate should be measured for an entire minute. If time does not allow it, or if the child is deteriorating, the respiratory rate should be measured for at least 30 seconds and multiplied by two to obtain the respiratory rate.

In addition to an increased work of breathing, the child in respiratory distress will initially have a slight decrease in the arterial carbon dioxide tension as the respiratory rate increases. However, as respiratory distress increases, the carbon dioxide tension will gradually increase.

The signs and symptoms of respiratory distress include:

- Normal mental status deteriorating to irritability or anxiety
- Tachypnea
- Retractions
- Nasal flaring (in infants)
- Poor muscle tone
- Tachycardia
- Head bobbing
- Grunting
- Cyanosis or hypoxia that improves with supplemental oxygen

If not corrected immediately, respiratory distress will lead to respiratory failure.

Respiratory Failure Respiratory failure occurs when the respiratory system is not able to meet the demands of the body for oxygen intake and for carbon dioxide removal. It is characterized by inadequate ventilation and oxygenation. During respiratory failure, the carbon dioxide level begins to rise because the body is not able to remove carbon dioxide. This ultimately leads to respiratory acidosis.

The signs and symptoms of respiratory failure include:

- Irritability or anxiety deteriorating to lethargy
- Marked tachypnea later deteriorating to bradypnea
- Marked retractions later deteriorating to agonal respirations
- Poor muscle tone
- Marked tachycardia later deteriorating to bradycardia
- Central cyanosis
- Hypoxia

Respiratory failure is a very ominous sign. If immediate intervention is not provided, the child will deteriorate to full respiratory arrest.

Respiratory Arrest The end result of respiratory impairment, if untreated, is respiratory arrest. The cessation of breathing typically follows a period of bradypnea and agonal respirations.

Signs and symptoms of respiratory arrest include:

- Unresponsiveness deteriorating to coma
- Bradypnea deteriorating to apnea
- Absent chest wall motion
- Bradycardia deteriorating to asystole
- Profound cyanosis

Respiratory arrest will quickly deteriorate to full cardiopulmonary arrest if appropriate interventions are not made. The child's chances of survival markedly decrease when cardiopulmonary arrest occurs.

Management of Respiratory Compromise

The management of respiratory compromise should be based on the severity of the problem. The goals of management include increasing ventilation and increasing oxygenation. You should try to identify the signs and symptoms of respiratory distress early so that you can intervene before the child deteriorates.

Your initial attention should be directed at the airway. Is it patent? Is it maintainable with simple positioning? Is endotracheal intubation required?

After assessing the airway, ensure continued maintenance of the airway by positioning, placement of an airway adjunct (oropharyngeal or nasopharyngeal airway), or endotracheal intubation.

For children in respiratory distress or early respiratory failure, administer high-concentration oxygen. Some children will tolerate a nonrebreather mask. Others may not and may require that someone (perhaps a parent) hold blow-by oxygen for them to breathe. If the child fails to improve with supplemental oxygen administration, the patient should be treated more aggressively. Often it is necessary to separate the parents

from the child so that you can provide the necessary care without interruption or distraction.

Pediatric patients with late respiratory failure or respiratory arrest require aggressive treatment. This includes:

CONTENT REVIEW

▶ Stages of Respiratory Compromise

- Respiratory distress
- Respiratory failure
- Respiratory arrest

- Establishment of an airway
- High-concentration, supplemental oxygen administration
- Mechanical ventilation with a BVM device attached to a reservoir delivering 100 percent oxygen
- Endotracheal intubation (or another acceptable airway) if mechanical ventilation does not rapidly improve the patient's condition
- Consideration of gastric decompression with an orogastric or nasogastric tube if abdominal distention is impeding ventilation
- Consideration of needle decompression of the chest if a tension pneumothorax is thought to be present
- Consideration of cricothyrotomy if complete airway obstruction is present and the airway cannot be obtained by any other method

In addition to the preceding treatments, you should obtain venous access. The child should be promptly transported to a facility staffed and equipped to handle critically ill children. While en route, continue to reassess the child. Signs of improvement include an improvement in skin color and temperature. As end-organ perfusion improves, the child will exhibit an increase in pulse rate, an increase in oxygen saturation, and an improvement in mental status. Provide emotional and psychological support to the parents and keep them abreast of the results of your care.

Specific Respiratory Emergencies

Respiratory problems typically arise from obstruction of a part of the respiratory tract or impairment of the mechanics of respiration. In the following discussion we present the common pediatric respiratory emergencies based on the part of the airway they most affect.

Upper Airway Obstruction

Obstruction of the upper airway can be caused by many factors. As previously mentioned, upper airway obstruction may be partial or complete. It can be caused by inflamed or swollen tissues resulting from infection or by an aspirated foreign body. Appropriate care depends on prompt and immediate identification of the disorder and its severity. Whenever you find an infant, toddler, or young child in respiratory or cardiac arrest, assume complete upper airway obstruction until proven otherwise.

Croup Croup, medically referred to as *laryngotracheobronchitis,* is a viral infection of the upper airway. It most commonly occurs in children six months to four years of age and is prevalent in the fall and winter. Croup causes an inflammation of the upper respiratory tract involving the subglottic region. The infection leads to edema beneath the glottis and larynx, thus narrowing the lumen of the airway. Severe cases of croup can lead to complete airway obstruction. Another form of croup, called *spasmodic croup,* occurs mostly in the middle of the night without any prior upper respiratory infection.

Assessment The history for croup is fairly classic. Often, the child will have a mild cold or other infection and be doing fairly well until evening. After dark, however, a harsh, barking, or brassy cough develops. The attack may subside in a few hours but can persist for several nights.

The physical exam will often reveal inspiratory stridor. There may be associated nasal flaring, tracheal tugging, or retraction. You should *never* examine the oropharynx. Often, in the prehospital setting, it is difficult to distinguish croup from epiglottitis (Table 4–12 and Figure 4-28 ●). If epiglottitis is present, examination of the oropharynx may result in laryngospasm and complete airway obstruction. If the attack of croup is severe and progressive, the child may develop restlessness, tachycardia, and cyanosis. Although croup can result in complete airway obstruction and respiratory arrest, this is a rare event.

Management Management of croup consists of appropriate airway maintenance. Place the child in a position of comfort and administer cool mist air or oxygen by facemask or blow-by method. If the attack is severe, the physician may order the administration of racemic epinephrine or albuterol. Recent studies have shown standard epinephrine by nebulizer just as effective, and in some cases better, in croup as is racemic epinephrine.[13] Some physicians also advocate the use of steroids, because they feel these drugs will shorten the course of the illness.

In preparing the patient for transport, remember that the journey from the house to the ambulance will often allow the child to breathe cool air. Because cool air causes a decrease in subglottic edema, the child may be clinically improved by the time you reach the ambulance. If appropriate, keep the parent or caregiver with the infant or child. Do not agitate the patient,

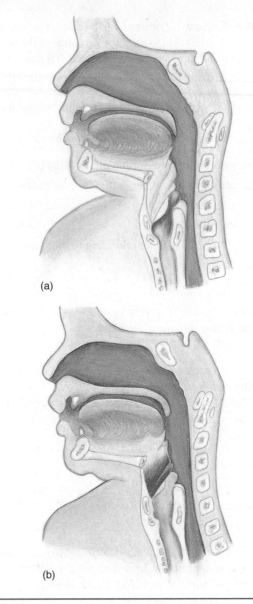

● **Figure 4-28** (a) Epiglottitis is characterized by inflammation of the epiglottis and supraglottic tissues. (b) Croup is characterized by subglottic edema.

which could worsen the croup, by administering nonessential measures such as IVs or blood pressure readings.

Epiglottitis **Epiglottitis** is an acute infection and inflammation of the epiglottis and is potentially life threatening. (Recall that the epiglottis is a flap of cartilage that protects the airway during swallowing.) Epiglottitis, unlike croup, is caused by a bacterial infection, usually *Haemophilus influenzae* type B. As a result of the availability of *H. influenzae* vaccination, epiglottitis has become an uncommon occurrence. When it does occur, it tends to strike children three to seven years old.

Assessment Epiglottitis presents similarly to croup. Often the child will go to bed feeling relatively well, usually with what parents or caregivers consider to be a mild infection of the respiratory tract. Later, the child awakens with a high temperature and a brassy cough. The progression of symptoms can be dramatic. There is often pain on swallowing, sore throat, high

TABLE 4–12 | Symptoms of Croup and Epiglottitis	
Croup	**Epiglottitis**
Slow onset	Rapid onset
Generally wants to sit up	Prefers to sit up
Barking cough	No barking cough
No drooling	Drooling; painful to swallow
Fever approximately 101°F–102°F (38.3°C–38.9°C)	Fever approximately 102°F–104°F (38.9°C–40.0°C)
	Occasional stridor

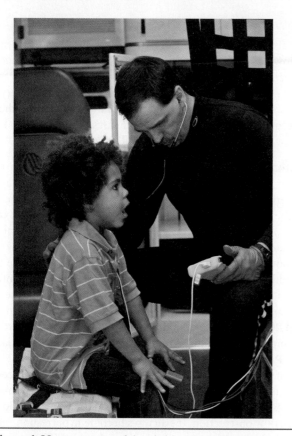

● **Figure 4-29** Posturing of the child with epiglottitis.

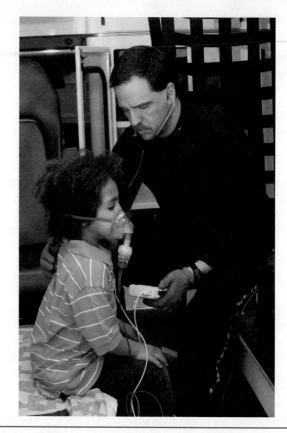

● **Figure 4-30** The child with epiglottitis should be administered humidified oxygen and transported in a comfortable position.

fever, shallow breathing, dyspnea, inspiratory stridor, and drooling (Figure 4-29 ●).

On physical examination, the child will appear acutely ill and agitated. *Never attempt to visualize the airway*. If the child is crying, the tip of the epiglottis can be seen posterior to the base of the tongue. In epiglottitis, the epiglottis is cherry red and swollen. As airway obstruction develops, the child will exhibit retractions, nasal flaring, and pulmonary hyperexpansion. As the epiglottis swells, he may not be able to swallow his saliva and will begin to drool. Often the child will want to remain seated. Patients will often assume the "tripod position" to help maximize their airway. If they lean backward or lie flat, the epiglottis can fall back and completely obstruct the airway.

Management Management of epiglottitis consists of appropriate airway maintenance and oxygen administration by facemask (Figure 4-30 ●) or the blow-by technique. Ideally, the oxygen should be humidified to minimize drying of the epiglottis and airway. To reduce the child's anxiety, you might ask the parent or caregiver to administer the oxygen. If the airway becomes obstructed, two-rescuer ventilation with BVM is almost always effective. Make sure that all intubation equipment is available, including an appropriately sized endotracheal tube. Remember, however, that intubation is contraindicated unless complete obstruction has occurred.

Also, do not intubate in settings with short transport times. If endotracheal intubation is required, it may be necessary to use a smaller endotracheal tube because of narrowing of the glottic opening. If you perform chest compression upon glottic visualization during intubation, a bubble at the tracheal opening may form. This may help to establish upper airway landmarks that are distorted by the disease. As a last resort, consider needle cricothyrotomy per medical direction.

Pediatric patients with epiglottitis require immediate transport. Handle the child gently, as stress could lead to total airway obstruction from spasms of the larynx and swelling tissues. Avoid IV sticks, do not take a blood pressure, and do not attempt to look into the mouth. During transport, reassure and comfort the child. Constantly monitor the child, and notify the hospital of any changes in status. Remember, if the patient is maintaining his airway, *do not put anything in the child's mouth*, including a thermometer. At all times, consider epiglottitis a critical condition.

Bacterial Tracheitis **Bacterial tracheitis** is a bacterial infection of the airway in the subglottic region. Although the condition is very uncommon, it is most likely to appear following episodes of viral croup. It afflicts mainly infants and toddlers one to five years of age.

Assessment In assessing this condition, parents or caregivers will typically report that the child has experienced an episode of croup in the preceding few days. They will also indicate the presence of a high-grade fever accompanied by coughing up of pus and/or mucus. The patient may exhibit a hoarse voice and, if able to talk, the child may complain of a sore throat. A physical examination may reveal inspiratory or expiratory stridor.

Management As with all respiratory emergencies, the child must be carefully monitored, because respiratory failure or arrest may be an end result. Carefully manage airway and breathing, providing oxygenation by facemask or blow-by technique. Keep in mind that ventilations may require high pressure in order to adequately ventilate the patient. This may require depressing the pop-off valve of the pediatric BVM device, if the valve is present. Consider intubation only in cases of complete airway obstruction. Transport guidelines are similar to those for cases of epiglottitis.

Foreign Body Aspiration Children—especially toddlers and preschoolers, one to four years old—like to put objects into their mouths. As a result, these children are at increased risk of aspirating foreign bodies, especially when they run or fall. In fact, foreign body aspiration is the number-one cause of in-home accidental deaths in children under six years of age. In addition, many children choke on, or aspirate, food given to them by their parents or other well-meaning adults. Young children have not yet developed coordinated chewing motions in their mouth and pharynx and cannot chew food adequately. Common foods associated with aspiration and airway obstruction in children include hard candy, nuts, seeds, hot dogs, sausages, and grapes. Nonfood items include coins, balloons, and other small objects.

Assessment The child with a suspected aspirated foreign body may present in one of two ways. If the obstruction is complete, the child will have minimal or no air movement. If the obstruction is partial, the child may exhibit inspiratory stridor, a muffled or hoarse voice, drooling, pain in the throat, retractions, and cyanosis.

Management Whenever you suspect that a child has aspirated a foreign body, immediately assess the patient's respiratory efforts. If the obstruction is partial, make the child as comfortable as possible and administer humidified oxygen. If the child is old enough, place him in a sitting position. Do not attempt to look in the mouth. Intubation equipment should be readily available because complete airway obstruction can occur. Transport the child to a hospital, where the foreign body can be removed by hospital personnel in a controlled environment.

If the obstruction is complete, clear the airway with accepted basic life support techniques. Sweep visible obstructions with your gloved finger. Do not perform blind finger sweeps, because this can push a foreign body deeper into the airway. Following BLS foreign body removal procedures, attempt ventilation with a BVM. If unsuccessful, visualize the airway with a laryngoscope. If the foreign body is seen and readily accessible, try to remove it with Magill forceps. Intubate if possible. Continue BLS foreign body removal procedures. If the airway cannot be cleared by routine measures, consider needle cricothyrotomy per medical direction and only as a last resort. Transport following appropriate guidelines, avoiding further agitation of the child.

Lower Airway Distress

As already discussed, suspect lower airway distress when the following conditions exist: an absence of stridor, presence of wheezing during exhalation, and increased work of breathing. Common causes of lower airway distress include respiratory diseases such as asthma, bronchiolitis, and pneumonia. Although infrequent, you may also encounter cases of foreign body lower airway aspiration, especially in toddlers and preschoolers.

Asthma Asthma is a chronic inflammatory disorder of the lower respiratory tract. The disease affects more than 6 million Americans. It occurs before age 10 in approximately 50 percent of the cases, and before age 30 in another 33 percent of cases. The disease tends to run in families. It is also commonly associated with atopic conditions, such as eczema and allergies. Although deaths from other respiratory conditions have been steadily declining, asthmatic deaths have risen significantly in recent decades. Hospitalization of children for treatment of asthma has increased by more than 200 percent during the past 20 years. Because children can readily succumb to asthma, prompt prehospital recognition and treatment are essential.[14]

Pathophysiology Asthma is a chronic inflammatory disorder of the airways, characterized by bronchospasm and excessive mucus production. In susceptible children, this inflammation causes widespread, but variable, airflow obstruction. In addition to airflow obstruction, the airways become hyperresponsive.

Asthma may be induced by one of many different factors, commonly called *triggers*. The triggers vary from one child to the next. Common triggers include environmental allergens, cold air, exercise, foods, irritants, emotional stress, and certain medications.

Within minutes of exposure to the trigger, a two-phase reaction occurs. The first phase of the reaction is characterized by the release of chemical mediators such as histamine. These cause bronchoconstriction and bronchial edema that effectively decrease expiratory airflow, causing the classic "asthma attack." If treated early, asthma may respond to inhaled bronchodilators. If the attack is not aborted, or does not resolve spontaneously, a second phase may occur. The second phase is characterized by inflammation of the bronchioles as cells of the immune system invade the respiratory tract. This causes additional edema and further decreases expiratory airflow. The second phase is typically unresponsive to inhaled bronchodilators. Instead, anti-inflammatory agents, such as corticosteroids, are often required.

As the attack continues, and swelling of the mucous membranes lining the bronchioles worsens, there may be plugging of the bronchi by thick mucus. This further obstructs airflow. As a result, sputum production increases. In addition, the lungs become progressively hyperinflated, because airflow is more restricted in exhalation. This effectively reduces vital capacity and results in decreased gas exchange by the alveoli, resulting in hypoxemia. If allowed to progress untreated, hypoxemia will worsen, and unconsciousness and death may ensue.

Assessment Asthma can often be differentiated from other pediatric respiratory illnesses by the history. In many cases, there is a prior history of asthma or reactive airway disease. The child's medications may also be an indicator. Children with asthma often have an inhaler or a nebulized beta-agonist preparation.

On physical examination, the child is usually sitting up, leaning forward, and tachypneic. Often, there is an associated unproductive cough. Accessory respiratory muscle usage is usually evident. Wheezing may be heard. However, in a severe attack, the patient may not wheeze at all. This is an ominous finding. Some children will not wheeze, but will cough, often continuously. Generally there is associated tachycardia; this should be monitored, as virtually all medications used to treat asthma increase the heart rate. Pulse oximetry and capnography can help assess the severity of asthma and guide treatment.

Management The primary therapeutic goals in the asthmatic patient are to correct hypoxia, reverse bronchospasm, and decrease inflammation. First, it is imperative that you establish an airway. Next, administer supplemental, humidified oxygen as necessary to correct hypoxia. Initial pharmacological therapy is the administration of an inhaled beta agonist (Figure 4-31 ●). All paramedic units should have the capability of administering nebulized bronchodilator medications such as albuterol, metaproterenol, or levalbuterol. Alternatively, a metered-dose inhaler (MDI) may be used. If the transport time is prolonged, the medical direction physician may also request administration of a steroid preparation.

Status Asthmaticus Status asthmaticus is defined as a severe, prolonged asthma attack that cannot be broken by aggressive pharmacological management. This is a serious medical emergency; prompt recognition, treatment, and transport are required. Often, the child suffering status asthmaticus will have a greatly distended chest from continued air trapping. Breath sounds, and often wheezing, may be absent. The patient is usually exhausted, severely acidotic, and often dehydrated. The management of status asthmaticus is basically the same as for asthma. However, you should recognize that respiratory arrest is imminent and remain prepared for endotracheal intubation. Transport should be immediate, with aggressive treatment continued en route.

Bronchiolitis Bronchiolitis is a respiratory infection of the medium-sized airways—the bronchioles—that occurs in early childhood. It should not be confused with bronchitis, which is an infection of the larger bronchi. Bronchiolitis is caused by a viral infection, most commonly *respiratory syncytial virus* (RSV) that affects the lining of the bronchioles.

Bronchiolitis is characterized by prominent expiratory wheezing and clinically resembles asthma. It most commonly occurs in winter in children less than two years of age. Bronchiolitis often spreads quickly through day care and preschool facilities. Most children will develop lifelong immunity to RSV following infection. The exception is the very young infant who has an immature immune system.

Assessment A history is necessary to distinguish bronchiolitis from asthma. Often, with bronchiolitis, there is a family history of asthma or allergies, although neither is yet present in the child. In addition, a low-grade fever often exists. A major distinguishing factor is age. Asthma rarely occurs before the age of one year, whereas bronchiolitis is more frequent in this age group.

Your physical examination should be systematic. Pay particular attention to the presence of crackles or wheezes. In addition, note any evidence of infection or respiratory distress.

Management Prehospital management of suspected bronchiolitis is much the same as with asthma. Place the child in a semisitting position, if old enough, and administer humidified oxygen by mask or blow-by method. Ventilations should be supported as necessary. Equipment for intubation should be readily available. If respiratory distress is present, consider administration of a bronchodilator such as albuterol (Ventolin, Proventil) or levalbuterol (Xopenex) by small-volume nebulizer. The cardiac rhythm should be monitored constantly. Pulse oximetry, if available, should be used continuously.

Pneumonia Pneumonia is an infection of the lower airway and lungs. Either a bacterium or a virus may cause it. Pneumonia can occur at any age, but in pediatric patients, it most commonly appears in infants, toddlers, and preschoolers aged one to five years. Most cases of pneumonia in children are viral and self-limited. As children get older, they can contract bacterial pneumonias as adults do. A pneumonia vaccine is available. However, its use is reserved for patients with an immune system problem or who are asplenic (lacking a spleen).

Assessment Persons with pneumonia often have a history of a respiratory infection, such as a severe cold or bronchitis. Signs and symptoms include a low-grade fever, decreased breath sounds, crackles, rhonchi, and pain in the chest area. Conduct a systematic assessment of a patient with suspected pneumonia, paying particular attention to evidence of respiratory distress.

Management Prehospital management of pneumonia is supportive. Place the patient in a position of comfort. Ensure a patent airway and administer supplemental oxygen via a nonrebreather device. If respiratory failure is present, support ventilations with a BVM device. If prolonged ventilation will be required, perform endotracheal intubation. Transport the patient in a position of comfort. Provide emotional and psychological support to the parents.

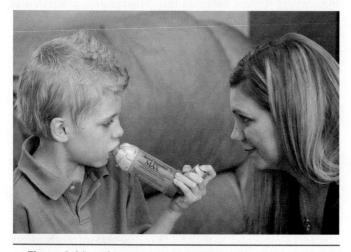

● **Figure 4-31** The young asthma patient may be making use of a prescribed inhaler to relieve symptoms.

CONTENT REVIEW

► Predisposing Factors of Pediatric Shock

- Hypothermia
- Dehydration (vomiting, diarrhea)
- Infection
- Trauma
- Blood loss
- Allergic reactions
- Poisoning
- Cardiac events (rare)

Foreign Body Lower Airway Obstruction The same pediatric patients that are at risk from upper airway obstruction are at risk for lower airway obstruction. A foreign body can enter the lower airway if it is too small to lodge in the upper airway. The object is often food (nuts, seeds, candy), small toys, or parts of toys. The child will take a deep breath or will fall and accidentally aspirate the foreign body. The foreign body will fall into the lower airway until it reaches the airway area that is smaller than the foreign body. Depending on positioning, the foreign body can act as a one-way valve and either trap air in distal lung tissues or prevent aeration of distal lung tissues, causing a ventilation/perfusion mismatch.

Assessment The history often includes information about the child having a foreign body in the mouth and then it suddenly disappears. The parents may be unsure whether the child swallowed it, aspirated it, or simply lost the object. If the object is fairly large and aspirated, then respiratory distress may be present. There is often considerable, often intractable, coughing. The child will be anxious and may have diminished breath sounds in the part of the chest affected by the foreign body. There may be crackles or rhonchi, usually unilateral. In some cases, there may be unilateral wheezing where some air is getting past the object. Unilateral wheezing should be considered to be due to an aspirated foreign body until proven otherwise.

Management The management of an aspirated foreign body is supportive. Place the child in a position of comfort and avoid agitation. Provide supplemental oxygen. Transport the child to a facility that has the capability of performing pediatric fiber-optic bronchoscopy. The bronchoscope can be used to visualize the airway and remove any foreign objects detected.

Shock (Hypoperfusion)

The second major cause of pediatric cardiopulmonary arrest—after respiratory impairment—is shock. Shock can most simply be defined as inadequate perfusion of the tissues with oxygen and other essential nutrients and inadequate removal of metabolic waste products. This ultimately results in tissue hypoxia and metabolic acidosis. Ultimately, if untreated, cellular death will occur.

When compared with the incidence of shock in adults, shock is an unusual occurrence in children because their blood vessels constrict so efficiently. However, when blood pressure does drop, it drops so far and so fast that the child may quickly develop cardiopulmonary arrest. A number of factors place infants and young children at risk of shock. As mentioned in Chapter 3, newborns and neonates can develop shock as a result of loss of body heat. Other causes include dehydration (from vomiting and/or diarrhea), infection (particularly septicemia), trauma (especially from abdominal injuries), and blood loss. Less common causes of shock in infants and children include allergic reactions, poisoning, and cardiac events (rare).

The definitive care of shock takes place in the emergency department of a hospital. Because shock is a life-threatening condition in pediatric patients, it is important to recognize early signs and symptoms—or even the possibility of shock in a situation when signs and symptoms have not yet developed. If you suspect a possibility of shock, provide oxygen to boost tissue perfusion and transport as quickly as possible. Also, keep the patient in a supine position and take steps to protect the child from hypothermia and agitation that might worsen the condition.

Severity of Shock

Shock is classified by degrees of severity as compensated, decompensated, and irreversible. The child responds to decreased perfusion by increasing heart rate and by increasing peripheral vascular resistance. The child has very little capacity to increase stroke volume. The key to early identification of shock is detecting the subtle signs that result from the body's various compensatory mechanisms.

Compensated Shock Early shock is known as *compensated shock* because the body is able to compensate for decreased tissue perfusion through various physiologic mechanisms. In compensated shock, the patient exhibits a normal blood pressure. The signs and symptoms of compensated shock include:

- Irritability or anxiety
- Tachycardia
- Tachypnea
- Weak peripheral pulses, full central pulses
- Delayed capillary refill (more than 2 seconds in children less than 6 years of age)
- Cool, pale extremities
- Systolic blood pressure within normal limits
- Decreased urinary output

Compensated shock is generally reversible if appropriate treatment measures are instituted. Again, the key to a good outcome is prompt detection of the early signs and symptoms and initiation of therapy based on this. Management is directed at correcting the underlying problem. High-concentration oxygen should be administered and venous access obtained. If the patient is hypovolemic, then fluid replacement should be initiated. If the cause is cardiogenic, then medications should be administered to support cardiac output and increase peripheral vascular resistance. Sometimes definitive care of shock is surgical. However, in these cases, fluid therapy and oxygen administration will help buy time until the patient can be taken to surgery.

Decompensated Shock *Decompensated shock* develops when the body can no longer compensate for decreased tissue perfusion. The hallmark of decompensated shock is a fall in blood pressure (an ominous sign in children). This results in hypoperfusion and inadequate end-organ perfusion. It is important to remember that a child's compensatory mechanisms are quite efficient. Thus, when a child develops decompensated shock, a significant loss of fluid or a significant impairment of

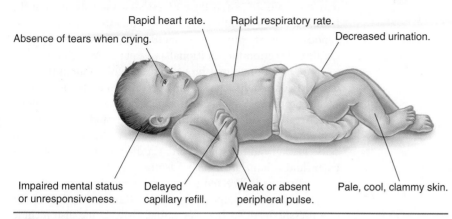

● **Figure 4-32** Signs and symptoms of shock (hypoperfusion) in a child.

cardiac output has occurred. The signs and symptoms of decompensated shock (Figure 4-32 ●) include:

- Lethargy or coma
- Marked tachycardia or bradycardia
- Absent peripheral pulses, weak central pulses
- Markedly delayed capillary refill
- Cool, pale, dusky, mottled extremities
- Hypotension
- Markedly decreased urinary output
- Absence of tears

Decompensated shock can become irreversible if aggressive treatment measures are not undertaken. In some cases, it may be irreversible despite the fact that aggressive treatment measures have been provided. Management is directed at treatment of the underlying cause. You should have a low threshold for initiating mechanical ventilation with a BVM device and 100 percent oxygen. Consider intubating the patient if mechanical ventilation will be prolonged.

Irreversible Shock *Irreversible shock* occurs when treatment measures are inadequate or too late to prevent significant tissue damage and death. Sometimes, blood pressure and pulse can be restored. However, the patient later succumbs as a result of organ failure. The best treatment for irreversible shock is prevention.

Categories of Shock

Shock can be categorized in a number of ways. Shock can be categorized as *cardiogenic* (caused by impaired pumping power of the heart), *hypovolemic* (caused by decreased blood or water volume), *obstructive* (caused by an obstruction that interferes with the return of blood to the heart, such as a pulmonary embolism, cardiac tamponade, or tension pneumothorax), and *distributive* (caused by abnormal distribution and return of blood resulting from vasodilation, vasopermeability, or both, as in septic, anaphylactic, or neurogenic shock).

Often, shock is classified into two general categories: cardiogenic and noncardiogenic. As noted earlier, **cardiogenic**

shock results from an inability of the heart to maintain an adequate cardiac output to the circulatory system and tissues. Cardiogenic shock in a pediatric patient is ominous and often fatal. **Noncardiogenic shock** includes types of shock that result from causes other than inadequate cardiac output. Causes may include hemorrhage, abdominal trauma, systemic bacterial infection, spinal cord injury, and others. In the following sections we first discuss types of noncardiogenic shock, then cardiogenic shock.

Noncardiogenic Shock

Noncardiogenic shock is more frequently encountered in prehospital pediatric care than cardiogenic shock. (Recall that children have a much lower incidence of cardiac problems than adults.) The forms that you will most commonly assess and manage are hypovolemic and distributive shock. (See also the discussion of metabolic problems in children later in the chapter.)

Hypovolemic Shock **Hypovolemic shock** results from loss of intravascular fluids. In pediatric patients, the most common causes include severe dehydration from vomiting and/or diarrhea and blood loss, usually as a result of trauma. Trauma may include blood loss into a body cavity (particularly the abdomen) or frank external hemorrhage. Children are also at risk of fluid loss as a result of burns, the second leading cause of pediatric deaths in the United States.

Treatment of hypovolemic shock involves administration of supplemental oxygen and establishment of intravenous access. This should be followed by a 20 mL/kg bolus of lactated Ringer's or normal saline. Following the bolus, the child should be reassessed. If signs and symptoms of compensated shock still exist, then administer a second bolus. Some children may require 80 to 100 mL/kg of fluid, depending on the volume of fluid lost.

Distributive Shock **Distributive shock** presents with a marked decrease in peripheral vascular resistance, usually owing to a loss of vasomotor tone. In pediatric patients, causes include sepsis from bacterial infection, anaphylactic reaction, and damage to the brain and/or spinal cord. Cardiac output and fluid volume are adequate.

Septic Shock This condition is caused by sepsis, an infection of the bloodstream by some pathogen, usually bacterial. Sepsis commonly occurs as a complication of an infection at some other site such as pneumonia, an ear infection, or a urinary tract infection. Meningitis is frequently associated with sepsis. The etiology can be varied, as can be the signs and symptoms.

The septic child is critically ill. Septic shock may develop when the pathogen causing the infection releases deadly toxins. These toxins cause peripheral vasodilation, leading to a drop in blood pressure and decreased tissue perfusion. Sepsis can be rapidly fatal if not promptly identified and treated.

Signs of sepsis include:

- Ill appearance
- Irritability or altered mental status
- Fever
- Vomiting and diarrhea
- Cyanosis, pallor, or mottled skin
- Nonspecific respiratory distress
- Poor feeding

Signs and symptoms of septic shock include:

- Very ill appearance
- Altered mental status
- Tachycardia
- Capillary refill time greater than 2 seconds
- Hyperventilation, leading to respiratory failure
- Cool and clammy skin
- Inability of child to recognize parents
- Acidosis (elevated lactate) and/or increasing CO_2 levels

Your goal in treating sepsis is to prevent the development of septic shock. Supplemental oxygen should be administered and intravenous access obtained. Administer a 20 mL/kg bolus of lactated Ringer's or normal saline. Consider initiating pressor therapy with epinephrine or dopamine. Begin at the designated starting dose and gradually increase the dose until the blood pressure improves or there is evidence of improved end-organ perfusion. Definitive treatment includes antibiotics and other therapy. Transport should be rapid with care provided en route.

Anaphylactic Shock Anaphylactic shock results from exposure to an antigen to which the patient has been previously exposed. Milder cases may simply result in an allergic reaction. More severe reactions can impair tissue perfusion. This primarily occurs as a result of the release of histamine and other similar chemicals. Histamine causes peripheral vasodilation and leakage of fluid from the intravascular space into the interstitial space. Anaphylactic shock can be differentiated from a severe allergic reaction by the presence of signs and symptoms of impaired end-organ perfusion. These include:

- Tachycardia
- Tachypnea
- Wheezing
- Urticaria (hives)
- Anxiousness
- Edema
- Hypotension

Treatment of a severe allergic reaction includes administration of intramuscular or subcutaneous epinephrine 1:1,000 and an antihistamine. Treatment of anaphylactic shock includes supplemental oxygen administration and intravenous access. If the patient is exhibiting decompensated shock, administer epinephrine 1:10,000 intravenously and diphenhydramine

(Benadryl) intravenously. Patients not exhibiting hypotension may be given an initial dose of epinephrine subcutaneously. If this does not rapidly improve the situation, then an intravenous dose of epinephrine should be considered. Contact medical direction for additional assistance. EMS systems with long transport times may be asked to administer an initial dose of a corticosteroid such as methylprednisolone (Solu-Medrol).

Neurogenic Shock Neurogenic shock is due to sudden peripheral vasodilation resulting from interruption of nervous control of the peripheral vascular system. The most common cause is injury to the spinal cord. Cardiac output and intravascular fluid volume are usually adequate.

Treatment is directed at increasing peripheral vascular resistance. This is accomplished primarily through administration of a pressor agent such as dopamine. Care should also include stabilization of the injury and administration of supplemental oxygen (if the patient is hypoxic).

Cardiogenic Shock

Cardiogenic shock results from inadequate cardiac output. In children, cardiogenic shock usually results from a secondary cause such as near drowning or a toxic ingestion. Children, unlike adults, rarely have primary cardiac disease. The exceptions are congenital heart disease and cardiomyopathy.

Congenital heart disease is an abnormality or defect in the heart that is present at birth. Many congenital cardiac problems are detected at birth. However, some may not be detected until later in life. Cardiomyopathy causes a decrease in cardiac output owing to impairment of cardiac muscle contraction. Arrhythmias, although rare in children, can cause a decrease in cardiac output. Rapid arrhythmias may impair ventricular filling and thus cause a decrease in cardiac output. Likewise, slow arrhythmias may cause decreased cardiac output simply because of their slow rate.

In the following sections we discuss in more detail congenital heart disease, cardiomyopathy, and arrhythmias, which, as noted, are primary causes of pediatric cardiogenic shock. Remember, however, that cardiogenic shock in children most often results from secondary causes.

Congenital Heart Disease

Congenital heart disease is the primary cause of heart disease in children. As noted earlier, although most congenital heart problems are detected at birth, some problems may not be discovered until later in childhood. A common symptom of congenital heart disease is cyanosis. This occurs when blood going to the lungs for oxygenation mixes with blood bound for other parts of the body. This may result from holes in the internal walls of the heart or from abnormalities of the great vessels.

The child with congenital heart disease may develop respiratory distress, congestive heart failure, or a "cyanotic spell." *Cyanotic spells* occur when oxygen demand exceeds that provided by the blood. They begin as irritability, inconsolable crying or altered mental status, and progressive cyanosis in conjunction with severe dyspnea. In severe and prolonged cases, seizures, coma, or cardiac arrest may result. Noncyanotic problems associated with congenital heart disease include respiratory distress, tachycardia, decreased end-organ perfusion, drowsiness, fatigue, and pallor.

Treatment includes the standard primary assessment. Administer high-concentration oxygen. If necessary, provide ventilatory support. If the patient is having a cyanotic spell, place the child in the knee–chest position facing downward or, in an older child, have him squat. This will help increase the cardiac return. Apply the ECG monitor, and start an intravenous line at a keep-open rate. Transport immediately.

Cardiomyopathy

Cardiomyopathy is a disease or dysfunction of the cardiac muscle. Although fairly rare, cardiomyopathy can result from congenital heart disease or infection. A frequent cause of infectious cardiomyopathy is *Coxsackie* virus. Cardiomyopathy causes mechanical pump failure, which is usually biventricular. It often develops slowly and is not detectable until heart failure develops.

The signs and symptoms of cardiomyopathy include early fatigue, crackles, jugular venous distention, engorgement of the liver, and peripheral edema. Later, as the disease progresses, the signs and symptoms of shock can develop.

The prehospital treatment of cardiomyopathy is supportive. Supplemental oxygen should be administered via a nonrebreather mask. Fluids should be restricted. If possible, IV access should be obtained. Severe cases resulting in the development of severe dyspnea should be treated with furosemide and pressor agents (dobutamine, dopamine). The child should be transported to a facility capable of managing critically ill children. Most cases of cardiomyopathy are managed with medication. Definitive care in severe cases may include cardiac transplantation.

Arrhythmias

Arrhythmias in children are uncommon. When arrhythmias occur, bradyarrhythmias are the most common. Supraventricular tachyarrhythmias are uncommon and ventricular tachyarrhythmias are very uncommon. Arrhythmias can cause pump failure, ultimately leading to cardiogenic shock. Children have a very limited capacity to increase stroke volume. The primary mechanism through which they increase cardiac output is through changes in the heart rate. The treatment of arrhythmias is specific for the arrhythmia in question.

Tachyarrhythmias Tachyarrhythmias are arrhythmias in which the rate is greater than the estimated maximum normal heart rate for the child. These can result from primary cardiac disease or from secondary causes. Tachyarrhythmias from any cause are relatively uncommon in children.

Supraventricular Tachycardia True supraventricular tachycardia (SVT) is a narrow-complex tachycardia (QRS ≤ 0.09 second) with a heart rate typically of 220 beats per minute or greater. Supraventricular tachycardia is usually caused by a problem in the cardiac conductive system. Rarely, it can be the result of a secondary cause such as drug ingestion. It is occasionally seen in infants with no prior history. The cause is uncertain but may be due to immaturity of the cardiac conductive system. Rapid heart rates often do not allow time for adequate cardiac filling, eventually causing congestive heart failure and cardiogenic shock.

The signs and symptoms of supraventricular tachycardia include irritability, poor feeding, jugular venous distention, hepatomegaly (enlarged liver), and hypotension. The ECG will show a narrow-complex (supraventricular) tachycardia with a rate greater than 220 beats per minute. Children can often tolerate the rapid rate well.

Prehospital treatment of supraventricular tachycardia depends on the clinical findings. Children who are tolerating the heart rate (normal blood pressure) and are stable should receive supplemental oxygen (if they are hypoxic) and transport. Vagal maneuvers may be attempted unless the patient is unstable. In older children, carotid sinus massage or Valsalva maneuvers are safe. Adenosine should be considered if the child is stable. If the child is exhibiting signs of decompensation (hypotension, mental status change, poor skin color), then synchronized cardioversion should be attempted at an initial energy dose of 0.5 to 1.0 joules per kilogram of body weight. This can be increased to 2 joules per kilogram if the initial shock is unsuccessful. Consider amiodarone 5 mg/kg IO/IV or procainamide 15 mg/kg IO/IV for a patient with SVT unresponsive to vagal maneuvers and adenosine and/or electric cardioversion. These medications must be administered slowly with all monitors in place. The child should be transported to the appropriate facility.

Ventricular Tachycardia with a Pulse Ventricular tachycardia (wide-complex tachycardia) and ventricular fibrillation are exceedingly rare in children. They are occasionally seen following near-drowning or following a prolonged resuscitation attempt. Unlike adults, in whom ventricular tachyarrhythmias result from primary heart disease, ventricular tachyarrhythmias in children are almost always due to a secondary cause. The exception is structural, congenital heart disease.

The signs and symptoms of ventricular tachycardia with a pulse include poor feeding, irritability, and a rapid, wide-complex tachycardia. Children are unable to tolerate this arrhythmia for very long. They soon develop signs of shock.

The prehospital management of ventricular tachycardia with a pulse includes supplemental oxygen and intravenous access. Stable patients who are not hypotensive should be transported. Unstable patients (hypotension) should be treated aggressively. Initially, amiodarone, procainamide, or lidocaine should be administered. However, ventricular tachycardia due to structural heart disease often does not respond to antiarrhythmic drugs.

- *Stable children with wide-complex tachycardia.* Adenosine may be used to help distinguish supraventricular tachycardia from ventricular tachycardia (if the rhythm is regular and monomorphic). It may also convert supraventricular rhythms. Electrical cardioversion at 0.5 to 1.0 J/kg should be considered. This can be increased to 2 J/kg if needed. Pharmacological therapy should be considered (amiodarone or procainamide).

- *Unstable children with wide-complex tachycardia.* Electrical cardioversion at 0.5 to 1.0 J/kg should be considered. This can be increased to 2 J/kg if needed.

Bradyarrhythmias Bradyarrhythmias are the most common type of pediatric arrhythmia. They most frequently result from hypoxia. Although rare, they can also result from vagal stimulation from such causes as marked gastric distention.

The signs and symptoms of bradycardia include a slow (usually <60 beats per minute), narrow-complex rhythm. The child may be lethargic, or exhibiting early signs of congestive heart failure.

- *Stable children with bradyarrhythmias.* Stable children with bradyarrhythmias should receive supportive care that addresses ventilation and oxygenation. If the heart rate falls below 60 beats per minute they should be considered unstable.

- *Unstable children with bradyarrhythmias.* Likewise, unstable children (hypotension, altered mental status, signs of shock) should be ventilated with a BVM unit and 100 percent oxygen. If the heart rate does not increase readily, consider epinephrine IV or IO. Atropine may be used for suspected increased vagal tone of primary AV block. If pulseless arrest develops, perform chest compressions. If necessary, consider epinephrine or atropine down the endotracheal tube until intravenous or intraosseous access can be obtained. Transport rapidly with care provided en route.[11]

Pulseless Arrest The absence of a cardiac rhythm is an ominous finding. Most cases are asystole. However, some cases may be a very fine ventricular fibrillation. If necessary, turn up the gain on the ECG to distinguish between the two.

Asystole Asystole is the absence of a rhythm and may be the initial rhythm seen in cardiopulmonary arrest. (Remember, children rarely develop ventricular fibrillation, which is often the precursor to arrest in adults.) Bradycardias can degenerate to asystole if appropriate intervention is not provided. The mortality rate associated with asystole in children is very high.

The child with asystole is pulseless and apneic. The cardiac rhythm is a straight line that should be confirmed in two leads. Treatment is often futile. However, CPR should be initiated, an IV or IO placed, and epinephrine administered every 3 to 5 minutes. The patient should receive an advanced airway and be ventilated with 100 percent oxygen. Chest compressions should be continued. Emergency resuscitative drugs (epinephrine, atropine) should be administered through the intraosseous or intravenous routes.[11]

Ventricular Fibrillation/Pulseless Ventricular Tachycardia Ventricular fibrillation and pulseless ventricular tachycardia are functionally the same rhythm. They are uncommon in children. Causes include electrocution and drug overdoses. The mortality rate is very high.

The child with ventricular fibrillation/pulseless ventricular tachycardia will be pulseless and apneic. The ECG will exhibit a wide-complex tachycardia or fibrillation. The child should receive uninterrupted CPR for 2 minutes and IV/IO access obtained. After 2 minutes of CPR, the rhythm should be checked. If the patient is shockable, an initial shock of 2 J/kg should be provided and CPR resumed. Epinephrine should be administered every 3 to 5 minutes; an advanced airway should be placed and mechanical ventilation with 100 percent oxygen provided. If the patient remains in a shockable rhythm, the second and subsequent shocks should be at 4 J/kg. Amiodarone should be considered after the second unsuccessful shock. Transport as soon as possible.[11]

Pulseless Electrical Activity Pulseless electrical activity (PEA) is the presence of a cardiac rhythm without an associated pulse. This is due to noncardiogenic causes such as hypoxia, pericardial tamponade, tension pneumothorax, trauma, acidosis, hypothermia, and hypoglycemia.

The patient with PEA is pulseless and apneic. Resuscitation should be directed toward correcting the underlying cause. Otherwise, treatment is the same as for asystole.[11]

Neurologic Emergencies

Neurologic emergencies in childhood are fairly uncommon. However, seizures can and do occur in children. In fact, they are a frequent reason for summoning EMS. In addition to seizures, meningitis tends to show up more often in children than in adults. Although your chances of encountering either of these two conditions are small, both are life threatening and should be promptly identified and treated.

Seizures

Seizures result from an abnormal discharge of neurons in the brain. Many people suffer seizures; it is a common reason for summoning EMS. People with chronic seizure disorders can often control their seizures with medications. A seizure can be an exceptionally scary event for both the parents and the child. This is especially true if the child has never had a seizure before.

Although the etiology for seizures is often unknown, several risk factors have been identified. They include:

- Fever
- Hypoxia
- Infections
- Idiopathic epilepsy (unknown origin)
- Electrolyte disturbances
- Head trauma
- Hypoglycemia
- Toxic ingestions or exposure
- Tumor
- CNS malformations

Seizures in pediatric patients may be either partial or generalized. (Recall that generalized seizures normally do not occur during the first month of life.) Simple partial seizures, sometimes called *focal motor seizures*, involve sudden jerking of a particular part of the body, such as an arm or a leg. Other characteristics include lip smacking, eye blinking, staring, confusion, and lethargy. There is usually no loss of consciousness. Generalized seizures involve sudden jerking of both sides of the body, followed by tenseness and relaxation of the body. In a generalized seizure, patients typically experience a loss of consciousness.

Keep in mind that children can have **status epilepticus**, a series of one or more generalized seizures, without any intervening periods of consciousness. Status epilepticus is a serious medical emergency because it involves a prolonged period of apnea, which in turn can cause hypoxia of vital brain tissues. The electrical discharges in the brain are harmful as well (see Volume 4, Chapter 3).

Most of the pediatric seizures that you will probably encounter are febrile seizures. **Febrile seizures** are seizures that occur as a result of a sudden increase in body temperature. They occur most commonly between the ages of six months and six years. Often, the parents or caregivers will report the recent onset of fever or cold symptoms. The diagnosis of febrile seizure should not be made in the field. All pediatric patients suffering a seizure must be transported to the hospital so that other etiologies can be excluded.

Assessment The history is a major factor in determining seizure type. Febrile seizure should be suspected if the temperature is above 39.2°C (103°F). The history of a previous seizure may suggest idiopathic epilepsy or another CNS problem. However, there is also a tendency for recurrence of febrile seizures in children.

When confronted with a seizing child, determine whether there is a history of seizures or seizures with fever. Has the child had a recent illness? Also, determine how many seizures occurred during the incident. If the child is not seizing on your arrival, elicit a description of the seizure activity. Note the condition and position of the child when found. Question parents, caregivers, or bystanders about the possibility of head injury. A history of irritability or lethargy prior to the seizure may indicate CNS infection. If possible, find out whether the child suffers from diabetes or has recently complained of a headache or a stiff neck. Note any current medications, as well as possible ingestions.

The physical examination should be systematic. Pay particular attention to the adequacy of respirations, the level of consciousness, neurologic evaluation, and signs of injury. Also inspect the child for signs of dehydration. Dehydration may be evidenced by the absence of tears or, in an infant, by the presence of a sunken fontanelle.

Management Management of pediatric seizures is essentially the same as for seizing adults. Place patients on the floor or on the bed. Be sure to lay them on their side, away from the furniture. Do not restrain patients, but take steps to protect them from injury. Maintain the airway, but do not force anything, such as a bite stick, between the teeth. Administer supplemental oxygen if the patient is hypoxic. Then take and record all vital signs. If the patient is febrile, remove excess layers of clothing, while avoiding extreme cooling. If status epilepticus is present, institute the following steps:

- Start an IV of normal saline or lactated Ringer's and perform a glucometer evaluation.

- Administer diazepam or lorazepam as directed.

- Contact medical direction for additional dosing. Diazepam or lorazepam can be administered rectally if an IV cannot be established. Intranasal midazolam may also be considered.

- If the seizure appears to be caused by fever and a long transport time is anticipated, medical direction may request the administration of acetaminophen to lower the fever. Acetaminophen is supplied as an elixir or as suppositories. The dose should be 15 mg/kg body weight.

As mentioned previously, all pediatric patients should be transported. Reassure and support the parents or caregivers, as this is a very stressful and frightening situation for them.[15]

Meningitis

Meningitis is an infection of the meninges, the lining of the brain and spinal cord. Meningitis can result from both bacteria and viruses. Viral meningitis is frequently called *aseptic meningitis,* because an organism cannot be routinely cultured from cerebrospinal fluid (CSF). Aseptic meningitis is generally less severe than bacterial meningitis and is self-limiting. Bacterial meningitis most commonly results from *Streptococcus pneumoniae, Haemophilus influenzae,* and *Neisseria meningitides.* These infections can be rapidly fatal if they are not promptly recognized and treated appropriately.

Assessment Meningitis is more common in children than in adults. Findings in the history that may suggest meningitis include a child who has been ill for one day to several days, a recent ear or respiratory tract infection, high fever, lethargy or irritability, a severe headache, or a stiff neck. Infants generally do not develop a stiff neck. They will generally become lethargic and will not feed well. Some babies may simply develop a fever.

On physical examination, the child with meningitis will appear very ill. With an infant, the fontanelle may be bulging or full unless accompanied by dehydration. Extreme discomfort with movement, owing to irritability of the meninges, may be present (Figure 4-33 ●).

Management Prehospital care of the pediatric patient with meningitis is supportive. Complete the primary assessment rapidly and transport the child to the emergency department. If shock is present, treat the child with intravenous fluids (20 mL/kg) and oxygen.

Gastrointestinal Emergencies

Childhood gastrointestinal problems almost always present with nausea and vomiting as a chief complaint. As a child gets older, other gastrointestinal system emergencies, such as appendicitis, become more common.

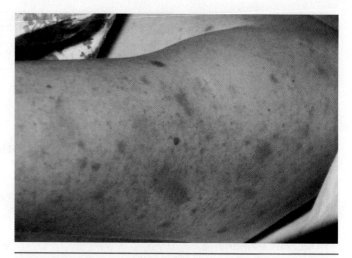

● **Figure 4-33** Petechial rash of meningococcal meningitis.

Nausea and Vomiting

Nausea and vomiting are not diseases themselves, but are symptoms of other disease processes. Virtually any medical problem can cause these conditions in an infant or child. The most common causes include fever, ear infections, and respiratory infections. In addition, many viruses and certain bacteria can infect the gastrointestinal system. These infections, collectively known as *gastroenteritis*, readily cause vomiting, diarrhea, or both.

The biggest risks associated with nausea and vomiting in children are dehydration and electrolyte abnormalities. Infants and toddlers can quickly become dehydrated from bouts of vomiting. If diarrhea or fever is also present, fluid loss is further accelerated, worsening the situation. Dehydration is more difficult to detect in infants and toddlers than in older children. (See Table 4–13 for a description of the signs and symptoms of dehydration.)

Treatment of pediatric nausea and vomiting is primarily supportive. If the child is dehydrated and unable to keep oral fluids down, intravenous fluid therapy may be indicated. Severe dehydration, as evidenced by prolonged capillary refill time, should be treated by 20 mL/kg fluid boluses of lactated Ringer's solution or 0.9 percent sodium chloride solution (normal saline).

Diarrhea

Diarrhea is a common occurrence in childhood. Often, what parents call diarrhea is actually loose bowel movements. Generally, 10 or more stools per day is considered diarrhea. As with nausea and vomiting, the main concern associated with diarrhea is dehydration. Most diarrhea is caused by viral infections of the gastrointestinal system or arises secondary to infections elsewhere in the body. However, certain bacterial infections can cause significant, even life-threatening, diarrhea.

Treatment of the child suffering from diarrhea is primarily supportive. If dehydration is evident, administer fluids. Oral hydration works quite well. Severe dehydration should be treated with 20 mL/kg boluses of intravenous fluids (lactated Ringer's or normal saline).[16]

Metabolic Emergencies

Metabolic problems are uncommon in children. However, diabetes can occur in very young children. It is rarely diagnosed until the child comes to the hospital in diabetic ketoacidosis. Diabetic children can have great swings in their blood glucose levels owing to diet, growth, and physical activity. Because of this, hypoglycemia and hyperglycemia are possible. It is important to remember that very young children, unlike adults, can develop hypoglycemia without having diabetes. This can occur with severe illnesses such as meningitis and pneumonia. The following sections will present the prehospital treatment of pediatric hypoglycemia and hyperglycemia.

Hypoglycemia

Hypoglycemia is an abnormally low concentration of sugar (glucose) in the blood. It is a true medical emergency that must be treated immediately. Without treatment, low blood sugar may progress to unconsciousness and convulsions.

In the prehospital setting, hypoglycemia in pediatric patients usually occurs in newborn infants and children with type I diabetes. Diabetic children increase their risk of hypoglycemia through overly strenuous exercise, too much insulin, and dehydration from illness. Nondiabetic children can develop hypoglycemia from physical activity, dietary changes, illness, and growth.

In known diabetics or hypoglycemics, preventive steps include:

- Taking extra snacks for extra activity
- Eating immediately after taking insulin if the blood sugar is less than 100 mg/dL
- Eating regular meals
- Regularly monitoring blood sugar
- Eating an extra snack of carbohydrate and protein if the blood sugar is less than 120 mg/dL at bedtime
- Replacing carbohydrates in the meal plan with things such as regular soda pop or regular popsicles on days when the child is sick

Assessment Suspect hypoglycemia when the patient exhibits the signs and symptoms listed in Table 4–14. Measure blood glucose with a glucometer and elicit a history of conditions known to cause hypoglycemia in infants and children. Treatment should be initiated whenever you have a high index of suspicion and/or blood sugar drops below 70 mg/dL (≤3.9 mmol/L).

Management As with all patients, continually monitor the ABCs. Be sure to find out whether parents or caregivers have given the patient any glucose tablets, gels, foods (cake icing, honey, maple syrup, sugar, raisins), or drinks (juice, regular soda pop, milk) to correct the situation. If

TABLE 4–13	Signs and Symptoms of Dehydration		
Signs/Symptoms	Mild	Moderate	Severe
Vital Signs			
Pulse	Normal	Increased	Markedly increased
Respirations	Normal	Increased	Tachypneic
Blood pressure	Normal	Normal	Hypotensive
Capillary refill	Normal	2–3 seconds	>2 seconds
Mental Status	Alert	Irritable	Lethargic
Skin	Normal	Dry and ashen	Dry, cool, mottled
Mucous Membranes	Dry	Very dry	Very dry/no tears

TABLE 4–14 | Signs and Symptoms of Hypoglycemia		
Mild	**Moderate**	**Severe**
Hunger	Sweating	Decreased level of consciousness
Weakness	Tremors	Seizure
Tachypnea	Irritability	Tachycardia
Tachycardia	Vomiting	Hypoperfusion
Shakiness	Mood swings	
Yawning	Blurred vision	
Pale skin	Stomachache	
Dizziness	Headache	
	Dizziness	
	Slurred speech	

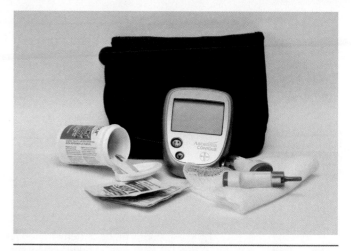

● **Figure 4-34**   Many diabetic children have home glucometers to test their blood glucose levels. Older children know what the readings mean and will be curious about any glucose testing device that you may use.

- Defective insulin pump, blockage of tubing, or disconnection of insulin pump infusion set
- Illness or stress

Hyperglycemia can occur with other severe illnesses and not necessarily mean that the child is developing diabetes mellitus.

Assessment   In cases of hyperglycemia, glucose is spilled into the urine, taking water with it through osmotic diuresis. This can result in a significant fluid loss with resultant dehydration.

Keep in mind that acidosis results from the accumulation of ketones, a by-product of fat metabolism. A continual increase in the ketones eventually leads to metabolic acidosis, which produces the fruity breath odor commonly associated with hyperglycemia. For other signs and symptoms, see Table 4–15.

As with hypoglycemia, elicit a history to determine causes linked with hyperglycemia. If possible, confirm your suspicions with a blood glucose test. A blood sugar reading of greater than 200 mg/dL typically indicates hyperglycemia.

Management   Carefully monitor the ABCs and vital signs. If you cannot confirm the presence of hyperglycemia with a blood glucose test, consider administering oral fluids with sugar or oral glucose in case the patient is hypoglycemic. If intravenous access is possible, consider initiating an IV of either normal saline or lactated Ringer's. Administer an IV bolus of 20 mL/kg, and repeat the bolus if the patient's vital signs do not change. Monitor the patient's mental status and be prepared to intubate if the respirations continue to decrease.

Remember, this is a potentially life-threatening situation. Consult with medical direction on all actions taken and transport immediately.

Poisoning and Toxic Exposure

Accidental poisoning or toxic exposure is a common reason for summoning EMS. Pediatric patients account for the majority of poisonings treated by EMS. Most poisonings result from accidental ingestion of a toxic substance, usually by a young child.

so, find out what was given, how much was given, and when it was given. Administer a blood glucose test, if possible.

In the conscious, alert patient, administer oral fluids with sugar or oral glucose. (Amounts are age and/or weight specific, so check with medical direction.) If there is no response, or if the patient exhibits an altered mental status, transport immediately. Consult your medical direction physician on orders for the administration of dextrose or IM glucagon. Twenty-five percent dextrose solution ($D_{25}W$) can be prepared by diluting 50 percent dextrose solution 1:1 with sterile water or saline. A 10 percent dextrose solution ($D_{10}W$) will also work. It is easier to dose children with this concentration and does not cause as much discomfort as with intravenous administration. Repeat blood glucose tests within 10 to 15 minutes of infusion or the administration of glucose.[17]

In treating diabetic pediatric patients, remember that most children have been taught about their condition and can participate, in varying degrees, in their care. Most understand how glucometers work, for example, and can hand you a test strip (Figure 4-34 ●). Also, they may be sensitive to their condition, so avoid labeling any tests as "good" or "bad."

Hyperglycemia

Hyperglycemia is an abnormally high concentration of blood sugar. For patients with type I diabetes, hyperglycemia may lead to dehydration and **diabetic ketoacidosis**, a very serious medical emergency. Left untreated, the condition will deteriorate to coma. Hyperglycemia and diabetic ketoacidosis are the most common findings in new-onset diabetics.

In the prehospital setting, pediatric hyperglycemia is commonly associated with type I diabetes. Causes include:

- Eating too much food relative to injected insulin
- Missing an insulin injection

TABLE 4–15	Signs and Symptoms of Hyperglycemia		
Early	**Late**	**Ketoacidosis**
Increased thirst	Weakness	Continued decreased level of consciousness progressing to coma
Increased urination	Abdominal pain	Kussmaul's respirations (deep and slow)
Weight loss	Generalized aches	Signs of dehydration
	Loss of appetite	
	Nausea	
	Vomiting	
	Signs of dehydration, except increased urinary output	
	Fruity breath odor	
	Tachypnea	
	Hyperventilation	
	Tachycardia	

Toddlers and preschoolers like to taste things, especially colorful objects and substances that look like food or beverages. They also mimic their parents or caregivers, swallowing pills or drinking alcohol "just like Mommy and Daddy." Teenagers on antidepressants are also at risk of misusing or abusing their prescriptions, especially if given a one- or two-month supply of a medication.

Poisonings are the leading cause of preventable death in children under age five (Figure 4-35 ●). Because of their immature respiratory and cardiovascular systems, even a single pill can poison or, in some cases, kill a child. Of all the substances ingested by young children, iron-containing supplements are the leading cause of poisonings, especially in toddlers and preschoolers.

The most dangerous rooms in a house in terms of poisons are the kitchen, where household cleaners are stored, and the bathroom, where many people keep their over-the-counter and prescription medications. Garages and utility rooms also contain toxic substances, made more attractive to children when they are poured into everyday containers such as coffee cans, soda bottles, or plastic cups. Living rooms may have poisonous plants and liquor bottles.

The best way to prevent pediatric poisonings is by helping the families in your communities learn how to "poison-proof" their homes. If your EMS system does not have information available on this topic, you can obtain guidelines from the U.S. Food and Drug Administration. Poisoning prevention should be a major goal of EMS prevention and community education programs. Many EMS systems will dedicate a specific month out of the year to poisoning awareness and prevention.

Assessment

Assessment of a pediatric poisoning depends on the type of poison ingested or the extent to which a child was exposed to a toxic substance (Figure 4-36 ●). Common substances involved in pediatric poisonings include:

- Alcohol, barbiturates, sedatives
- Amphetamines, cocaine, hallucinogens
- Anticholinergic agents (jimson weed, belladonna products)
- Aspirin, acetaminophen
- Lead
- Vitamins and iron-containing supplements
- Corrosives
- Digitalis and beta-blockers
- Hydrocarbons
- Narcotics

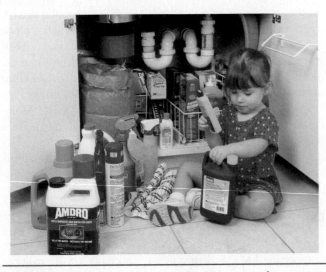

● **Figure 4-35** Poisonings are the leading cause of preventable death in children under age five.

Possible Indicators of Ingested Poisoning in Children

PAY PARTICULAR ATTENTION TO:

The child who has swallowed a poison before.

The level of responsiveness, including any behavioral changes (clumsiness, drowsiness, coma, convulsions, mental disturbances, confusion)

Skin and mucosa findings (color, temperature of skin, lips, mucous membranes)

Temperature, blood pressure, pulse rate, respiratory alterations

Constriction   Dilation

The size and reaction of pupils (constriction, dilation)

Mouth signs (burns, discoloration, dryness, excessive salivation, stains, characteristic breath odors, pain on swallowing)

Nausea, vomiting (Examine the vomitus. Make note of pill fragments if present.)

Diarrhea (blood present)

● **Figure 4-36**   Possible indicators of ingested poisoning in children.

- Organic solvents (inhaled)
- Organophosphates (insecticides)

Poisoning can cause many different signs and symptoms, depending on the poison ingested, the route of exposure, and the time since exposure. Narcotics and some of the hydrocarbons can cause respiratory system depression. Digitalis, beta-blockers, calcium-channel blockers, and many of the antihypertensive agents can cause circulatory depression or collapse. A great many agents can impair the central nervous system. These include alcohol, barbiturates, narcotics, and cocaine. Virtually any substance can affect thought and behavior. Common agents are the anticholinergics, alcohol, narcotics, hydrocarbons, and many others. Aspirin, corrosives, and hydrocarbons can irritate or destroy the gastrointestinal system. Acetaminophen can cause liver necrosis and, eventually, liver failure.

Management

Although scenarios vary, take these general steps in managing a pediatric poisoning patient:

Responsive Poisoning Patient

- Administer oxygen (if the patient is hypoxic).
- Contact medical direction and/or the poison control center.
- Consider the need for activated charcoal (rarely indicated).
- Transport. (Be sure to take any pills, substances, and containers to the hospital.)
- Monitor the patient continuously in case the child suddenly becomes unresponsive.

Unresponsive Poisoning Patient

- Ensure a patent airway. Apply suctioning, if necessary.
- Administer oxygen (if the patient is hypoxic).
- Be prepared to provide artificial ventilations if respiratory failure or cardiac arrest is present.
- Contact medical direction and/or the poison control center.
- Transport. (Be sure to take any pills, substances, and containers to the hospital.)
- Monitor the patient continuously, and rule out trauma as a cause of altered mental status.

For more on poisonings and toxic exposure, see Volume 4, Chapter 8.

TRAUMA EMERGENCIES

Trauma is the number-one cause of death in infants and children. Most pediatric injuries result from blunt trauma. As mentioned previously, children have thinner body walls that allow forces to be more readily transmitted to body contents, increasing the possibility of injury to internal tissues and organs. If you serve in an urban area, you can expect to see a higher incidence of penetrating trauma, mostly intentional and mostly from gunfire or knife wounds. Significant incidences of penetrating trauma are also seen outside the cities—mostly unintentional, from hunting accidents and agricultural accidents.

CONTENT REVIEW

▶ Most Common Pediatric
Mechanisms of Injury

• Falls
• Motor vehicle collisions
• Car vs. pedestrian
  collisions
• Drownings
• Penetrating injuries
• Burns
• Physical abuse

Mechanisms of Injury

Although pediatric patients can be injured in the same way as adults, children tend to be more susceptible to certain types of injuries than adults are. The following categories describe the most common mechanisms of injury among infants and children.

Falls

Falls are the single most common cause of injury in children (Figure 4-37 ●). Fortunately, serious injury or death from accidental falls is relatively uncommon, unless the fall is from a significant height. Falls from bicycles account for a significant number of injuries. The incidence of head injuries is declining, primarily because of bicycle safety helmets.

Motor Vehicle Collisions

Approximately 25,000 American children die annually from trauma. Approximately one-third of these die from motor vehicle collisions, making motor vehicle collisions the leading cause of traumatic death in children. In addition, motor vehicle collisions are the leading cause of permanent brain injury and new-onset epilepsy. Improperly seated children are at increased risk of sustaining injury or death from automobile air bags when they deploy (Figure 4-38 ●). This is an area in which EMS prevention strategies can make a difference. Public education

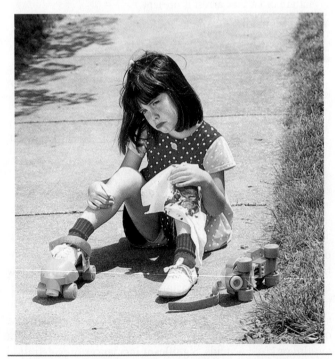

● **Figure 4-37**   Falls are the most common cause of injury in young children.

● **Figure 4-38**   A deploying air bag can propel a child safety seat back into the vehicle's seat, seriously injuring the child secured in it.

programs on drunk driving, safe driving, air bags, and proper use of children's car seats can be a major focus of EMS personnel. Some states have given paramedics the ability to issue citations to persons who do not correctly buckle their children or place them in child safety seats.

Car-versus-Pedestrian Injuries

Car-versus-child pedestrian injuries are more common in cities where children play close to the street. Car-versus-pedestrian injuries are a particularly lethal form of trauma in children because their short stature tends to push them down under the car. There are two phases of injury in car-versus-pedestrian collisions. The first group of injuries occurs when the auto contacts the child. Because of the energy present, the child may be propelled away from the car or pushed down underneath the car. It is at this point that the second group of injuries occurs, as the child contacts the ground or other objects. Head and spinal injuries often occur with the secondary impact. The best treatment for car-versus-child-pedestrian collisions is prevention. This, too, can be a major area of emphasis for prehospital prevention programs.

Drownings and Near-Drownings

Drowning is the third leading cause of death in children between birth and four years of age, with approximately 2,000 deaths occurring in the United States annually. The term *drowning* is used to describe deaths that occur within 24 hours of the incident. *Near-drowning* refers to injuries in which the child did not die or where the death occurred more than 24 hours after the injury. Many children who do not die from drowning suffer severe and irreversible brain injuries as a result of anoxia. Approximately 20 to 25 percent of near-drowning survivors exhibit severe neurologic deficits. The outcomes are better when the water is cold, because the body's protective mechanisms protect against brain injury.

Again, as with the other injury processes, the best treatment is prevention. EMS personnel, in conjunction with local building inspectors, can inspect pools for safety. A pool should be fenced off with a gate that closes automatically. Essential rescue equipment (pole, life preserver) should be immediately available and the local emergency number posted. The best time for drowning prevention programs is late spring and early summer. Encourage parents to enroll their children in water safety classes as early as possible.

Penetrating Injuries

Until 20 years ago, penetrating injuries in children were fairly uncommon. Since then, an increase in violent crime (although violent crime rates have both risen and fallen within that period) has resulted in an increasing number of children sustaining penetrating trauma. Stab wounds and firearm injuries account for approximately 10 to 15 percent of all pediatric trauma admissions. The risk of death increases with age. Children are usually innocent victims of crimes perpetrated against adults. However, children are sometimes the intended victims of gunfire and stabbings, as in the shootings that have taken place in schools.

It is important to remember that visual inspection of external injuries does not provide adequate evaluation of internal injuries. This is especially true with high-energy, high-velocity weapons that can cause massive internal injury with only minimal external trauma.

Paramedics can play a major role in preventing pediatric shootings. During public education and community service programs, it is prudent to talk about gun safety, including such measures as using trigger locks or locking weapons in places where children cannot reach them. You might emphasize the fact that children have an uncanny ability to find and gain access to weapons that adults think they have hidden and secured. As with many other pediatric emergencies, the best treatment is prevention.

Burns

Burn injuries are the leading cause of accidental death in the home for children under 14 years of age. Children can sustain both burn injuries and smoke inhalation in house fires. Unsupervised children with matches or cigarette lighters are responsible for many fires that result in pediatric injury.

Fire prevention programs are a major area of emphasis for fire departments. The importance of smoke detectors cannot be overemphasized. Citizens should be encouraged to change the batteries in their smoke detectors when the clock is moved backward or forward when daylight saving time changes. Many fire departments and EMS systems replace smoke detector batteries as a part of their fire prevention programs. Part of the fire prevention program should be specifically directed at children. It is especially important to teach children how to exit their houses in case fire erupts.

Physical Abuse

Unfortunately, children are at risk for physical abuse by adults and older children. Factors leading to child abuse are known to include social phenomena such as poverty, domestic disturbances, younger parents, substance abuse, and community violence. Paramedics are often the first members of the health care team to come into contact with the abused child. It is very important to not accuse the parents or confront a suspected abuser. Instead, document all pertinent findings, treatments, and interventions and report these to the proper authorities. (Child abuse is discussed in more detail later in this chapter.)

Special Considerations

As emphasized previously, children are not small adults. You should keep this in mind and modify treatment accordingly. Specific items to consider will be discussed next.

Airway Control

Special considerations are related to characteristics of the child's airway. These include the following:

- Maintain in-line stabilization in neutral instead of the sniffing position to prevent possible pinching of the trachea (Figure 4-39 ●).
- Administer oxygen if the patient is hypoxic.
- Maintain a patent airway with suctioning and the jaw-thrust maneuver.
- Be prepared to assist ineffective respirations. Remember that airway pressures can be high in children and it may be necessary to depress the pop-off valve to ventilate the child adequately.
- Intubate the child when the airway cannot be maintained, while simultaneously maintaining cervical spine stabilization (Figure 4-40 ●).
- A gastric tube should be placed following intubation to decompress the stomach.
- Needle cricothyrotomy is rarely indicated for traumatic upper airway obstruction.

Immobilization

Use appropriately sized pediatric immobilization equipment, including:

- Rigid cervical collar
- Towel or blanket roll
- Child safety seat
- Pediatric immobilization device
- Vest-type device (Kendrick extrication device)
- Short wooden backboard
- Straps and cravats
- Tape
- Padding

Keep infants, toddlers, and preschoolers supine with the cervical spine in a neutral in-line position by placing padding from the shoulders to the hips. (Review the discussion of pediatric immobilization earlier in this chapter.)

Fluid Management

Management of the airway and breathing takes priority over management of circulation, because circulatory compromise is less common in children than in adults. When obtaining vascular access, remember the following:

- If possible, insert a large-bore intravenous catheter into a peripheral vein.
- Do not delay transport to gain venous access.

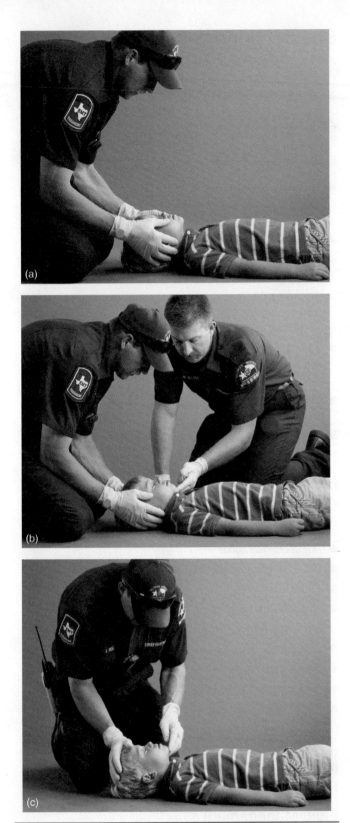

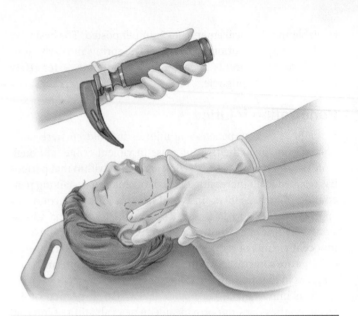

● **Figure 4-40** Simultaneous cervical spine stabilization and intubation in a pediatric patient.

● Intraosseous access in children is an alternative when a peripheral IV cannot be obtained.

● Administer an initial fluid bolus of 20 mL/kg of lactated Ringer's solution or normal saline.

● Reassess the vital signs and give another bolus of 20 mL/kg if there is no improvement.

● If improvement does not occur after the second bolus, there is likely to be a significant blood loss that may require surgical intervention. Rapid transport is essential.

Pediatric Analgesia and Sedation

An often-overlooked aspect of prehospital pediatric care is pain control. Many pediatric injuries are painful and analgesics are indicated. These include burns, long-bone fractures, dislocations, and others. Unless there is a contraindication, pediatric patients should receive analgesics. Commonly used analgesics include morphine and fentanyl. Also, certain pediatric emergencies may benefit from sedation. These include such problems as penetrating eye injuries, prolonged rescue from entrapment in machinery, cardioversion, and other painful procedures. The intranasal administration of fentanyl is an effective route of administering analgesia in the prehospital setting without first obtaining IV access. Always consult medical direction if you feel that pediatric analgesia or sedation may be indicated.

Traumatic Brain Injury

Children, because of the relatively large size of their heads and weak neck muscles, are at increased risk for traumatic brain injury. These injuries can be devastating and are often fatal. Early recognition and aggressive management can reduce both morbidity and mortality. Pediatric head injuries can be classified as follows:

● *Mild*—Glasgow Coma Scale score is 13–15
● *Moderate*—Glasgow Coma Scale score is 9–12
● *Severe*—Glasgow Coma Scale score is less than or equal to 8

● **Figure 4-39** In the pediatric trauma patient, use the combination jaw-thrust/spine stabilization maneuver to open the airway. (a) Single paramedic kneels above child's head, holds head in neutral position while thrusting jaw forward with fingers. (b) Two paramedics working together; one holds head in neutral position while the other thrusts the jaw forward. (c) Single paramedic uses alternative technique to hold head in neutral position while thrusting jaw forward.

Traumatic head injuries can cause intracranial bleeding or swelling. This ultimately results in an increase in intracranial pressure. The signs of increased intracranial pressure can be subtle. They include:

- Elevated blood pressure
- Bradycardia
- Rapid, deep respirations progressing to slow, deep respirations
- Bulging fontanelle in infants

Increased intracranial pressure will eventually lead to herniation of a portion of the brain through the foramen magnum. This is an ominous development that is often associated with irreversible injury. Signs and symptoms of herniation include:

- Asymmetrical pupils
- Decorticate posturing
- Decerebrate posturing

Specific management of traumatic head injuries in children is similar to that for adults. As a rule, follow these steps:

- Administer supplemental oxygen (if the patient is hypoxic).
- Provide ventilation. Consider intubation in children with a Glasgow Coma Scale score of less than or equal to 8 (severe head injury) and ventilate at a normal rate.
- Consider rapid sequence intubation (RSI) for children with a Glasgow Coma Scale score of less than or equal to 8 who have too much muscle tone to allow endotracheal intubation.

Consider hyperventilation only if there is a deterioration in the child's condition as evidenced by asymmetric pupils, active seizures, or neurologic posturing (indicating herniation). Children with traumatic head injuries do best at facilities that treat a great number of children and who have pediatric neurosurgeons on staff. Consider diverting to a pediatric trauma facility if a moderate or severe traumatic head injury is present.

Specific Injuries

As previously mentioned, more pediatric patients die of trauma than of any other cause. Statistics reveal that nearly 50 percent of these deaths occur within the first hour of injury. The quick arrival of EMS at the scene can literally mean the difference between life and death for a child. Although management of trauma is basically the same for children as for adults, anatomic and physiologic differences cause pediatric patients to have different patterns of injury.

Head, Face, and Neck

The majority of children who sustain multiple trauma will suffer associated head and/or neck injuries. As previously mentioned, the larger relative mass of the head and lack of neck muscle strength provide for increased momentum in acceleration–deceleration injuries and a greater stress on the cervical spine. The fulcrum of cervical mobility in the younger child is at the C2–C3 level. As a result, nearly 60 to 70 percent of pediatric fractures occur in C1–C2.[18]

Injuries to the head are the most common cause of death in pediatric trauma victims. School-age children tend to sustain head injuries from bicycle collisions, falls from trees, or car–pedestrian collisions. Older children most commonly suffer head injuries from sporting events. Head injuries in all age groups may result from abuse.

In treating head injuries, remember that diffuse injuries are common in children, whereas focal injuries are rare. Because the skull is softer and more compliant in children than in adults, brain injuries occur more readily in infants and young children. Because of open fontanelles and sutures, infants up to an average age of 16 months may be more tolerant to an increase in intracranial pressure and can have delayed signs. (Keep this fact in mind when taking the history of children in the one-month to two-year age range.)[19]

Children also frequently injure their faces. The most common facial injuries are lacerations secondary to falls. Young children are very clumsy when they first start walking. A fall onto a sharp object, such as the corner of a coffee table, can result in a laceration. Older children sustain dental injuries in falls from bicycles, skateboard accidents, fights, and sports activities.

Spinal injuries in children are not as common as in adults. However, as noted earlier, a child's proportionately larger and heavier head makes the cervical spine vulnerable to injury. Any time a child sustains a severe head injury, always assume that a neck injury may also be present.

Chest and Abdomen

Most injuries to the chest and abdomen result from blunt trauma. As noted earlier, infants and young children lack the rigid rib cages of adults. Therefore, they suffer fewer rib fractures and more intrathoracic injuries. Likewise, their relatively undeveloped abdominal musculature affords minimal protection to the viscera.

Because of the high mortality associated with blunt trauma, children with significant blunt abdominal or chest trauma should be transported immediately to a pediatric trauma center with appropriate care provided en route.

Injuries to the Chest Chest injuries are the second most common cause of pediatric trauma deaths. Because of the compliance of the chest wall, severe intrathoracic injury can be present without signs of external injury. Pneumothorax and hemothorax can occur in the pediatric patient, especially if the mechanism of injury was a motor vehicle collision.

Tension pneumothorax can also occur in children. Pediatric patients poorly tolerate the condition and a needle thoracostomy may be lifesaving. Tension pneumothorax presents with the following signs and symptoms:

- Diminished breath sounds over the affected lung
- Shift of the trachea to the opposite side
- Progressive decrease in ventilatory compliance

Keep in mind that children with cardiac tamponade may have no physical signs of tamponade other than hypotension. Also remember that flail chest is an uncommon injury in children. When chest injury is noted without a significant mechanism of injury, suspect child abuse.

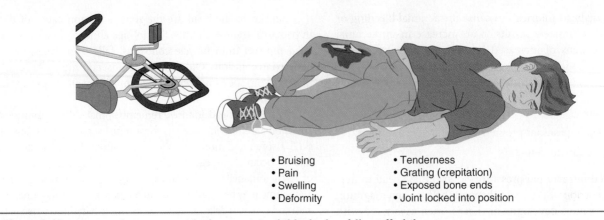

- Bruising
- Pain
- Swelling
- Deformity
- Tenderness
- Grating (crepitation)
- Exposed bone ends
- Joint locked into position

● **Figure 4-41** Signs and symptoms of a fracture in a child who has fallen off a bike.

Injuries to the Abdomen Significant blunt trauma to the abdomen can result in injury to the spleen or liver. In fact, the spleen is the most commonly injured organ in children. Signs and symptoms of a splenic injury include tenderness in the left upper quadrant of the abdomen, abrasions on the abdomen, and hematoma of the abdominal wall. Symptoms of liver injury include right upper quadrant abdominal pain and/or right lower chest pain. Both splenic and hepatic injuries can cause life-threatening internal hemorrhage.

In treating blunt abdominal trauma, keep in mind the small size of the pediatric abdomen. Be certain to palpate only one quadrant at a time. In cases of both chest and abdominal trauma, treat for shock with positioning, fluids, and maintenance of body temperature.

Extremities

Extremity injuries in children are typically limited to fractures and lacerations. Children rarely sustain amputations and other serious extremity injuries. An exception includes farm children who may become entangled in agricultural equipment.

The most common injuries are fractures, usually resulting from falls (Figure 4-41 ●). Because children have more flexible bones than adults, they tend to have incomplete fractures, such as **bend fractures**, **buckle fractures**, and **greenstick fractures**. In younger children, the bone growth plates have not yet closed. Some types of growth plate fractures can lead to permanent disability if not managed correctly. Whenever indicated, perform splinting to decrease pain and prevent further injury and/or blood loss.

Burns

Burns are the second leading cause of death in children. They are the leading cause of accidental death in the home for children under 14. Burns may be chemical, thermal, or electrical. The most common type of burn injury encountered by EMS personnel is

scalding. Children can scald themselves by pulling hot liquids off tables or stoves. In cases of abuse, they can be scalded by immersion in hot water.

Estimation of the burn surface area is slightly different for children than for adults (Figure 4-42 ●). In adults, the "rule of nines" assigns 9 percent of the body surface area (BSA) to each of 11 body regions: the entire head and neck; the anterior chest; the anterior abdomen; the posterior chest; the lower back (posterior abdomen); the anterior surface of each lower extremity; the posterior surface of each lower extremity; and the entirety of each upper extremity. The remaining 1 percent is assigned to the genitalia.

In a child, the head accounts for a larger percentage of BSA, whereas the legs make up a smaller percentage. Thus, for children the rule of nines is modified to take away 8 percent from the lower extremities (2 percent from the front and 2 percent from the back of each leg) plus the 1 percent assigned to

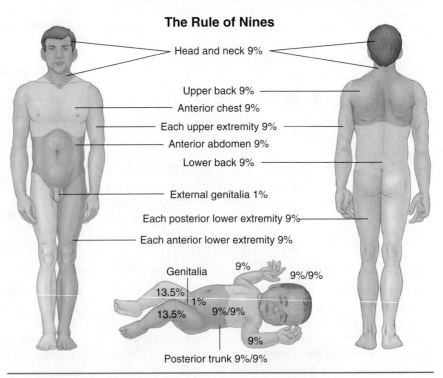

The Rule of Nines

Head and neck 9%

Upper back 9%
Anterior chest 9%
Each upper extremity 9%
Anterior abdomen 9%
Lower back 9%

External genitalia 1%

Each posterior lower extremity 9%
Each anterior lower extremity 9%

Genitalia
13.5%
13.5%

9%
9%/9%
1%
9%/9%
9%

Posterior trunk 9%/9%

● **Figure 4-42** The rule of nines helps to estimate the extent of a burn in adults and children. Note the modifications for the child.

the adult genitalia. This 9 percent that is taken from the lower part of the body is reassigned to the head. Therefore, whereas the adult's entire head and neck are counted as 9 percent, in the child the anterior head and neck count as 9 percent and the posterior head and neck count as another 9 percent.

You can also use the child's palm as a guide (the "rule of palm"). The palm equals about 1 percent of the body surface area. You can calculate a burn area by estimating how many palm areas it equals. Usually, the rule of nines works best for more extensive burns and the rule of palm for less extensive ones.

Management considerations for pediatric burn patients include the following:

- Provide prompt management of the airway, because swelling can develop rapidly.

- If intubation is required, you may need to use an endotracheal tube up to two sizes smaller than normal because of the swelling.

- Thermally burned children are very susceptible to hypothermia. Be sure to maintain body heat.

- When treating serious electrical burn patients, suspect musculoskeletal injuries and perform spinal immobilization.

Sudden Infant Death Syndrome

Sudden infant death syndrome (SIDS) is defined as the sudden death of an infant during the first year of life from an illness of unknown etiology. The incidence of SIDS in the United States is approximately 0.57 deaths per 1,000 births. SIDS is the leading cause of death between two weeks and one year of age. It is responsible for a significant number of deaths between one month and six months, with peak incidence occurring at two to four months.

SIDS occurs most frequently in the fall and winter months. It tends to be more common in boys than in girls. It is more prevalent in premature and low-birth-weight infants, in infants of young mothers, and in infants whose mothers did not receive prenatal care. Infants of mothers who used cocaine, methadone, or heroin during pregnancy are at greater risk. Occasionally, a mild upper respiratory infection will be reported prior to the death. SIDS is not caused by external suffocation from blankets or pillows, nor is it related to allergies to cow's milk or regurgitation and aspiration of stomach contents. It is not thought to be hereditary.

Current theories vary about the etiology of SIDS. Some authorities feel that it may result from an immature respiratory center in the brain that leads the child to simply stop breathing. Others think there may be an airway obstruction in the posterior pharynx as a result of pharyngeal relaxation during sleep, a hypermobile mandible, or an enlarged tongue. Studies strongly link SIDS to a prone sleeping position. Soft bedding, waterbed mattresses, smoking in the home, and/or an overheated environment are other potential associations. A small percentage of SIDS may be abuse related.

Although research into SIDS continues, the American Academy of Pediatrics suggests that infants be placed supine unless medical conditions prevent this. In addition, the Academy urges parents or caregivers to avoid placing infants in overheated environments, overwrapping them with too many clothes or blankets, smoking before and after pregnancy, and filling the crib with soft bedding.

Assessment

Infants suffering SIDS have similar physical findings. From an external standpoint, there is a normal state of nutrition and hydration. The skin may be mottled. There are often frothy, occasionally blood-tinged, fluids in and around the mouth and nostrils. Vomitus may be present. Occasionally, the infant may be in an unusual position as a result of muscle spasm or high activity at the time of death. Common findings noted at autopsy include intrathoracic petechiae (small hemorrhages) in 90 percent of cases. There is often associated pulmonary congestion and edema. Sometimes, stomach contents are found in the trachea. Microscopic examination of the trachea often reveals the presence of inflammatory changes.

Management

The immediate needs of the family with a SIDS baby are many. Unless the infant is obviously dead, undertake active and aggressive care of the infant to assure the family that everything possible is being done. A first responder or other personnel should be assigned to assist the parents and to explain the procedures. At all points, use the baby's name.

After arrival at the hospital, direct management at the parents or caregivers, as nothing can be done for the child. Allow the family to see the dead child. Expect a normal grief reaction. Initially, there may be shock, disbelief, and denial. Other times, the parents or caregivers may express anger, rage, hostility, blame, or guilt. Often, there is a feeling of inadequacy as well as helplessness, confusion, and fear. The grief process is likely to last for years. SIDS has major long-term effects on family relations. It may also affect you, the on-scene paramedic. If so, do not be reluctant to seek counseling.

Apparent Life-Threatening Event

The term *apparent life-threatening event* (ALTE) is defined as a sudden event, often characterized by apnea or other abrupt changes in the child's behavior. Symptoms of an ALTE include one or more of the following:

- Apnea
- Change in color (cyanosis)
- Loss of muscle tone
- Coughing
- Gagging

These episodes may necessitate stimulation or resuscitation to arouse the child and reinitiate regular breathing. ALTE was once referred to as "near-miss SIDS." The true incidence is unknown. ALTE is often a result of another condition and is not an entity of its own. However, in some instances, the cause cannot be identified. Child abuse should be considered if other medical causes have been excluded. Home monitoring technology may be beneficial. From an EMS standpoint, the care provided should be based on your assessment and immediate life threats.[20, 21]

CHILD ABUSE AND NEGLECT

A tragic truth is that some people cause physical and psychological harm to children, either through intentional abuse or through intentional or unintentional neglect. The estimated child mortality rate for child abuse and neglect is 18.4 per 100,000.

Abused children share several common characteristics. Often, the child is seen as "special" and different from others. Premature infants and twins stand a higher risk of abuse than other children. Many abused children are less than five years of age. Children with physical and mental handicaps, as well as those with other special needs, are at greater risk. So are uncommunicative (autistic) children. Boys are more often abused than girls. A child who is not what the parents wanted (e.g., the "wrong" gender) is at increased risk of abuse, too.

Perpetrators of Abuse or Neglect

A parent, a legal guardian, or a foster parent may instigate abuse or neglect. A person, an institution, or an agency or program entrusted with custody can carry it out. Abuse or neglect can also result from the actions of a caretaker, such as a babysitter or nanny.

The person who abuses or neglects a child can come from any geographic, religious, ethnic, racial, occupational, educational, or socioeconomic background. Despite their diversity, people who abuse children tend to share certain traits. The abuser is usually a parent or a full-time caregiver. When the mother spends the majority of the time with the child, she is the parent most frequently identified as the abuser. Most abusers were abused themselves as children.

Three conditions can alert you to the potential for abuse:

- A parent or adult who seems capable of abuse, especially one who exhibits evasive or hostile behavior
- A child in one of the high-risk categories noted in the preceding section
- The presence of a crisis, particularly financial stress, marital or relationship stress, or physical illness in a parent or child

Types of Abuse

Child abuse can take several forms, including:

- Psychological abuse
- Physical abuse
- Sexual abuse
- Neglect (either physical or emotional)

Abused children suffer every imaginable kind of mistreatment. They are battered with fists, belts, broom handles, hairbrushes, baseball bats, electric cords, and any other objects that can be used as weapons (Figure 4-43 ●). They are locked in closets, denied food, or deprived of access to a toilet. They are intentionally burned or scalded with

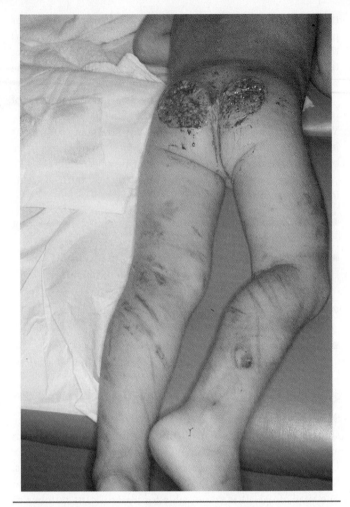

● **Figure 4-43**   An abused child. Note the marks on the legs associated with beatings with an electric wire. The burns on the buttocks are from submersion in hot water. *(Courtesy of Scott and White Healthcare)*

anything from hot water to cigarette butts to open flames (Figure 4-44 ●). They are severely shaken, thrown into cribs, pushed down stairs, or shoved into walls. Some are shot, stabbed, or suffocated.

Sexual abuse ranges from adults exposing themselves to children to overt sexual acts to sexual torture. Sexual abuse can occur at any age, and the victims may be either male or female. Generally, the sexual abuser is someone the child knows and, perhaps, trusts. Stepchildren or adopted children face a greater risk for sexual abuse than biological children. Cases in which sexual abuse causes physical harm may get reported. Other cases, especially those with emotional and minor physical injury, may go undetected.

Assessment of the Potentially Abused or Neglected Child

Signs of abuse or neglect can be startling. As a guide, the following findings should trigger a high index of suspicion:

- Any obvious or suspected fractures in a child under two years of age

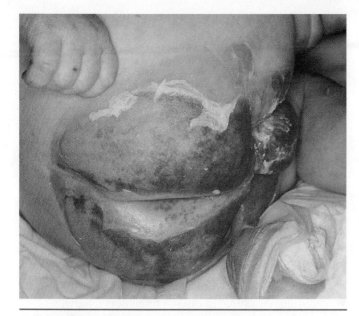

● **Figure 4-44** Burn injury from placing a child's buttocks in hot water as a punishment. *(Courtesy of Scott and White Healthcare)*

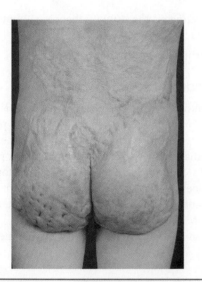

● **Figure 4-45** The effects of child abuse, both physical and mental, can last a lifetime. *(Courtesy of Scott and White Healthcare)*

- Multiple injuries in various stages of healing, especially burns and bruises (Figure 4-45 ●)
- More injuries than usually seen in children of the same age or size
- Injuries scattered on many areas of the body
- Bruises or burns in patterns that suggest intentional infliction
- Increased intracranial pressure in an infant
- Suspected intraabdominal trauma in a young child
- Any injury that does not fit with the description of the cause given

Information in the medical history may also raise the index of suspicion. Examples include:

- A history that does not match the nature or severity of the injury
- Vague parental accounts or accounts that change during the interview
- Accusations that the child injured himself intentionally
- Delay in seeking help
- Child dressed inappropriately for the situation
- Revealing comments by bystanders, especially siblings

Suspect child neglect if you spot any of the following conditions:

- Extreme malnutrition
- Multiple insect bites
- Long-standing skin infections
- Extreme lack of cleanliness
- Verbal or social skills far below those you would expect for a child of similar age and background
- Lack of appropriate medical care

Management of the Potentially Abused or Neglected Child

In cases of child abuse or neglect, the goals of management include appropriate treatment of injuries, protection of the child from further abuse, and notification of proper authorities. You should obtain as much information as possible, in a nonjudgmental manner. Document all findings or statements in the patient report. Do not "cross-examine" the parents—this job belongs to the police or other authorities. Try to be supportive toward the parents, especially if it helps you to transport the child to the hospital. Remember: Never leave transport to the alleged abuser.

On arrival at the emergency department, report your suspicions to the appropriate personnel. Complete the patient report and all available documentation at this time, as delay may inhibit accurate recall of data.

Child abuse and neglect are particularly stressful aspects of emergency medical services. You must recognize and deal with your feelings, perhaps by seeking counseling.

Resources for Abuse and Neglect

You can contact your local child protection agency for additional information on child abuse. Consider taking a course in the recognition of child abuse and neglect. These are often offered by children's hospitals. The Internet has several sites that provide up-to-date information on child abuse.[22, 23]

INFANTS AND CHILDREN WITH SPECIAL NEEDS

For most of human history, infants and children with devastating congenital conditions or diseases either died or remained confined to a hospital. In recent decades, however, medical technology has lowered infant mortality rates and allowed a greater number of children with special needs to live at home. (See more about home care in Volume 6, Chapter 6.) Some of these infants and children include:

- Premature babies
- Infants and children with lung disease, heart disease, or neurologic disorders
- Infants and children with chronic diseases, such as cystic fibrosis, asthma, childhood cancers, and cerebral palsy
- Infants and children with altered functions from birth, such as cerebral palsy, spina bifida, and other congenital birth defects

In caring for these children, family members receive education relative to the special equipment required by the infant or child. Even so, they may feel a great deal of apprehension when care moves from the hospital to the home. As a result, they may summon EMS at the first indication of trouble. This is especially true in the initial weeks following discharge.

Common Home Care Devices

Devices you might commonly find in the home include tracheostomy tubes, apnea monitors, home artificial ventilators, central intravenous lines, gastric feeding tubes, gastrostomy tubes, and shunts. In treating children with special needs, remember that the parents and caregivers are often very knowledgeable about their children and the devices that sustain their lives. Listen to them. They know their children better than anybody else.

Tracheostomy Tubes

Patients who are on prolonged home ventilators or who have chronic respiratory problems may have surgically placed tubes in the inferior trachea (Figure 4-46 ●). A **tracheostomy** (trach) tube may be used as a temporary or a permanent device.

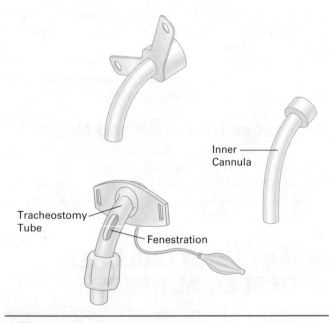

● **Figure 4-46**   Tracheostomy tubes. Top: Plastic tube. Bottom: Metal tube with inner cannula.

Inner Cannula

Tracheostomy Tube

Fenestration

Although various types of tubes are used, you might encounter some common complications. They include:

- Obstruction, usually by a mucus plug
- Site bleeding, either from the tube or around the tube
- An air leakage
- A dislodged tube
- Infection—a condition that will worsen an already impaired breathing ability

Management steps for a patient with a tracheostomy include:

- Maintaining an open airway
- Suctioning the tube, as needed
- Allowing the patient to remain in a position of comfort, if possible
- Administering oxygen in cases of respiratory distress
- Assisting ventilations in cases of respiratory failure/ arrest by:
  - Using the tracheostomy to ventilate
  - Intubating orally in the absence of an upper airway obstruction
  - Intubating via the **stoma** if there is an upper airway obstruction
- Transporting the patient to the hospital

Apnea Monitors

Apnea monitors are used to alert parents or caregivers to the cessation of breathing in an infant, especially a premature infant. Some types of monitors signal changes in heart rate, such as bradycardia or tachycardia. They operate via pads attached to the baby's chest and connected to the monitor by wires. If the device does not detect a breath within a specific time frame or if the infant's heart rate is too slow or too fast, an alarm will sound (Figure 4-47 ●).

When an apnea monitor is placed in a home, the parents are typically instructed on what to do if the alarm sounds

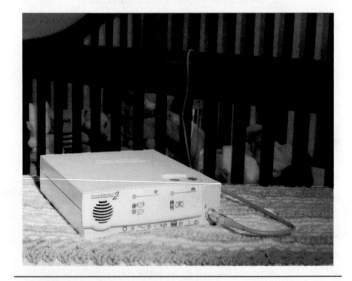

● **Figure 4-47**   Home apnea monitor.

(stimulate the child, provide artificial respirations, and so on). If these fail, EMS may be summoned. Also, nervous parents who have just brought a baby home on an apnea monitor may panic the first couple of times the alarm sounds and call 911. Be patient and kind while instructing them on what to do when the alarm sounds.

Home Artificial Ventilators

Various configurations exist for home ventilators. *Demand ventilators* sense the rate and quality of a patient's respiration as well as several other parameters, including pulse oximetry. They typically respond to preset limits. Other devices provide a constant PEEP (positive end-expiratory pressure) and a set oxygen concentration for the patient.

Two complications commonly result in EMS calls: (1) a device's mechanical failure and (2) shortages of energy during an electrical failure. Treatment typically includes:

- Maintaining an open airway
- Administering artificial ventilations via an appropriately sized BVM with oxygen
- Transporting the patient to a hospital until the home ventilator is working

Central Intravenous Lines

Children who require long-term IV therapy will often have central lines placed into the superior vena cava near the heart. If IV therapy is necessary for only several weeks, percutaneous intravenous catheter (PIC) lines may be placed in the arm and threaded into the superior vena cava. Otherwise, the lines are placed through subclavian venipuncture. **Central IV lines** are commonly used to administer intravenous nutrition, antibiotics, or chemotherapy for cancer.

Possible complications for central IV lines include:

- Cracked line
- Infection, either at the site or at more distal aspects of the line
- Loss of patency (e.g., clotting)
- Hemorrhage, which can be considerable
- Air embolism

Emergency medical care steps include control of any bleeding through direct pressure. If a large amount of air is in the line, try to withdraw it with a syringe. If this fails, clamp the line and transport. In cases of a cracked line, place a clamp between the crack and the patient. If the patient exhibits an altered mental status following the cracked line, position the child on the left side with head down. Transport the child to the hospital as quickly as possible.

Gastric Feeding Tubes and Gastrostomy Tubes

Children who are not capable of swallowing or eating receive nutrition through either a gastric feeding tube or a gastrostomy tube (Figure 4-48 ●). (A gastric feeding tube is placed through the nostrils into the stomach. A gastrostomy tube is placed through the abdominal wall directly into the stomach.) These

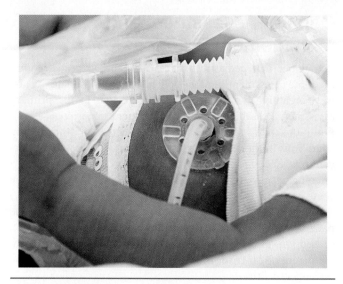

● **Figure 4-48**   Infant with feeding tube.

special devices are commonly used in disorders of the digestive system or in situations in which the developmental ability of the patient hinders feeding. Food consists of nutritious liquids.

Possible emergency complications include:

- Bleeding at the site
- Dislodged tube
- Respiratory distress, particularly if a tube feeding backs up into the esophagus and is aspirated into the trachea and lungs
- In the case of diabetics, altered mental status due to missed feedings

Emergency medical care involves supporting the ABCs, including possible suctioning and administration of supplemental oxygen. Patients should be transported to a definitive care facility, either in a sitting position or lying on the right side with the head elevated. The goal is to reduce the risk of aspiration, a serious condition.

Shunts

A **shunt** is a surgical connection that runs from the brain to the abdomen. It removes excess cerebrospinal fluid from the brain through drainage. A subcutaneous reservoir is usually palpable on one side of the patient's head. A pathologic rise in intracranial pressure, secondary to a blocked shunt, is a primary complication. Shunt failure may also result when the shunt's connections separate, usually because of a child's growth.

Cases of shunt failure present as altered mental status. The patient may exhibit drowsiness, respiratory distress, or the classic signs of pupil dysfunction or posturing. Be aware that an altered mental status may be caused by infection—a distinction to be made in a hospital setting.

Care steps involve maintenance of an open airway, administration of ventilations as needed, and immediate transport. Shunt failures require correction in the operating room, where the cerebrospinal fluid can be drained or, in rare cases, an infection identified and treated.

General Assessment and Management Practices

Remember that pediatric patients with special needs require the same assessment as other patients. Always evaluate the airway, breathing, and circulation. (Recall that in the primary assessment, "disability" refers to the patient's neurologic status, not to the child's special need.) If you discover life-threatening conditions in the primary assessment, begin appropriate interventions. Keep in mind that the child's special need is often an ongoing process. In most cases, you should concentrate on the acute problem.

During the assessment, ask pertinent questions of the patient, parent, or caregiver, such as "What unusual situation caused you to call for an ambulance?" As already mentioned, the parent or caregiver is usually very knowledgeable about the patient's condition.

In most cases, the physical examination is essentially the same as with other patients. It is important to explain everything that is being done, even if the patient does not seem to understand. Do not be distracted by the special equipment. Be aware of the help that the patient, parent, or caregiver may be able to provide in handling home care devices.

In managing patients with special needs, try to keep several thoughts in mind:

● Avoid using the term *disability* in reference to the child's special need. Instead, think of the patient's many abilities.

● Never assume that the patient cannot understand what you are saying.

● Involve the parents, caregivers, or the patient, if appropriate, in treatment. They manage the illness or congenital condition on a daily basis.

● Treat the patient with a special need with the same respect as any other patient.

MULTIPLE-CASUALTY INCIDENTS INVOLVING CHILDREN

The criteria routinely used for triage of injured or ill patients at a multiple-casualty incident (MCI) are based on adult anatomic and physiologic data. However, as detailed earlier, children respond to injuries and illnesses somewhat differently because their anatomy and physiology are different. Recognizing this deficiency, noted pediatric emergency physician Lou Romig, MD, FAAP, FACEP, developed the JumpSTART™ system for pediatric triage.[21]

The *JumpSTART Pediatric MCI Triage Tool* is an objective tool developed specifically for the triage of children in the multicasualty/disaster setting. JumpSTART was developed in 1995 to parallel the structure of the START system—the adult MCI triage tool most commonly used in the United States and adopted in many countries around the world. JumpSTART's objectives are:

1. To optimize the primary triage of injured children in the MCI setting

2. To enhance the effectiveness of resource allocation for *all* MCI victims

3. To reduce the emotional burden on triage personnel who may have to make rapid life-or-death decisions about the injured

JumpSTART provides an objective framework that helps to ensure that injured children are triaged by responders using their heads instead of their hearts, thus reducing overtriage that might siphon resources from other patients who need them more. In addition, this system minimizes physical and emotional trauma to children from unnecessary painful procedures and separation from loved ones. Undertriage is addressed by recognizing the key differences between adult and pediatric physiology and using appropriate pediatric physiologic parameters at decision points.

JumpSTART was designed for use in disaster/multicasualty settings and not for daily EMS or hospital triage. The triage philosophies in the two settings are different and require different guidelines. JumpSTART is also intended for the triage of children with acute injuries and may not be appropriate for the primary triage of children with medical illnesses in a disaster setting.

Using the JumpSTART System

The entry category for the JumpSTART system is simple. That is, if the victim "appears to be a child," use the JumpSTART algorithm. If the victim appears to be a young adult or older, use the START system. (The START triage system is detailed in Volume 5, Chapter 9.)

To use the JumpSTART system, follow this algorithm (see Figure 4-49 ●):

1. *Identify and direct all ambulatory patients to the designated minor (GREEN) area for secondary triage and treatment.* Begin assessment of nonambulatory patients as you come to them. Because children less than one year of age cannot walk, they should be carried to the minor (GREEN) area by other ambulatory victims and *must* be the first assessed by medical personnel in that area.

2. *Assess breathing.* If the child is breathing spontaneously, go on to the next step (assessing respiratory rate). If the child is apneic or with very irregular breathing, open the airway using standard positioning techniques. If positioning results in resumption of spontaneous respirations, tag the patient *immediate* (RED) and move on. If the child is not breathing after airway opening, check for peripheral pulse. If no pulse, tag the patient *deceased/ nonsalvageable* (BLACK) and move on. If there is a peripheral pulse, give five mouth-to-barrier

JumpSTART Pediatric MCI Triage

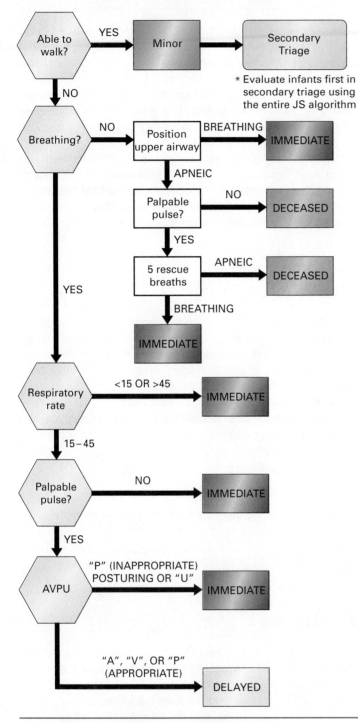

* Evaluate infants first in secondary triage using the entire JS algorithm

● **Figure 4-49**   JumpSTART Pediatric MCI Triage Algorithm.

ventilations. If apnea persists, tag the patient *deceased/ nonsalvageable* (BLACK) and move on. If breathing resumes after the "jumpstart" (ventilation attempt), tag the patient *immediate* (RED) and move on.

3. ***Assess respiratory rate.*** If the child's respiratory rate is 15 to 45 per minute, proceed to the next step (assess perfusion). If respiratory rate is 45 per minute or irregular, tag patient as *immediate* (RED) and move on.

4. ***Assess perfusion.*** If a peripheral pulse is palpable, proceed to the next step (assess mental status). If no peripheral pulse is present (in the least injured limb), tag the patient *immediate* (RED) and move on.

5. ***Assess mental status.*** Use the AVPU scale to assess mental status. If the patient is **a**lert, responsive to **v**erbal stimuli, or appropriately responsive to **p**ain, tag as *delayed* (YELLOW) and move on. If the patient is inappropriately responsive to **p**ain or is **u**nresponsive, tag as *immediate* (RED) and move on.

Modifications for Nonambulatory Children

All nonambulatory children must be immediately evaluated using the JumpSTART algorithm. Nonambulatory children include those who are too young to walk, children with a developmental delay, children with acute injuries that prevented them from walking *before* the incident, and children with chronic disabilities. If any are *immediate* (RED) criteria, tag as RED. If the child meets the *delayed* (YELLOW) criteria, further classify:

● *Delayed* (YELLOW) if significant external signs of injury are found (i.e., deep penetrating wounds, severe bleeding, severe burns, amputations, distended tender abdomen).

● *Minor* (GREEN) if no significant external injury.

Reassessing Dead/Nonsalvageable (BLACK) Victims

Unless clearly suffering from injuries incompatible with life, victims tagged in the *dead/nonsalvageable* (BLACK) category should be reassessed once critical interventions have been completed for *immediate* (RED) and *delayed* (YELLOW) patients. Care should be taken to preserve the dignity of the dead, at the same time being careful to not disturb any forensic evidence present.

SUMMARY

Pediatric emergencies can be stressful for both you and the adults responsible for the child's well-being. Many of the pediatric emergencies for which you will be called will be the results of trauma, respiratory distress, ingestion of poisons, or febrile seizure activity. Keep in mind that pediatric medical emergencies are often caused by airway or breathing problems, so focus on these first.

With all pediatric calls, you must be on the lookout for signs and symptoms of child abuse or neglect and report them when found. Remember to never accuse or engage a family member or caregiver. Simply document your objective findings and relay the information to the receiving facility and to local law enforcement.

Keep in mind that the approach and management of pediatric emergencies must be modified for the age and size of the child. Certain skills generally considered routine, such as IV administration, become difficult in the pediatric patient because of size and other factors. As long as you remember that children are not "small adults" and approach them knowing that they have special considerations—both physical and emotional—that must be managed accordingly, you will be successful in assessing and appropriately treating your pediatric patient.

YOU MAKE THE CALL

Dispatch sends you to a residence in an affluent neighborhood. The call reports that "a child is hurt and bleeding." On arrival at the scene, the parents greet you and your crew with controlled anger. Apparently, the neighbors dialed 911 when they heard a child's loud cries coming from the house. The mother tells you that her 24-month-old son fell off the kitchen counter while trying to reach the cookie jar. "He's always climbing after something," she snaps. "I can't watch him 24 hours a day."

As you listen, the child remains strangely quiet. He avoids all eye contact and does not seek comfort from either his mother or father. You observe that a scalp laceration is bleeding profusely. You also observe a number of bruises and abrasions in various stages of healing on the patient's upper torso and arms.

1. What are your assessment priorities for this patient?

2. What interventions would you perform on scene and en route to the receiving hospital?

3. Describe possible transport considerations, including a potential refusal of transport by the angry parents.

4. What are the important factors in reporting this incident and documenting the call?

See Suggested Responses at the back of this book.

REVIEW QUESTIONS

1. The _____ was formed for the express purpose of improving the health of pediatric patients who suffer potentially life-threatening illnesses or injuries.
   a. DHHS   c. AHA
   b. EMSC   d. NHTSA

2. The term *neonate* describes infants from birth to _____ of age.
   a. one week   c. one month
   b. two weeks   d. two months

3. Children in which age group should be examined in toe-to-head order?
   a. infants, ages 1–5 months
   b. infants, ages 6–12 months
   c. preschoolers, ages 3–5 years
   d. school-age children, ages 6–12 years

4. Children in which age group worry about their physical image more than those in any other pediatric age group?
   a. toddlers, ages 1–3 years
   b. adolescents, ages 13–18 years
   c. school-age children, ages 6–12 years
   d. infants, ages 1–5 months

5. The combination of increased oxygen requirements and decreased oxygen reserves makes infants and children especially susceptible to _____.
   a. trauma
   b. hypoxia
   c. epilepsy
   d. diabetes

6. Evaluation of breathing includes assessment of all of the following conditions *except* _____.
   a. color
   b. heart rate
   c. respiratory rate
   d. respiratory effort

7. Capillary refill time is considered reliable as a sign of perfusion primarily in children less than _____ years of age.
   a. six
   b. seven
   c. eight
   d. nine

8. _____ in a distressed infant or child may indicate hypoxia and is an ominous sign of cardiac arrest.
   a. Retraction
   b. Bradycardia
   c. Tachycardia
   d. Head bobbing

9. Conditions that place a pediatric patient at risk of cardiopulmonary arrest include all of the following *except* _____.
   a. respiratory rate greater than 40
   b. respiratory rate greater than 60
   c. heart rate greater than 180 or less than 80 (under five years of age)
   d. heart rate greater than 180 or less than 60 (over five years of age)

10. The only alternative airway that can be used in the pediatric patient is the _____.
    a. EOA
    b. PtL
    c. ETC
    d. LMA

11. Which of the following medications is not used in pediatric cardiac arrest?
    a. epinephrine
    b. amiodarone
    c. lidocaine
    d. oxygen

12. An example of a commonly used neuromuscular blocker is _____.
    a. fentanyl
    b. diazepam
    c. thiopental
    d. succinylcholine

13. The initial dosage of fluid in hypovolemic shock should be _____ mL/kg of an isotonic solution such as lactated Ringer's or normal saline.
    a. 10
    b. 20
    c. 25
    d. 30

14. You are administering amiodarone to a pediatric patient. You know that the proper dosage of this medication is _____ mg/kg per dose.
    a. 1.0
    b. 0.5
    c. 2.5
    d. 5.0

15. You have elected to use electrical therapy for your pediatric patient. You realize that you will administer an initial dose of _____ of body weight.
    a. 2 joules per pound
    b. 4 joules per pound
    c. 2 joules per kilogram
    d. 4 joules per kilogram

16. The majority of childhood medical emergencies involve the _____ system.
    a. nervous
    b. endocrine
    c. respiratory
    d. cardiovascular

17. The mildest form of respiratory impairment is classified as respiratory _____.
    a. arrest
    b. failure
    c. distress
    d. compromise

18. _____ shock develops when the body can no longer compensate for decreased tissue perfusion.
    a. Compensated
    b. Irreversible
    c. Anaphylactic
    d. Decompensated

19. Bradyarrhythmias are the most common pediatric arrhythmias. They most frequently result from _____.
    a. anoxia
    b. hypoxia
    c. acidosis
    d. hypothermia

20. _____ are the single most common cause of injury in children.
    a. MVCs
    b. Burns
    c. Falls
    d. Drownings

See Answers to Review Questions at the back of this book.

REFERENCES

1. Viner, R., C. Coffey, C. Mathers, et al. "50-year Mortality Trends in Children and Young People: A Study of 50 Low-Income, Middle-Income, and High-Income Countries." *Lancet* 377 (2011): 1162–1174.

2. Wood, D., E. J. Kalinowski, D. R. Miller, et al. "Pediatric Continuing Education for Emergency Medical Technicians. The National Council of State Emergency Medical Services Training Coordinators." *Prehosp Emerg Care* 20 (2004): 261–268.

3. U.S. Department of Health and Human Services. *Emergency Medical Services for Children.* [Available at http://bolivia.hrsa.gov/emsc/]

4. Richard, J., M. H. Osmond, L. Nesbitt, and I. G. Stiell. "Management and Outcomes of Pediatric Patients Transported by Emergency Medical Services in a Canadian Prehospital System." *CJEM* 8 (2006): 6–12.

5. Diekmann, R. A., D. Brownstein, and M. Gausche-Hill. "The Pediatric Assessment Triangle: A Novel

Approach for the Rapid Evaluation of Children." *Pediatr Emerg Care* 26 (2010): 312–315.

6. Corrales, A. Y. and M. Starr. "Assessment of the Unwell Child." *Aust Fam Physician* 39 (2010): 270–275.

7. Singh, S., W. D. Allen, Jr., S. T. Venkataraman, and M. S. Bhende. "Utility of a Novel Quantitative Handheld Microstream Capnometer during Transport of Critically Ill Children." *Am J Emerg Med* 24 (2006): 302–307.

8. Bhende, M. S. and W. D. Allen, Jr. "Evaluation of a Capno-Flo Resuscitator during Transport of Critically Ill Children." *Pediatr Emerg Care* 18 (2002): 414–416.

9. Moynihan, R. J., J. G. Brock-Utne, J. H. Archer, L. H. Feld, and T. R. Kreitzman. "The Effect of Cricoid Pressure on Preventing Gastric Insufflation in Infants and Children." *Anesthesiology* 78 (1993): 652–656.

10. Gausche, M., R. J. Lewis, S. J. Stratton, et al. "Effect of Out-of-Hospital Pediatric Endotracheal Intubation on Survival and Neurologic Outcome: A Controlled Clinical Trial." *JAMA* 283 (2000): 783–790.

11. Kleinman, M. E., L. Chameides, S. M. Schexnayder, et al. "Part 14: Pediatric Advanced Life Support: 2010 American Heart Association Guidelines for Cardiopulmonary Resuscitation and Emergency Cardiovascular Care." *Circulation* 122 (2010): S876–S908.

12. Ritter, S. C. and F. X. Guyette. "Prehospital Pediatric King LT-D Use: A Pilot Study." *Prehosp Emerg Care* 15 (2011): 401–404.

13. Bjornson, C., K. F. Russell, B. Vandermeer, et al. "Nebulized Epinephrine for Croup in Children." *Cochrane Database Syst Rev* 16 (2011): CD006649.

14. Stranges, E., C. T. Merrill, and C. A. Steiner. "Hospital Stays Related to Asthma, 2006 HCUP Statistical Brief # 58," August 2008.

15. Sharieff, G. Q. and P. L. Hendry. "Afebrile Pediatric Seizures." *Emerg Med Clin North Am* 29 (2011): 95–108.

16. Colletti, J. E., K. M. Brown, G. Q. Sharieff, et al. "The Management of Children with Gastroenteritis and Dehydration in the Emergency Department." *J Emerg Med* 38 (2010): 686–698.

17. Clarke, W., T. Jones, A. Rewers, et al. "Assessment and Management of Hypoglycemia in Children and Adolescents with Diabetes." *Pediatr Diabetes* 10 (Suppl) (2009): 134–145.

18. Klimo, P., Jr., M. L. Ware, N. Gupta, and D. Brockmeyer. "Cervical Spine Trauma in the Pediatric Patient." *Neurosurg Clin N Am* 18 (2007): 599–620.

19. Scaife, E. R. and K. D. Statler. "Traumatic Brain Injury: Preferred Methods and Targets for Resuscitation." *Curr Opin Pediatr* 22 (2010): 339–345.

20. Hall, K. L. and B. Zalman. "Evaluation and Management of Apparent Life-Threatening Events in Children." *Am Fam Physician* 15 (2005): 2301–2308.

21. Sanddal, T. L., T. Loyacono, and N. D. Sanddal. "Effect of JumpSTART Training on Immediate and Short-Term Pediatric Triage Performance." *Pediatr Emerg Care* 20 (2004): 749–753.

22. Child Abuse. "Medline Plus/United States National Library of Medicine." [Available at http://www.nlm.nih.gov/medlineplus/childabuse.html]

23. Child Abuse. "ChildAbuse.com." [Available at http://www.childabuse.com/]

FURTHER READING

American Academy of Pediatrics. *Pediatric Education for Prehospital Professionals*. 2nd ed. Sudbury, MA: Jones and Bartlett Publishers, 2006.

American Heart Association. *2010 American Heart Association Guidelines for CPR and ECC*. Dallas, TX: American Heart Association, 2010.

American Heart Association and American Academy of Pediatrics. *PALS Provider Manual*. Dallas, TX: American Heart Association, 2011.

Gausche-Hill, M., et al. *Pediatric Airway Management for the Prehospital Professional*. Sudbury, MA: Jones and Bartlett Publishers, 2004.

Markenson, D. S. *Pediatric Prehospital Care*. Upper Saddle River, NJ: Pearson/Prentice Hall, 2002.

Porter, R. S., et al. *The Merck Manual of Diagnosis and Therapy*. 19th ed. Whitehouse Station, NJ: Merck, Sharp, and Dohme, 2011.

Romig, L. E. The JumpSTART Pediatric MCI Triage Tool and Other Pediatric and Disaster Emergency Management Resources. [Available at http://www.jumpstarttriage.com/]

Strange, G., et al. *Pediatric Emergency Medicine*. 3rd ed. New York: McGraw-Hill, 2009.

5 Geriatrics

Bryan Bledsoe, DO, FACEP, FAAEM, EMT-P

STANDARD
Special Patient Populations (Geriatrics)

COMPETENCY
Integrates assessment findings with principles of epidemiology and pathophysiology and knowledge of psychosocial needs to formulate a field impression and implement a comprehensive treatment/disposition plan for patients with special needs.

OBJECTIVES

Terminal Performance Objective
After reading this chapter, you should be able to integrate patient assessment findings, patient history, and knowledge of anatomy, physiology, pathophysiology, and basic and advanced life support interventions to recognize and manage emergencies in geriatric patients.

Enabling Objectives
To accomplish the terminal performance objective, you should be able to:

1. Define key terms introduced in this chapter.
2. Describe the epidemiology and demographics of aging.
3. Anticipate psychosocial challenges in the elderly population.
4. Identify government and community resources for the elderly.
5. Anticipate complex interactions between the effects of aging on the body systems and multiple disease processes in elderly patients.
6. Explain the special considerations that necessitate maintaining a high index of suspicion for toxicologic emergencies in the elderly, including specific classes of medications that commonly result in toxicity.
7. Describe special considerations for the elderly patient regarding mobility and falls, communication difficulties, and continence and elimination.
8. Describe the importance of performing a general health assessment when caring for elderly patients.
9. Adapt the scene size-up, primary assessment, patient history, secondary assessment, and use of monitoring technology to meet the needs of geriatric patients.
10. Anticipate common medical problems in the elderly.
11. Describe special considerations in the elderly that necessitate maintaining a high index of suspicion for environmental emergencies.
12. Describe special considerations in the elderly that necessitate maintaining a high index of suspicion for behavioral and psychiatric problems, including risk of suicide.
13. Describe special considerations in the elderly that increase the risk of particular injuries and impair the elderly patient's physiologic response to injuries.

14. Relate the pathophysiology of specific geriatric problems to the priorities of patient assessment and management.

15. Adapt equipment and techniques of management to meet the needs of geriatric patients.

16. Recognize indications of abuse or neglect of a geriatric patient.

17. Communicate relevant patient information orally and in writing when transferring care of the geriatric patient to hospital personnel.

KEY TERMS

acute respiratory distress syndrome (ARDS), p. 176
advance directive, p. 142
ageism, p. 140
Alzheimer's disease, p. 164
aneurysm, p. 161
ankylosing spondylitis, p. 169
anorexia nervosa, p. 149
anoxic hypoxemia, p. 153
aortic dissection, p. 161
aphasia, p. 164
assisted living, p. 141
autonomic dysfunction, p. 162
brain ischemia, p. 163
cataracts, p. 150
comorbidity, p. 146
congregate care, p. 141
delirium, p. 164
dementia, p. 164
dysphagia, p. 146
dysphoria, p. 175
elderly, p. 140
epistaxis, p. 162
fibrosis, p. 154
functional impairment, p. 145
geriatric abuse, p. 177
geriatrics, p. 140

gerontology, p. 140
glaucoma, p. 150
glomerulonephritis, p. 170
heatstroke, p. 170
hepatomegaly, p. 161
herpes zoster, p. 167
hiatal hernia, p. 156
hypertrophy, p. 154
hypochondriasis, p. 175
immune senescence, p. 157
incontinence, p. 147
intracerebral hemorrhage, p. 163
intractable, p. 163
kyphosis, p. 153
life-care community, p. 141
maceration, p. 168
Marfan syndrome, p. 155
melena, p. 167
Ménière's disease, p. 150
mesenteric ischemia or infarct, p. 166
nephrons, p. 156
nocturia, p. 161
old-old, p. 140
osteoarthritis, p. 168
osteoporosis, p. 156
Parkinson's disease, p. 165

personal-care home, p. 141
pill-rolling motion, p. 165
polycythemia, p. 163
polypharmacy, p. 146
pressure ulcer, p. 167
pruritus, p. 167
retinopathy, p. 166
senile dementia, p. 164
Shy-Drager syndrome, p. 165
sick sinus syndrome, p. 162
silent myocardial infarction, p. 160
spondylosis, p. 179
Stokes-Adams syndrome, p. 162
stroke, p. 162
subarachnoid hemorrhage, p. 163
substance abuse, p. 174
tinnitus, p. 150
transient ischemic attack (TIA), p. 148
two-pillow orthopnea, p. 161
urosepsis, p. 170
Valsalva maneuver, p. 162
varicosities, p. 162
vertigo, p. 163

CASE STUDY

"Turnpike Rescue, respond Priority One to 957 Homestead Road for a 79-year-old female with abdominal pain."

You've just arrived on duty when this call comes in to the station. "The day is starting early," you say to a coworker. Oh well, you think. It's a good chance to teach Andrew, the paramedic student intern assigned to your crew, about elderly patients. "Hey, Andy," you call out. "What are the causes of abdominal pain in an elderly patient?"

Andy tells you that the pain could be related to any number of bowel complaints—from obstruction to simple constipation. He also mentions problems such as ulcers, urinary infections, and even trauma. He ends with a quip: "Probably isn't related to too many beers and a taco, huh?"

You've just pulled up to the house, so you let Andy's remark slide for now. A man standing in the doorway calls out: "Come quickly—I think my mother may be dying."

You and your partner allow Andy to conduct a complete scene survey. You concur with his decision that the scene is safe at the present time and enter what appears to be a well-kept home.

"Does your mother live alone?" you ask. The son, who identifies himself as Michael, replies: "Yes, Mom lives alone. She's extremely independent. She drives everywhere, even at night. She does volunteer work and still likes to travel. This past summer, she took a cruise to the Bahamas all by herself." Michael then adds, "That's why I'm so worried. I stopped in to visit, and there was Mom still in bed, crying out in pain."

On entering the patient's bedroom, you see a well-nourished elderly woman, tossing and turning on her bed. "My stomach hurts so much," she sobs. Between cries of anguish, she manages to tell you that the pain woke her up early this morning. She has not gotten out of bed since. When you ask if she has fallen recently, she says "No."

You notice that Andy has instructed your partner to place the appropriate monitors. You nod in approval and ask him to begin the primary assessment. Meanwhile, you obtain a history from the son.

Michael explains that his mom, Mrs. Hildegaard, has been very healthy. She has hypertension, but is compliant with her medication of lisinopril and hydrochlorothiazide. When you ask about allergies, Michael mentions aspirin. He knows of no changes in his mother's diet and her appetite has been good. In fact, she and his brother Allen went out to dinner last night. Michael explains that Mrs. Hildegaard was clinically depressed after the death of her husband seven years ago, but "bounced back" after therapy. She has taken no antidepressants for more than five years.

After performing a primary assessment, Andy reports: "Airway is open and clear. Breathing is slightly fast at 22 per minute, but is interspersed with crying. Lungs are clear. Skin is cool, but dry. No overt bleeding. Pupils equal and reactive, with no neuro deficits noted." He then states the vital signs as BP 154/90, pulse 110 and irregular, respirations 22 and nonlabored. SpO_2 is 97 percent on room air. On examination of the patient's abdomen, Andy found no evidence of guarding and no specific area of tenderness. Mrs. Hildegaard told him: "My stomach hurts all over, everywhere you touch."

Your partner has also established an IV line of normal saline and placed the patient on the cardiac monitor. The monitor shows atrial fibrillation with an average rate of 110 bpm.

The patient is packaged and transported to the emergency department. En route, you contact the receiving hospital.

In the ED, the attending physician orders blood work, a chest film, and an abdominal CT. Following an exploratory laparotomy, the physician admits Mrs. Hildegaard to the surgical intensive care unit. The diagnosis is an infarcted bowel. The patient's prognosis is poor.

Back at the station, you take time to address Andy's quip about the "beers and a taco." You say: "You probably know that as people age they often lose lifelong support systems, like a job or a spouse. But did you realize that the elderly sometimes turn to alcohol to relieve the pain, just like people our own age?"

You then offer some pointers for providing quality EMS care to the elderly. "The most important thing to remember about the elderly patient is that although many changes occur as a result of aging, you must avoid jumping to conclusions. Give proper attention to assessment and think about normal changes of aging versus changes as a result of disease. Provide prompt treatment because the elderly patient has less physiologic reserve than a younger patient. Once the elderly patient starts to deteriorate, the process is difficult to stop. Always remember that when complaints of abdominal pain are out of proportion to your exam, you should suspect a serious medical condition—in this case, bowel infarct."

As you walk away, you say: "So, Andy, do you want to talk about what went right with this call, and what we could have done better, while we restock the ambulance?"

"You bet," he replies.

INTRODUCTION

Aging—the gradual decline of biological functions—varies widely from one individual to another. Most people reach their biological peak in the years before age 30. For practical purposes, however, the aging process does not affect their daily lives until later years. Many of the decrements commonly ascribed to aging are caused by other factors, such as lifestyle, diet, behavior, or environment. The aging process becomes even more complicated if we remember that age-related changes in organ functions also occur at different rates. For example, a person's kidneys may decline rapidly with age while the heart remains strong, or vice versa.

As people age, they actually become less like one another, both physiologically and psychologically. Although some functional losses in old age are caused by normal age-related changes, many others result from abnormal changes, particularly disease. In assessing and treating older patients, it is important to distinguish, when possible, normal age-related changes from abnormal changes. The purpose of this chapter is to present some of the most common physiologic changes associated with aging and the implications of these changes to the quality of EMS care provided to the elderly, one of the fastest growing segments of our population.

EPIDEMIOLOGY AND DEMOGRAPHICS

The twentieth century—with its tremendous medical and technological advances—witnessed both a reduction in infant mortality rates and an increase in life expectancies. The cumulative effect was a population boom worldwide, with the greatest gains seen among people age 65 or older. During the 1900s, the population of the United States increased threefold, with the number of elderly increasing tenfold. Today, in the twenty-first century, the growing number of elderly patients presents a challenge to all health care services, including EMS, not only in terms of resources, but also in the enormous impact that aging has on our society.

Population Characteristics

America is getting older. Between 1960 and 1990, the number of elderly people in the United States nearly doubled. By late 2009, the total reached more than 40 million, with approximately 337,000 people age 95 and older. As the twenty-first century opened, demographers talked about the "graying of America," a process in which the number of elderly people is pushing up the average age of the U.S. population as a whole. The percentage of elderly Americans is expected to increase by 19 percent by 2030. Reasons for this trend include:

- The mean survival rate of older persons is increasing.
- The birth rate is declining.
- There has been an absence of major wars and other catastrophes.
- Health care and standards of living have improved significantly since World War II.

In 2030, when the post–World War II baby boomers enter their 80s, more than 70 million people will be age 65 or older. By 2040, the elderly will represent roughly 20 percent of the population. In other words, one in five Americans will be age 65 or older.

Not only will the elderly population increase in size, but its members also will live longer, which in turn will swell the number of the old-old. By 2040, the number of people age 85 and older is expected to rise by 17 percent. Whether longer life spans mean longer years of active living or longer years of disease and disability is unknown (Figure 5-1 ●).

Gerontology—the study of the effects of aging on humans—is a relatively new science. (The Gerontological Society of America was formed in 1945.) Gerontologists still do not fully understand the underlying causes of aging. However, most believe that some form of cellular damage or loss, particularly of nerve cells (neurons), is involved. The result is a general decline in the body's efficiency, such as a reduction in the size and function of most internal organs.

To treat age-related changes, physicians and other health care workers have increasingly specialized in the care of the elderly. This aspect of medicine, known as geriatrics, is essential in caring for our aging population.

The demographic changes will also affect your EMS career. Today nearly 36 percent of all EMS calls involve the elderly. The percentage is expected to grow. Therefore, you will need to be familiar with the fundamental principles of geriatrics, especially those related to advanced prehospital care. You will also need to be aware of the social issues that can affect the health and mental well-being of the elderly patients that you will be treating.

Societal Issues

For a typical working person, the retirement years can be up to one-quarter of an average life span. The years include a series of transitions, such as reduced income, relocation, and loss of friends, family members, spouse, or partner.[1]

After years of working and/or raising a family, an elderly person must not only find new roles to fulfill but, in many cases, must also overcome the societal label of "old person." Many elderly people disprove ageism—and all the stereotypes it engenders—by living happy, productive, and active lives (Figure 5-2 ●). Others, however, feel a sense of social isolation or uselessness. Physical and financial difficulties reinforce these feelings and help create an emotional context in which illnesses can occur. Therefore, successful medical treatment of elderly patients involves an understanding of the broader social situation in which they live.

Living Environments

The elderly live in both independent and dependent living environments. Many continue to live alone or with their partner well into their 80s or 90s. The "oldest" old are the most likely to live alone—and, in fact, nearly half of those age 85 and older live by themselves. The great majority of these people—an estimated 78 percent—are women. This is because married men tend to die before their wives, and widowed men tend to remarry more often than widowed women.

Poverty and Loneliness   Elderly persons living alone can be one of the most impoverished and vulnerable parts of society. Death

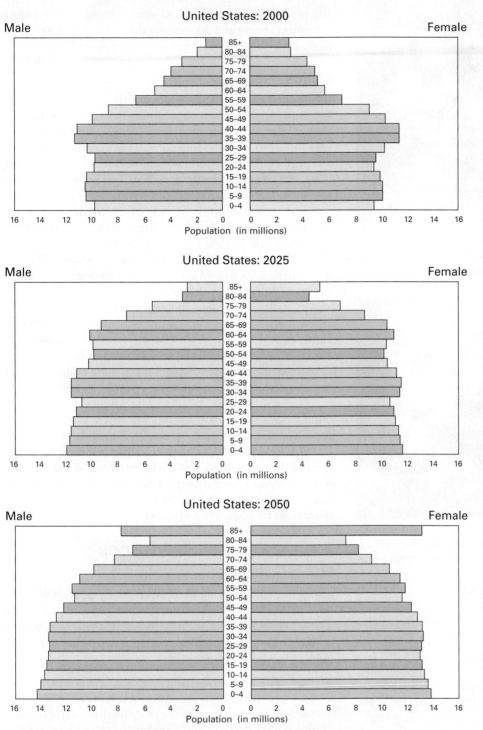

United States: 2000

Male / Female

Population (in millions)

United States: 2025

Male / Female

Population (in millions)

United States: 2050

Male / Female

Population (in millions)

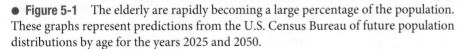

● **Figure 5-1** The elderly are rapidly becoming a large percentage of the population. These graphs represent predictions from the U.S. Census Bureau of future population distributions by age for the years 2025 and 2050.

among those who are both poor and alone.

Despite these difficulties, nearly 90 percent of the elderly who live alone choose to maintain their independence. Many fear any situation in which they would be treated as helpless human beings. Others do not want to burden family, friends, or even society with their problems. Some see their situation, including illness, as an inevitable part of aging and refuse to complain or ask for help. Keep this fact in mind whenever you question an elderly patient: The elderly often do not reveal problems beyond the chief complaint, either because they fear the loss of independence or because they consider the illnesses as "normal" for their age.

Social Support Of the elderly people who live alone and who cannot perform some everyday tasks, nearly 74 percent receive no form of assistance. To avoid the dangers of social isolation, doctors encourage the elderly to interact with other people. This helps them to build a network of social support, a factor critical to mental health and physical well-being (Figure 5-3 ●). Interaction may be with family members, neighbors, or other elderly people at senior centers. Levels of interaction can be gauged by questions such as "Is there anyone you can call if you have trouble with your medications tonight?" "Can someone stay with you when you return from the hospital?"

Among the elderly who receive help, more than 43 percent rely on paid assistance. Another 54 percent use unpaid assistance, and 3 percent use both types of help. Elderly people who turn to dependent care arrangements may choose among a variety of options, including live-in nursing, **assisted living**, **life-care communities**, **congregate care**, or **personal-care homes**. Approximately 5 percent of the elderly live in nursing homes.

of a partner reduces income sharply, especially for women whose savings are depleted by long illnesses and/or who relied on their husbands' retirement benefits. Such low incomes force the elderly to choose among such basic necessities as food, shelter, or medicine.

In addition to poverty, many of the elderly who live alone, especially the old-old, have few or no living family members. Not surprisingly, more than 60 percent of those over age 75 report feelings of loneliness. Depression is also common, particularly

Both independent and dependent living arrangements have benefits and drawbacks. Independence is an important concept. Older persons with the desire and ability to do so should be allowed to remain in their homes. Keep in mind, however, that tight finances and limited mobility may prevent an independent elderly person from maintaining adequate nutrition and safety. As a result, elderly patients may be at increased risk of accidental hypothermia, carbon monoxide

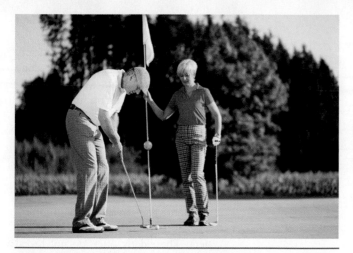

● **Figure 5-2** Many older adults live active lives, participating in sports and exercises popular among people of all ages.

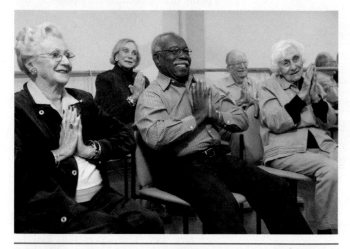

● **Figure 5-3** Many elderly people form social networks by joining a senior center or by taking part in volunteer programs.

poisoning, or fires. They may also reduce their medications, or "half dose," to save money.

Many states have few or no restrictions on personal-care aides or others who provide assistance in the home. The elderly can be at risk for criminal activities. Living in an adult community or nursing home removes some of the concerns of self-care. Trade-offs include the loss, in varying degrees, of independence; exposure to illnesses found in an institutional setting; and a lack of contact with people of varying ages, particularly the young.

As a paramedic, you may be called on to assist elderly patients in any number of environments, both independent and dependent. These conditions will be a part of the patient's history and often will play a key role in your assessment of the elderly patient. For example, a deterioration in independence is not necessarily a function of aging. It may well be a sign of an untreated illness.

Whenever you treat elderly patients, remember that illness carries a special meaning for them. They are more aware than any other age group of the potential of death. They also realize that many "curable" injuries or diseases can lead to functional impairment and a reduction in self-sufficiency. An elderly patient may recover, but be unable to meet his own needs. An EMS call is almost always a stressful event for the elderly person. Communication

and psychological support are of utmost importance in reducing patient anxiety and determining the underlying causes of the medical condition that brought you to the patient's home.

Ethics

In the course of caring for elderly patients, ethical concerns frequently arise. You may be confronted with multiple decision makers, particularly in dependent living environments. You may also have a question about the patient's competency to give informed consent or refusal of treatment. Finally, you may be faced with **advance directives**, such as "living wills" and do not resuscitate (DNR) orders (Figure 5-4 ●).[2]

These situations may be confusing to emergency care providers. In cases of multiple decision makers, you should usually honor the wishes of the patient, if he is judged competent. If a caregiver opposes treatment, keep in mind the possibility of abuse. This also applies to institutionalized settings, such as nursing homes, where an elderly patient may have been subjected to neglect.

In matters of consent, follow the same general guidelines as you would with any other patient (see Volume 1, Chapter 7). However, remain aware of the high incidence of depression and suicide in the elderly. (The topic of suicide will be discussed in greater detail later in this chapter.) If you think a patient should be transported to the hospital, make every effort to get him there.

Whenever you are presented with advance directives, you should follow state laws and local EMS system protocols. Some states have standard legal forms for DNR orders to prevent confusion. Cases in which you receive an advance directive are truly life-and-death situations. If you have any doubt about what the directive says or its legality, begin treatment and contact medical direction. In all situations involving ethical decisions, document the reasons for your choice of action.

Financing and Resources for Health Care

Caring for an increasing number of elderly patients places a huge demand on traditional health care resources, including EMS. Currently, Social Security pays a significant portion of monthly bills, with medical support provided by various major publicly funded programs:

● *Medicare.* This program basically operates as a two-part complementary system. Part A covers in-hospital care; Part B provides medical insurance to cover physicians, outpatient care, therapy, and durable medical equipment. About 95 percent of all people over age 65 are enrolled in Part A; nearly all of them are also enrolled in Part B, which is voluntary. Under Medicare, people may enroll in health maintenance organizations (HMOs) that accept Medicare benefits. In 2006 the Medicare program was expanded to cover certain prescription drugs. This program, called Part D, made it easier for Medicare beneficiaries to receive needed prescription drugs.

● *Medicaid.* Under Medicaid, the federal and state governments share responsibility for providing health care to the aged poor, people who are blind, people with disabilities, and low-income families with dependent children. Although Medicaid was created to help the poor, the high cost of medical care has

PREHOSPITAL DO NOT RESUSCITATE ORDER

ATTENDING PHYSICIAN

In completing this prehospital DNR form, please check part A if no intervention by prehospital personnel is indicated. Please check Part A and options from Part B if specific interventions by prehospital personnel are indicated. To give a valid prehospital DNR order, this form must be completed by the patient's attending physician and must be provided to prehospital personnel.

A) _____ **Do Not Resuscitate (DNR):**
No Cardiopulmonary Resuscitation or Advanced Cardiac Life Support should be performed by prehospital personnel

B) _____ **Modified Support:**
Prehospital personnel administer the following checked options:
_____ Oxygen administration
_____ Full airway support: intubation, airways, bag-valve-mask
_____ Venipuncture: IV crystalloids and/or blood draw
_____ External cardiac pacing
_____ Cardiopulmonary resuscitation
_____ Cardiac defibrillator
_____ Pneumatic anti-shock garment
_____ Ventilator
_____ ACLS meds
_____ Other interventions/medications (physician specify)
_____

Prehospital personnel are informed that (print patient name)_____
should receive no resuscitation (DNR) or should receive Modified Support as indicated. This directive is medically appropriate and is further documented by a physician's order and a progress note on the patient's permanent medical record. Informed consent from the capacitated patient or the incapacitated patient's legitimate surrogate is documented on the patient's permanent medical record. The DNR order is in full force and effect as of the date indicated below.

_____   _____
Attending Physician's Signature

_____   _____
Print Attending Physician's Name   Print Patient's Name and Location
                                           (Home Address or Health Care Facility)

_____
Attending Physician's Telephone

_____   _____
Date   Expiration Date (6 Mos from Signature)

● **Figure 5-4** An example of a do not resuscitate order.

---

brought large numbers of elderly people into the program. Today Medicaid provides the largest share of public funding for long-term care. It contributes approximately 45 percent of the financing for nursing home services.

● *Veterans Administration (VA).* The Veterans Administration offers health care to veterans with disabilities or service-related problems. It operates more than 170 hospitals and more than 100 nursing homes. Services may be provided free or on a sliding scale.

● *Local government.* In many communities, publicly funded hospitals and clinics provide care for those unable to find health care. In many instances, persons less than 65 years of age and those who do not have legal resident status are not

eligible for Medicare or Medicaid. In these instances, health care needs are met by public hospitals and clinics typically funded through taxes.

With the number of younger taxpaying workers shrinking, publicly funded medical programs face an uncertain future. A growing number of private insurers have started offering policies for long-term care during a person's older years. These policies, however, may be too expensive for many of the elderly, and younger people may not be willing to purchase them when they are young and premiums are low. Many experts worry that the booming elderly population projected for the 2030s and 2040s may have to rely increasingly on private savings, retirement plans, and state assistance in whatever form it exists.

Hospital Alternatives

One of the biggest health care debates of the early twenty-first century centers around the question of preventing death at all costs. A significant amount of health care dollars is spent during a person's last month of life, much of which is spent during the final ten days. Governmental and independent agencies have advised that it might be better to spend money on preventing disease rather than preventing death.

In an effort to bring down the cost of acute medical care, hospitals have shifted patient care increasingly to the home. The emphasis on home care, with appropriate medical and nursing assistance, has become a recognized medical practice. (See Chapter 8.) This development has gone hand in hand with the hospice movement, which allows terminally ill patients to live the remainder of their lives outside a hospital. Both trends have a deep impact on EMS personnel, who will be called on to provide more complicated care for more patients, particularly the elderly, in an out-of-hospital setting.

Prevention and Self-Help

In treating the elderly, remember that the best intervention is prevention (Table 5–1). The goal of any health care service, including EMS, should be to help keep people from becoming sick or injured in the first place. As previously mentioned, disease and disability in later life are often linked to unhealthy or unsafe behavior. As a paramedic, you can reduce morbidity among the elderly by taking part in community education programs and by cooperating with agencies or organizations that support the elderly. Some possible resources are described in the following sections.

Senior Centers   Many communities have senior centers, which provide a social atmosphere for education, recreation, and entertainment. These centers also support health care endeavors such as flu shots, blood pressure monitoring, and transport to clinics. Meals on Wheels, a program that provides from one to three meals a day, may be part of a senior volunteer organization (Figure 5-5 ●).

Religious Organizations   Religious organizations commonly serve as a resource for the elderly. Some provide services, including dependent living environments, for their members. Others keep in touch with governmental agencies, provide food or clothing for the aged poor, and offer volunteer programs in which the elderly can make useful contributions, thus reducing their sense of isolation.

National and State Associations   A number of associations serve as clearinghouses for information to aid the elderly. Some of these groups include AARP, the Alzheimer's Association, and the Association for Senior Citizens. These organizations provide significant advocacy for retired persons. They

TABLE 5–1	Prevention Strategies for the Older Person	
Issues	**Strategies**
Lifestyle	
Exercise	Weight-bearing and cardiovascular exercise (walking) for 20–30 minutes at least three times a week
Nutrition	Varies, but generally low fat, adequate fiber (complex carbohydrates), reduced sugar (simple carbohydrates), moderate protein; adequate calcium, especially for women*
Alcohol/tobacco	Moderate alcohol, if any; abstinence from tobacco
Sleep	Generally 7–8 hours a night
Accidents	
	Maintain good physical condition; add safety features to home (handrails, nonskid surfaces, lights, etc.); modify potentially dangerous driving practices (driving at night with impaired night vision, traveling in hazardous weather, etc.)
Medical Health	
Disease/illness	Routine screening for hearing, vision, blood pressure, hemoglobin, cholesterol, etc.; regular physical examinations; immunizations (tetanus booster, influenza vaccine, once-in-a-lifetime pneumococcal vaccine)
Pharmacologic	Regular review of prescriptive and over-the-counter medications, focusing on potential interactions and side effects
Dental	Regular dental checkups and good oral hygiene (important for nutrition and general well-being)
Mental/emotional	Observe for evidence of depression, disrupted sleep patterns, psychosocial stress; ensure effective support networks and availability of psychotherapy; compliance with prescribed antidepressants

*Vitamin supplements may be required, but should be taken only after other medications are reviewed and in correct dosages. Excessive doses of vitamin A or D, for example, can be toxic.

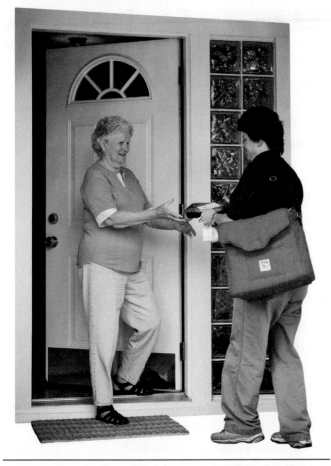

● **Figure 5-5** Meals on Wheels helps ensure that elderly people receive adequate nutrition by providing from one to three meals a day.

often have local chapters within a county or region and usually maintain web pages where elderly patients can access information from their homes. AARP is one of the largest, most visible, and most politically connected nonprofit organizations in the world today advocating for the elderly.

Governmental Agencies   A wide range of services can be found through governmental agencies, such as the Department of Health and Human Services. Many areas maintain an office for the aging, which refers the elderly to a wide range of community programs, including nutrition centers, senior citizen law projects, home-care services, senior citizen discount programs, and transportation services.

Familiarize yourself with agencies and organizations in your area that work with the elderly. They can be found through use of the Internet, the Department of Health, or special pages in the telephone book, usually at the front or in the Yellow Pages under the heading "Senior Citizens." You can either pass this information on to elderly patients, as needed, or work with one of these groups to initiate programs such as free blood pressure checks (Figure 5-6 ●). You might also start a prevention program that helps the elderly to safeguard their environment against fires, theft, carbon monoxide poisoning, or extremes in temperature.

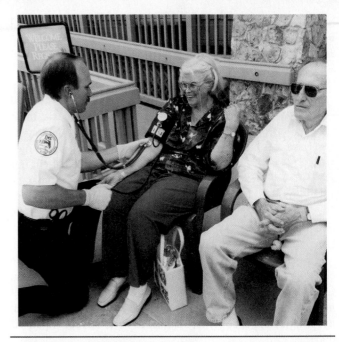

● **Figure 5-6**   In some communities, paramedics offer free medical screening programs, such as blood pressure checks, to the elderly. (© *Craig Jackson/In the Dark Photography*)

GENERAL PATHOPHYSIOLOGY, ASSESSMENT, AND MANAGEMENT

In treating elderly patients, it is important to recall several facts. First, medical disorders in the elderly often present as **functional impairment** and should be treated as an early warning of a possibly undetected medical problem. Second, signs and symptoms do not necessarily point to the underlying cause of the problem or illness. For example, whereas confusion often indicates a brain disease in younger patients, this may not be the case in an elderly patient. The confused patient may be suffering from a wide range of disorders, including drug toxicity, malnutrition, or accidental hypothermia.

A thorough evaluation must always be done to detect possible causes of an impairment. If identified early, an environmental- or disease-generated impairment can often be reversed. Your success depends on a knowledge of age-related changes and the implications of these changes for patient assessment and management.

Pathophysiology of the Elderly Patient

As mentioned, patients become less like one another as they enter their elderly years. Even so, certain generalizations can be made about age-related changes and the disease process in the elderly.

Multiple-System Failure

There is no escaping the fact that the body becomes less efficient with age, increasing the likelihood of malfunction. The body is susceptible to all the disorders of young people, but its

CONTENT REVIEW

► Common Complaints in the Elderly

- Fatigue/weakness
- Dizziness/vertigo/syncope
- Falls
- Headaches
- Insomnia
- Dysphagia
- Loss of appetite
- Inability to void
- Constipation/diarrhea

maintenance, defense, and repair processes are weaker. As a result, the elderly often suffer from more than one illness or disease at a time. On average, six medical disorders may coexist in an elderly person—and perhaps even more in the old-old. Neither the patient nor the patient's doctor may be aware of all these problems. Furthermore, disease in one organ system may result in the deterioration of other systems, compounding existing acute and/or chronic conditions.

Because of concomitant diseases (comorbidity) in the elderly, complaints may not be specific to any one disorder. Common complaints of the elderly include fatigue and weakness, dizziness/vertigo/syncope, falls, headaches, insomnia, dysphagia, loss of appetite, inability to void, and constipation/diarrhea.

Elderly patients often accept medical problems as a part of aging and fail to monitor changes in their condition. In some cases, such as a silent myocardial infarction, pain may be diminished or absent. In others, an important complaint, such as constipation, may seem trivial.

Although many medical problems in the young and middle-aged populations present with a standard set of signs and symptoms, the changes involved in aging lead to different presentations. In pneumonia, for example, the classic symptom of fever is often absent in the elderly. Chest pain and a cough are also less common. Finally, many cases of pneumonia among the elderly are caused by aspiration, not infection. The presentation of pneumonia and other diseases commonly found in the elderly will be covered later in this chapter.

Pharmacology in the Elderly

The existence of multiple chronic diseases in the elderly leads to the use of multiple medications. Persons age 65 and older use one-third of all prescription drugs in the United States, taking an average of 4.5 medications per day. This does not include over-the-counter (OTC) medications, vitamin supplements, or herbal remedies.

If medications are not correctly monitored, polypharmacy can lead to a number of problems among the elderly. In general, a person's sensitivity to drugs increases with age. When compared with younger patients, the elderly experience more adverse drug reactions, more drug–drug interactions, and more drug–disease interactions. Because of age-related pharmacokinetic changes such as a loss of body fluid and atrophy of organs, drugs concentrate more readily in the plasma and tissues of elderly patients. As a result, drug dosages often must be adjusted to prevent toxicity.[3] (The problem of toxicity is discussed in more detail later in this chapter.)

In taking a medical history of an elderly patient, remember to ask questions to determine whether a patient is taking a prescribed medication as directed. Noncompliance with drug therapy—usually underadherence—is common among

the elderly. Up to 40 percent do not take medications as prescribed. Of these individuals, 35 percent experience some type of medical problem. Factors that can decrease compliance in the elderly include:

- Limited income
- Memory loss owing to decreased or diseased neural activity
- Limited mobility
- Sensory impairment (cannot hear/read/understand directions)
- Multiple or complicated drug therapies
- Fear of toxicity
- Childproof containers (especially with arthritic patients)
- Duration of drug therapy (the longer the therapy, the less likely a patient will stick with it)

Factors that can increase compliance among the elderly include:

- Good patient–physician communication
- Belief that a disease or illness is serious
- Drug calendars or reminder cards
- Compliance counseling
- Blister-pack or other easy-to-open packaging (Figure 5-7 ●)
- Multiple-compartment pillboxes
- Transportation services to pharmacy
- Clear, simple directions written in large type
- Ability to read

Problems with Mobility and Falls

Regular exercise and a good diet are two of the most effective preventive measures for ensuring mobility among the elderly. However, not all elderly people take these measures. They may suffer from severe medical problems, such as crippling arthritis. They may fear for their personal safety, either from accidental

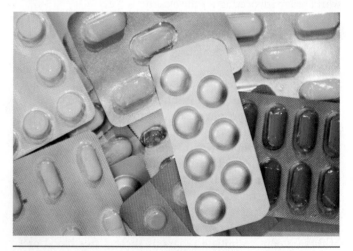

● **Figure 5-7** "Childproof" pill vials are sometimes "elder-proof" as well. Blister-pack packaging makes it easier for elderly patients, especially those suffering from arthritis, to take their medicines, thus furthering compliance.

injury or intentional injury, such as robbery. Certain medications also may increase their lethargy. Whatever the cause, a lack of mobility can have detrimental physical and emotional effects. Some of these include:

- Poor nutrition
- Difficulty with elimination
- Poor skin integrity
- A greater predisposition for falls
- Loss of independence and/or confidence
- Depression from "feeling old"
- Isolation and lack of a social network

Falls present an especially serious problem for the elderly. Fall-related injuries represent the leading cause of accidental death among the elderly and the seventh highest cause of death overall. Only children and young adults have a higher incidence of falls. However, unlike the elderly, children and young adults rarely die from fall-related injuries.

Falls may be either intrinsic (related to the patient) or extrinsic (related to the environment). Intrinsic factors include a history of repeated falls, dizziness, a sense of weakness, impaired vision, an altered gait, CNS problems, decreased mental status, or use of certain medications. Extrinsic factors include environmental hazards such as slippery floors, a lack of handrails, or loose throw rugs (Table 5–2).

In assessing an elderly patient who has fallen, remember that a fall can result from any of multiple causes. An overmedicated patient, for example, may trip over a throw rug. A fall may also be a presenting sign of an acute illness, such as a myocardial infarction, or a sign that a chronic illness has worsened. Bear in mind the possibility of physical abuse, especially if the injury does not match the story.

Communication Difficulties

Most elderly patients suffer from some form of age-related sensory changes. Normal physiologic changes may include impaired vision or blindness, impaired or loss of hearing, an altered sense of taste or smell, and/or a lower sensitivity to pain (touch). Any of these conditions can affect your ability to communicate with the patient. Table 5–3 lists some communication strategies you can use with elderly patients. (A discussion on the implications of sensory impairment on patient assessment appears later in this chapter.)

Problems with Continence and Elimination

The elderly often find it embarrassing to talk about problems with continence and elimination. They may feel stigmatized, isolated, and/or helpless. When confronted with these problems, *do not* make a big deal out of them. Respect the patient's dignity and assure the person that, in many cases, the problem is treatable.

Incontinence The problem of incontinence can affect nearly any age group, but is most commonly associated with the elderly. Incontinence may be either urinary or fecal. An estimated 15 percent of the elderly who live at home experience

TABLE 5–2	Making a Home Safe for the Elderly		
Hazard	**Intervention**	**Reason**
Torn or slippery rugs	Repair or replace.	To prevent tripping or slipping
Chair without armrests	Install armrests.	To provide leverage in getting out of chair
Chair with low back	Replace with chair with high backs.	To support neck; prevent falling backward for patients who must rock to get out of a chair
Chair with wheels	Replace with chair with sturdy legs.	To prevent chair from sliding when elder is getting into or out of it
Obstructing furniture	Move items so that clutter is minimized and pathways are clear.	To help those with poor mobility and poor peripheral vision
Slippery bathtub	Install skid-resistant strips or mat.	To provide more stable footing
Dim lighting	Provide adequate lighting in all areas, perhaps with automatic timers.	To improve ability to see, especially in darkened rooms and at night
High cabinet shelves	Place frequently used items on lower shelves or in easy-to-reach places.	To eliminate unnecessary reaching or climbing
Missing handrails on stairways	Install handrail.	To allow elder to grab onto railing for support
High steps on stairways	Rebuild for a rise of less than 6 inches between steps or install a ramp.	To reduce the risk of tripping, falling, or overexertion (especially for cardiac or pulmonary patients)

TABLE 5–3 | Age-Related Sensory Changes and Implications for Communication

Sensory Change	Result	Communication Strategy
Clouding and thickening of lens in eye	Cataracts; poor vision, especially peripheral vision	Position yourself in front of patient where you can be seen; put hand on arm of blind patient to let patient know where you are; locate a patient's glasses, if necessary.
Shrinkage of structure in ear	Decreased hearing, especially ability to hear high-frequency sounds; diminished sense of balance	Speak clearly; check hearing aids as necessary; write notes if necessary; allow the patient to put on the stethoscope, while you speak into it like a microphone.
Deterioration of teeth and gums	Patient needs dentures, but they may inflict pain on sensitive gums, so patient doesn't always wear them	If patient's speech is unintelligible, ask patient to put in dentures, if possible.
Lowered sensitivity to pain and altered sense of taste and smell	Patient underestimates the severity of the problem or is unable to provide a complete pertinent history	Probe for significant symptoms, asking questions aimed at functional impairment.

some form of urinary incontinence. Nearly 30 percent of the hospitalized elderly and 50 percent of those living in nursing homes suffer from the same condition. Although fecal, or bowel, incontinence is less common, it seriously impairs activity and may lead to dependent care. Between 16 and 60 percent of the institutionalized elderly have some kind of fecal incontinence.

Incontinence can lead to a variety of conditions, such as rashes, skin infections, skin breakdown (ulcers), urinary tract infections, sepsis, and falls or fractures. The condition can also take a high emotional toll on both the patient and the caregiver. Management of incontinence costs billions of dollars each year.

In general, effective continence requires several physical conditions. These include:

● An anatomically correct GI/GU tract

● Competent sphincter mechanism

● Adequate cognition and mobility

Although incontinence is not necessarily caused by aging, several factors predispose older patients to this condition. As mentioned, the elderly tend to have several medical disorders, each of which may require drug therapy. These disorders and/or the drugs used to treat them may compromise the integrity of either the urinary or bowel tracts. In addition, bladder capacity, urinary flow rate, and the ability to postpone voiding appear to decline with age. Certain diseases, such as diabetes and autonomic neuropathy, may also cause sphincter dysfunction. Diarrhea or lack of physical sensation may produce bowel incontinence as well.

Management of incontinence depends on the cause, which cannot be easily diagnosed in the field. Some cases of incontinence can be managed surgically. In most cases, however, patients use some type of absorptive devices, such as leakproof underwear or panty liners. Indwelling catheters are less common and may cause infections when used, particularly if not properly managed. Of critical importance is respect for the patient's modesty and dignity.

Elimination   Difficulty with elimination can be a sign of a serious underlying condition (Table 5–4). It can also lead to other complications. Straining to eliminate may have serious effects on the cerebral, coronary, and peripheral arterial circulations. In elderly people with cerebrovascular disease or impaired baroreceptor reflexes, efforts to force a bowel movement can lead to a **transient ischemic attack (TIA)** or syncope. In the case of prolonged constipation, the elderly may experience colonic ulceration, intestinal obstruction, and urinary retention.

In assessing a patient with difficulty eliminating, remember to inquire about his medications. Any of the following drugs can cause constipation:

● Opioids

● Anticholinergics (e.g., antidepressants, antihistamines, muscle relaxants, antiparkinsonian drugs)

TABLE 5–4 | Possible Causes of Elimination Problems

Difficulty in Urination	Difficulty with Bowel Movements
Enlargement of the prostate in men	Diverticular disease
Urinary tract infection	Constipation*
Acute or chronic renal failure	Colorectal cancer

*Constipation may be related to dietary, medical, or surgical conditions. It could also be the result of a malignancy, intestinal obstruction, or hypothyroidism. Treat constipation as a serious medical problem.

- Cation-containing agents (e.g., antacids, calcium supplements, iron supplements)
- Neurally active agents (e.g., opiates, anticonvulsants)
- Diuretics

Assessment Considerations

As with all patients, be sure to take Standard Precautions when assessing an elderly patient. Because of the increased risk of tuberculosis in patients who are in nursing homes, consider wearing a HEPA or N-95 respirator. Remain alert to the environment, particularly the temperature of the surroundings and evidence of prescription medications.

In general, assessment of the elderly patient follows the same basic approach used with any patient. However, you need to keep in mind several factors that will improve the quality of your evaluation and make subsequent treatment more successful.

General Health Assessment

As already mentioned, you need to set a context for illness when assessing an elderly patient. When performing a general health assessment, take into account the patient's living situation, level of activity, network of social support, level of independence, medication history (both prescription and nonprescription), and sleep patterns.

Pay particular attention to the patient's nutrition. Elderly patients often have a decreased sense of smell and taste, which decreases their pleasure in eating. They also may be less aware of internal cues of hunger and thirst. Although caloric requirements generally decrease with age, an elderly patient can still suffer from malnutrition. Conditions that may complicate or discourage eating among the elderly include:

- Breathing or respiratory problems
- Abdominal pain
- Nausea/vomiting, sometimes a drug-induced condition as with antibiotics or aspirin
- Poor dental care
- Medical problems, such as hyperthyroidism, hypercalcemia, and chronic infections (e.g., cancer or tuberculosis)
- Medications (e.g., digoxin, vitamin A, fluoxetine)
- Alcohol or drug abuse
- Psychological disorders, including depression and **anorexia nervosa**
- Poverty
- Problems with shopping or cooking

As with any person, nutrition greatly affects a patient's overall health. For the reasons just cited, patients may suffer from a number of by-products of malnutrition, including vitamin deficiencies, dehydration, and hypoglycemia. Also remember that when a malnourished elderly person is fed, the food may produce other side effects, including electrolyte abnormalities, hyperglycemia, aspiration pneumonia, and a significant drop in blood pressure.

Pathophysiology and Assessment

Assessment of the elderly reflects the pathophysiology of this age group. As already mentioned, the chief complaint of the elderly patient may seem trivial or vague at first. Also, the patient may fail to report important symptoms. Therefore, you should try to distinguish the patient's chief complaint from the patient's primary problem. A patient may report nausea, which is the chief complaint. The primary problem, however, may be the rectal bleeding that the patient neglected to mention.

The presence of multiple diseases also complicates the assessment process. The presence of chronic problems may make it more difficult to assess an acute problem. It is easy to confuse symptoms from a chronic illness with those of an acute condition. When confronted with an elderly patient who has chest pain, for example, it is difficult to determine whether the presence of frequent premature ventricular contractions is acute or chronic. If you lack access to the patient's medical record, you should treat the patient on a "threat-to-life" basis.

Other complications stem from age-related changes in an elderly patient's response to illness and injury. Pain may be diminished, causing both you and the patient to underestimate the severity of the primary problem. In addition, the temperature-regulating mechanism may be altered or depressed. This

CONTENT REVIEW

▶ Factors in Forming a General Assessment

- Living situation
- Level of activity
- Network of social support
- Level of independence
- Medication history
- Sleep patterns

CULTURAL CONSIDERATIONS

How Well Are They Living?

Unfortunately, many elderly persons are economically disadvantaged. In fact many, especially elderly women, live at or below the poverty line. The reasons for this are many. Most important, these persons are likely to live on a fixed income—from retirement pensions and/or Social Security benefits. Although this income remains fixed, the cost of living continues to increase. Thus, some elderly persons must make decisions as to what they can and cannot afford. Some will forgo certain medications. Others will try to live with reduced heating or cooling to save energy costs. Unfortunately, others will forgo food to maintain their independence.

When called to assess geriatric patients, try to get an idea about how well they are living. Is the house unusually hot or cold? Are they forgoing certain medications that they consider to be too expensive? Is the house safe and clean? Are they eating well? Are they able and motivated to prepare meals for themselves? Most important, do family members or friends periodically check in on them? If you have any concerns, you should notify the proper authorities or the hospital staff so that social services can provide an evaluation to ensure that these persons can live safely in their present setting.

can result in the absence of fever, or a minimal fever, even in the face of a severe infection. Alterations in the temperature-regulating mechanism, coupled with changes in the sweat glands, also makes the elderly more prone to environmental thermal problems.

Because of the complexity of factors that can affect assessment, you must probe for significant symptoms and, ultimately, the primary problem. Patience, respect, and kindness will elicit the answers needed for a pertinent medical history.

History

You should be prepared to spend more time obtaining histories from elderly patients. You may need to split the interview into sessions. For example, you might need to allow patients time to rest if they become fatigued during the interview, or you might take a break to talk with caregivers.

When gathering the history, keep in mind the complications that arise from multiple diseases and multiple medications. Medications can be an especially important indicator of the patient's diseases. Therefore, you should find the patient's medications and take them to the hospital with the patient. Try to determine which of the medications, including OTC medications, are currently being taken. In cases of multiple medications, there is an increased incidence of medication errors, drug interactions, and noncompliance.

Communication Challenges As previously mentioned, communication may be more difficult when dealing with the aged. **Cataracts** (Figure 5-8 ●) and **glaucoma** can diminish sight. Cataracts cause clouding of the lens, leading to impairments in

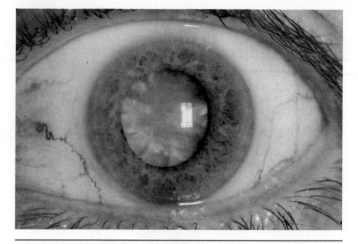

● **Figure 5-9**   A clearly visible mature cataract. (*National Eye Institute, National Institutes of Health*)

vision (Figure 5-9 ●). Blindness, often resulting from diabetes and stroke, is more common in the elderly. The level of anxiety increases when a patient is unable to see his surroundings clearly. As a result, you should talk calmly to patients with visual impairments. Yelling does not help. Instead, position yourself so the patient can see (if he is not totally blind) or touch you.

Age also affects hearing. Overall hearing decreases and patients may suffer from auditory disorders such as **tinnitus** or **Ménière's disease**. Diminished hearing or deafness can make it virtually impossible to obtain a history. In such cases, try to determine the history from a friend or family member. *Do not* shout at the patient. This will not help if the patient is deaf, and it may distort sounds and make it difficult for the patient who still has some hearing to understand you. Write notes if necessary. If the patient can lip-read, speak slowly and directly toward the patient. Whenever possible, verify the history with a reliable source. Also, because loss of hearing may result from other causes (such as a buildup of earwax), confirm whether deafness is a preexisting condition.

Patients may also have trouble with speech. They find it difficult to retrieve words. They will often speak slowly and exhibit changes in voice quality, which may be a normal age-related change. If a patient has forgotten to put in dentures, politely ask him to do so.

To improve your skill at communicating with the elderly, keep these techniques in mind:

● Always introduce yourself.

● Speak slowly, distinctly, and respectfully.

● Speak to the patient first, rather than to family members, caregivers, or bystanders.

● Speak face to face, at eye level with eye contact (Figure 5-10 ●).

● Locate the patient's hearing aid or eyeglasses, if needed (Figure 5-11 ●).

● Allow the patient to put on the stethoscope, while you speak into it like a microphone.

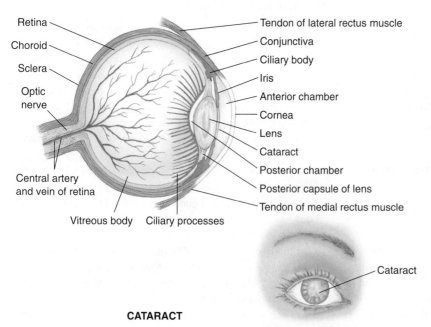

Retina
Choroid
Sclera
Optic nerve
Central artery and vein of retina
Vitreous body   Ciliary processes
Tendon of lateral rectus muscle
Conjunctiva
Ciliary body
Iris
Anterior chamber
Cornea
Lens
Cataract
Posterior chamber
Posterior capsule of lens
Tendon of medial rectus muscle

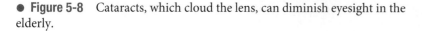

Cataract

CATARACT

● **Figure 5-8**   Cataracts, which cloud the lens, can diminish eyesight in the elderly.

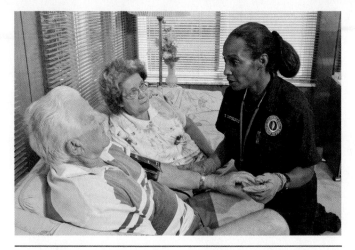

● **Figure 5-10**   If possible, talk *to* the elderly patient rather than talking about the patient to others.

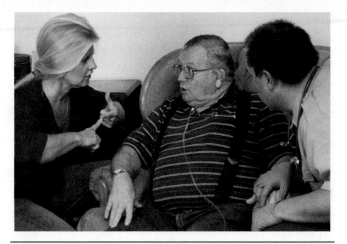

● **Figure 5-11**   Make sure the elderly patient is wearing his eyeglasses and hearing aids, if required.

- Turn on the room lights.
- Display verbal and nonverbal signs of concern and empathy.
- Remain polite at all times.
- Preserve the patient's dignity.
- Do not be afraid to rephrase a question or ask the patient again if you could not understand or hear the patient.
- Always explain what you are doing and why.
- Use your power of observation to recognize anxiety—tempo of speech, eye contact, tone of voice—during the telling of the history.

Altered Mental Status and Confusion Remember that age sometimes diminishes mental status. The patient can be confused and unable to remember details. In addition, the noise of radios, ECG equipment, and strange voices may add to the confusion. Both senility and organic brain syndrome may manifest themselves similarly. Common symptoms include:

- Delirium
- Confusion
- Distractibility
- Restlessness
- Excitability
- Hostility

When confronted with a confused patient, try to determine whether the patient's mental status represents a significant change from normal. *Do not* assume that a confused, disoriented patient is "just senile," thus failing to assess for a serious underlying problem (Figure 5-12 ●). Alcoholism, for example, is more common

in the elderly than was once recognized. It can further complicate taking the history.

Another complication results from depression, which can be mistaken for many other disorders. It can often mimic senility and organic brain syndrome. Depression may also inhibit patient cooperation. The depressed patient may be malnourished, dehydrated, overdosed, contemplating suicide, or simply imagining physical ailments to gain attention. If you suspect depression, question the patient regarding drug ingestion or suicidal ideation. It is important to remember that suicide is a common cause of death among the elderly in the United States.

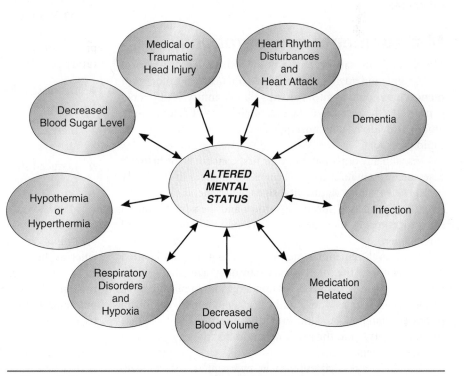

● **Figure 5-12**   *Do not* assume that an altered mental status is a normal age-related change. A number of serious underlying problems may be responsible for changes in consciousness.

Concluding the History After obtaining the history, and if time allows, try to verify the patient's history with a credible source. This will often be less offensive to the patient if done out of his presence. While at the scene, it is important to observe the surroundings for indications of the patient's self-sufficiency. Look for evidence of drug or alcohol ingestion and for MedicAlert tags, Vial of Life, or similar medical identification items. It is also important to spot signs of abuse or neglect, particularly in dependent living arrangements.

Physical Examination

Certain considerations must be kept in mind when examining the elderly patient. Remember that some patients may be easily fatigued and unable to tolerate a long examination. Also, because of the problems with temperature regulation, the patient may be wearing several layers of clothing, which can make examination difficult. Be sure to explain all actions clearly before initiating the examination, especially to patients with impaired vision. Be aware that the patient may minimize or deny symptoms because of a fear of becoming institutionalized or a loss of self-sufficiency.

Try to distinguish signs of chronic disease from an acute problem. Peripheral pulses may be difficult to evaluate, because of peripheral vascular disease and arthritis. The elderly may also have nonpathologic crackles (rales) on lung auscultation. In addition, the elderly often exhibit an increase in mouth breathing and a loss of skin elasticity, which may be easily confused with dehydration. Dependent edema may be caused by inactivity, not congestive heart failure. Only experience and practice will allow you to distinguish acute from chronic physical findings.

Management Considerations

Elderly patients can present a unique challenge in terms of assessment and management. You will need to tailor your management plan to fit a patient's illness, injury, and overall general health. Because of the potential for rapid deterioration among the elderly, you must quickly spot conditions requiring rapid transport.

As with any other patient, your first concern is the primary assessment. Remain alert at all times for changes in an elderly patient's neurologic status, vital signs, and general cardiac status. (Management of specific disorders and the administration of medications to the elderly are covered in other sections of this chapter.)

In general, remember that transport to a hospital is often more stressful for the elderly than to any other age group, except for the very young. Avoid lights and sirens in all but the most serious cases, such as when you suspect a pulmonary embolism or bowel infarction. A calm, smooth transport helps to reduce patient anxiety—and the resulting strain that anxiety places on an elderly patient's heart.

Provide emotional support at every phase of the call. Nearly any serious illness or injury in the elderly can provoke a sense of impending doom. Death is a very real possibility to this age group. To help reduce patient fears, keep these guidelines in mind:

- Encourage patients to express their feelings.
- *Do not* trivialize their fears.
- Acknowledge nonverbal messages.
- Avoid questions that are judgmental.
- Confirm what the patient says.
- Recall all you have learned about communicating with the elderly, thus avoiding communication breakdowns.
- Assure patients that you understand that they are adults on an equal footing with their care providers, including you.

SYSTEM PATHOPHYSIOLOGY IN THE ELDERLY

Although aging begins at the cellular level, it eventually affects virtually every system in the body (Figure 5-13 ●). Age-related changes in the structure and function of organs increase the probability of disease, modify the threshold at which signs and symptoms appear, and affect assessment and treatment of the elderly patient (Table 5–5). You should be familiar with normal systemic changes related to aging so that you can more easily identify the abnormal changes that may point to a serious underlying problem.

Respiratory System

The effects of aging on the respiratory system begin as early as age 30. Without regular exercise and/or training, the lungs start to lose their ability to defend themselves and to carry out their prime function of ventilation. Age-related changes in the respiratory system include:

- Decreased chest wall compliance
- Loss of lung elasticity
- Increased air trapping due to collapse of the smaller airways
- Reduced strength and endurance of the respiratory muscles

Functionally, by the time we reach age 65, vital capacity may be reduced by as much as 50 percent. In addition, the maximum breathing capacity may decrease by as much as 60 percent, whereas the maximum oxygen uptake may decrease by as much as 70 percent. These changes ultimately result in decreased ventilation and progressive hypoxemia. Any presence of underlying pulmonary diseases, such as emphysema and chronic bronchitis, further reduces respiratory function.

In addition, a decrease is seen in the effective cough reflex and the activity of the cilia, the small hair-like fibers that trap particles and infectious agents. The decline of these two defense mechanisms leaves the lungs more susceptible to recurring infection.

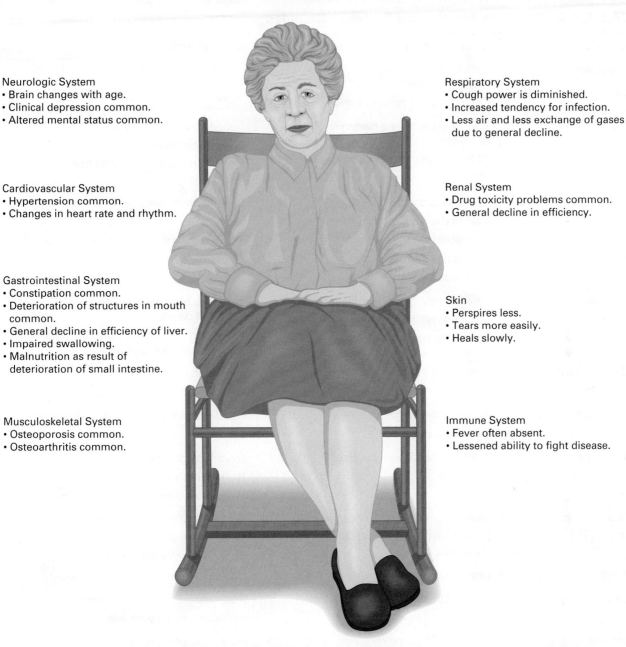

Neurologic System
• Brain changes with age.
• Clinical depression common.
• Altered mental status common.

Cardiovascular System
• Hypertension common.
• Changes in heart rate and rhythm.

Gastrointestinal System
• Constipation common.
• Deterioration of structures in mouth common.
• General decline in efficiency of liver.
• Impaired swallowing.
• Malnutrition as result of deterioration of small intestine.

Musculoskeletal System
• Osteoporosis common.
• Osteoarthritis common.

Respiratory System
• Cough power is diminished.
• Increased tendency for infection.
• Less air and less exchange of gases due to general decline.

Renal System
• Drug toxicity problems common.
• General decline in efficiency.

Skin
• Perspires less.
• Tears more easily.
• Heals slowly.

Immune System
• Fever often absent.
• Lessened ability to fight disease.

● **Figure 5-13**   Some changes in the body systems of the elderly.

Other factors that may affect pulmonary function in the elderly include:

● **Kyphosis**

● Chronic exposure to pollutants

● Long-term cigarette smoking

The management of respiratory distress in elderly patients is essentially the same as for all age groups. Position the patient for adequate breathing, usually upright or sitting. Teach breathing patterns that assist in exhalation, such as pursed-lip breathing. (Tell patients to pretend they are blowing out a candle with each exhalation.) Use bronchodilators as needed, and provide supplemental oxygen to correct hypoxia.

At all times, remain attentive for possible complications, such as **anoxic hypoxemia**. Monitor ventilations closely because an elderly patient can become easily fatigued from any increase in the work of breathing. Remember that many elderly patients with respiratory disease have underlying cardiac disease. With this in mind, drugs such as beta agonists should be used with extreme caution. Monitor cardiovascular status and administer IV fluids judiciously. *Do not* overload fluids. When infusing fluids, frequently reassess lung sounds to check for the pressure of pulmonary edema.

TABLE 5–5 | Common Age-Related Systemic Changes

Body System	Changes with Age	Clinical Importance
Respiratory	Loss of strength and coordination in respiratory muscles Cough and gag reflex reduced	Increased likelihood of respiratory failure
Cardiovascular	Loss of elasticity and hardening of arteries Changes in heart rate, rhythm, efficiency	Hypertension common Greater likelihood of strokes, heart attacks Great likelihood of bleeding from minor trauma
Neurologic	Brain tissue shrinks Loss of memory Clinical depression common Altered mental status common Impaired balance	Delay in appearance of symptoms with head injury Difficulty in patient assessment Increased likelihood of falls
Endocrine	Lowered estrogen production (women) Decline in insulin sensitivity Increase in insulin resistance	Increased likelihood of fractures (bone loss) and heart disease Diabetes mellitus common with greater possibility of hyperglycemia
Gastrointestinal	Diminished digestive functions	Constipation common Greater likelihood of malnutrition
Thermoregulatory	Reduced sweating Decreased shivering	Environmental emergencies more common
Integumentary (skin)	Thins and becomes more fragile	More subject to tears and sores Bruising more common Heals more slowly
Musculoskeletal	Loss of bone strength (osteoporosis) Loss of joint flexibility and strength (osteoarthritis)	Greater likelihood of fractures Slower healing Increased likelihood of falls
Renal	Loss of kidney size and function	Increased problems with drug toxicity
Genitourinary	Loss of bladder function	Increased urination/incontinence Increased urinary tract infection
Immune	Diminished immune response	More susceptible to infections Impaired immune response to vaccines
Hematologic	Decrease in blood volume and/or RBCs	Slower recuperation from illness/injury Greater risk of trauma-related complications

Cardiovascular System

A number of variables unrelated to aging influence cardiovascular function. They include diet, smoking and alcohol use, education, socioeconomic status, and even personality traits. Of particular importance is the level of physical activity. Even though maximum exercise capacity and maximum oxygen consumption decline with age, a well-trained elderly person can match—or even exceed—the aerobic capacity of an unconditioned younger person.

This said, the cardiovascular system still experiences age-related deterioration, in varying degrees. The wall of the left ventricle may thicken and enlarge (**hypertrophy**), often by as much as 25 percent. This is even more pronounced if there is associated hypertension. In addition, **fibrosis** develops in the heart and peripheral vascular system, resulting in hypertension, arteriosclerosis, and decreased cardiac function.

The aorta also becomes stiff and lengthens. This results from deposits of calcium and changes in the connective tissue.

These changes predispose the aorta to partial tearing, resulting in dissection (thoracic) or aneurysm (abdominal).

As a person ages, the pattern of ventricular filling changes. Less blood enters the left ventricle during early diastole when the mitral valve is open. Therefore, filling and stretch (preload) depend on atrial contraction. Loss of the atrial kick (as will occur with atrial fibrillation) is not well tolerated in the elderly.

Over time, the conductive system of the heart degenerates, often causing arrhythmias and varying degrees of heart block. Ultimately, the stroke volume declines and the heart rate slows, leading to decreased cardiac output. Because of this, the heart's ability to respond to stress diminishes. In such situations, expect exercise intolerance—that is, an inability of the heart to meet an exercising muscle's need for oxygen.

To adequately manage complaints related to the cardiovascular system, ask the patient to stop all activity. This reduces the myocardial oxygen demand. *Do not* walk a patient with a cardiovascular complaint to your ambulance. Take the following basic steps per local protocols:

- Administer oxygen if the patient is hypoxic
- Start an IV for medication administration. Medications will vary with the complaint, but may include:
  - Antianginal agents
  - Aspirin
  - Diuretics
  - Antiarrhythmics
- Inquire about age-related dosages.
- Monitor vital signs and rhythm.
- Acquire a 12-lead ECG.
- Remain calm, professional, and empathetic. A heart attack is one of the most fear-inducing situations for the elderly.

Nervous System

Unlike cells in other organ systems, nerve cells in the central nervous system cannot significantly reproduce. The brain can lose as much as 45 percent of its cells in certain areas of the cortex. Overall, people experience an average 10 percent reduction in brain weight from age 20 to age 90. Keep in mind that reductions in brain weight and ventricular size are not well correlated with intelligence, and elderly people may still be capable of highly creative and productive thought. Once again, *do not* assume that an elderly person possesses less cognitive skill than a younger person. Slight changes that may be expected include:

- Difficulty with recent memory
- Psychomotor slowing
- Forgetfulness
- Decreased reaction times

Although brain size may not have clinical implications in terms of intelligence, it does have implications for trauma.

A reduction in brain size allows mass effects (bleeding, tumors) to become larger before they become clinically significant. Thus, following a blow to the head, a subdural hematoma may take longer to manifest when compared with one in a younger person. In cases of altered mental status or seizure, maintain a suspicion of trauma, especially when an accident has been reported.

Whenever you assess an elderly patient for mental status, determine a baseline. Presume your patient to have been mentally sharp unless proven otherwise. (Talk with partners, caregivers, family members, and so on.) Focus on the patient's perceptions, thinking processes, and communication. In questioning an elderly patient, provide an environment with minimal distractions. As already mentioned, ask clear and unhurried questions.

In forming a patient plan, observe for weakness, chronic fatigue, changes in sleep patterns, and syncope or near syncope. If you suspect a stroke, assign the patient a priority status. (Additional material on strokes appears later in this chapter.) Consider blood pressure control per local protocol, but remember that perfusion of the brain tissue depends on an adequate blood pressure. In most cases, *do not* plan to reduce the blood pressure in stroke because raising the blood pressure is the body's response to increase cerebral blood flow to ensure brain perfusion. Consider the causes of changes in mental status, keeping in mind the possibility of trauma. Apply oxygen if the patient is hypoxic, monitor ventilations with capnography (if available), and continually reassess the patient.

Endocrine System

Early diagnosis of disorders in the endocrine system offers some of the greatest opportunities to prevent disabilities through appropriate hormonal therapy and/or lifestyle changes. Diabetes mellitus, for example, is extremely common among the elderly. However, normalization of glucose levels through diet, exercise, and/or drug therapy can reduce some of the devastating vascular and neurologic complications.

Thyroid disorders are "clinical masqueraders," especially in the elderly. Common signs and symptoms may be absent or diminished. When signs and symptoms are present, they may be attributed to aging or tied to other diseases, such as cardiovascular, GI, or neuromuscular disorders. However, it has been shown that thyroid disorders, especially hypothyroidism and thyroid nodules, increase with age. (For more on thyroid disorders, see the section Metabolic and Endocrine Disorders later in this chapter.)

With the exception of glucose disorders, most endocrine disorders cannot be easily determined in the field. Many endocrine emergencies will present as altered mental status, especially with insulin-related diseases. Monitor for cardiovascular effects of endocrine changes such as aortic aneurysm in a patient with **Marfan syndrome**, a disorder resulting in abnormal growth of distal tissues and a dilation of the root of the aorta. Also remain alert to blood pressure swings in thyroid disorders such as hyperthyroidism and hypothyroidism.

Gastrointestinal System

Age affects the gastrointestinal system in various ways. The volume of saliva may decrease by as much as 33 percent, leading to complaints of dry mouth, nutritional deficiencies, and a predisposition to choking. Gastric secretions may decrease to as little as 20 percent of the quantity present in younger people. Esophageal and intestinal motility also decrease, making swallowing more difficult and delaying digestive processes. The production of hydrochloric acid also declines, further disrupting digestion and, in some adults, contributing to nutritional anemia. Gums atrophy and the number of taste buds decreases, reducing even further the desire to eat.

Other conditions may also develop. **Hiatal hernias** are not age related per se, but can have serious consequences for the elderly. They may incarcerate or strangulate the contents of the hernia (esophagus, stomach), or, in the most severe cases, result in massive GI hemorrhage. Diminished liver function, which is associated with aging, can delay or impede detoxification. A common drug toxicity problem for EMS personnel is the use of various medications (e.g., amiodarone) for ventricular arrhythmias. (See the section Toxicologic Emergencies later in this chapter.) Diminished liver function can also reduce the production of clotting proteins, which in turn leads to bleeding abnormalities.

Complications in the gastrointestinal system can be life threatening. Use shock protocols as necessary, and remember that not all fluid loss occurs outside the body.

Thermoregulatory System

The elderly and infants are highly susceptible to variations in environmental temperatures. This occurs in the elderly because of altered or impaired thermoregulatory mechanisms. Aging seems to reduce the effectiveness of sweating in cooling the body. Older persons tend to sweat at higher core temperatures and have less sweat output per gland than younger people. As people age, they also experience deterioration of the autonomic nervous system, including a decrease in shivering and a lower resting peripheral blood flow. In addition, the elderly may have a diminished perception of the cold. Drugs and disease can further affect an elderly patient's response to temperature extremes, resulting in hyperthermia or accidental hypothermia.

Environmental emergencies are common causes of EMS calls, especially among the elderly living alone or in poverty. For more on these emergencies, see the discussion of heatstroke, hypothermia, and hyperthermia later in this chapter.

Integumentary System

As people age, the skin loses collagen, a connective tissue that gives elasticity and support to the skin. Without this support, the skin is subject to a greater number of injuries from bumping or tearing. The lack of support also makes it more difficult to start an IV, because the veins tend to "roll away." Furthermore, the assessment of tenting skin becomes an inaccurate indicator of fluid status in the elderly. Without elasticity, the skin often will remain tented regardless of water balance.

As the skin thins, cells reproduce more slowly. In the elderly, injury to skin is often more severe than in younger patients and healing time is increased. As a rule, the elderly are at a higher risk of secondary infection, skin tumors, drug-induced eruptions,

and fungal or viral infections. Decades of exposure to the sun also makes the elderly vulnerable to melanoma and other sun-related carcinomas (e.g., basal cell carcinoma, squamous cell carcinoma).

Musculoskeletal System

An aging person may lose as much as 2 to 3 inches of height from narrowing of the intervertebral disks and osteoporosis. Much of the height loss is caused by vertebral fractures.[4] **Osteoporosis** is the loss of mineral from the bone, resulting in softening of the bones. This is especially evident in the vertebral bodies, thus causing a change in posture. The posture of the aged individual often reveals an increase in the curvature of the thoracic spine, commonly called kyphosis, and slight flexion of the knee and hip joints. The demineralization of bone makes the patient much more susceptible to hip and other fractures. Some fractures may even occur from simple actions such as sneezing.

In addition to skeletal changes, a decrease in skeletal muscle weight commonly occurs with age, especially with sedentary individuals. To compensate, elderly women develop a narrow, short gait, whereas older men develop a wide gait. These changes make the elderly more susceptible to falls and, consequently, a possible loss of independence.

Because of the changes in the musculoskeletal system, simple trauma in the elderly can lead to complex injuries. In treating musculoskeletal disorders, supply supplemental oxygen (if the patient is hypoxic), initiate an IV line, and consider pain control. Many extremity injuries should be splinted as found because of changes in the bone and joint structure of the elderly. To determine the cause of any injury, be sure to look beyond the obvious. Keep in mind the possibility of underlying medical conditions, drug complications, abuse or neglect, and ingestion of alcohol or drugs.

Renal System

Aging affects the renal system through a reduction in the number of functioning **nephrons**, which may be decreased by 30 to 40 percent. Renal blood flow may also be reduced by up to 45 percent, increasing the waste products in the blood and upsetting the fluid and electrolyte balance. Because the kidneys are responsible for the production of erythropoietin (which stimulates the production of red blood cells in the bone marrow) and renin (which stimulates vasoconstriction), a decrease in renal function may result in anemia or hypertension in the older patient.

Prehospital treatment of complaints involving the renal and urinary systems is directed toward adequate oxygenation, fluid status, monitoring output, and pain control. Pay attention to the airway because nausea and vomiting are complications of pain secondary to renal obstruction. Monitor vital signs to detect changes in blood pressure and pulse.

Genitourinary System

As people age, they experience a progressive loss of bladder sensation and tone. The bladder does not empty completely and, consequently, the patient may sense a frequent need to urinate. This urge increases the risk of falls, especially during the middle of the night when lighting is dim or the patient is sleepy. Furthermore, the lack of emptying increases the likelihood of urinary tract infection and perhaps sepsis. In the male, the prostate often becomes enlarged (benign prostatic hypertrophy), causing difficulty in urination or urinary retention. As already mentioned, the elderly also commonly develop, in varying degrees, problems with incontinence.

Treatment for a complaint in the genitourinary system is described in the preceding section on the renal system and in the earlier discussion of incontinence.

Immune System

As a person ages, the function of T cells declines, making them less able to notify the immune system of invasion by antigens. A diminished immune response, sometimes called **immune senescence**, increases the susceptibility of the elderly to infections. It also increases the duration and severity of an infection.

Barring contraindications, the elderly should receive vaccinations suggested by the health department. However, keep in mind that aging impairs the immune response to vaccines. The best prevention is adequate nutrition, infection control measures (e.g., washing hands), and exercise. Recognition and treatment of diseases such as diabetes mellitus, heart failure, thyroid disease, and occult malignancy also reduce the risk and severity of infections. As a paramedic, you should treat alterations in immune status as life threats and seek to prevent exposure of patients to infectious agents. Take necessary precautions so that you *do not* transmit an illness—even a mild cold—to an elderly patient.

Hematologic System

The hematologic system is affected by a failure of the renal system to stimulate the production of red blood cells (RBCs). Changing coagulation factors and vessel damage increase the chance of thromboembolic events in the elderly. Nutritional abnormalities may also produce abnormal RBCs. Because the elderly have less body water, blood volume is decreased. This makes it difficult for an elderly patient to recuperate from an illness or injury. Intervention must be started early in order to make a lasting difference.

In addition to providing supplemental oxygen if the patient is hypoxic, you should prepare for increases in bleeding time. Monitor the elderly patient closely because deterioration is difficult to stop.

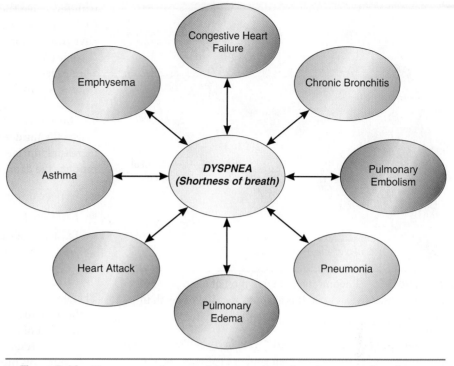

● **Figure 5-14** Dyspnea can be caused by a number of respiratory and cardiac problems in the elderly.

COMMON MEDICAL PROBLEMS IN THE ELDERLY

In general, the elderly suffer from the same kinds of medical emergencies as younger patients. However, illnesses may be more severe, complications more likely, and classic signs and symptoms absent or altered. In addition, the elderly are more likely to react adversely to stress and deteriorate much more quickly than young or middle-aged adults. The following are some of the medical disorders that you may encounter.

Pulmonary/Respiratory Disorders

Respiratory emergencies are some of the most common reasons elderly persons summon EMS or seek emergency care. Most elderly patients with a respiratory disorder present with a chief complaint of dyspnea. However, coughing, congestion, and wheezing are also common chief complaints.

Many factors can trigger respiratory distress among the elderly (Figure 5-14 ●). Descriptions of the most common ones follow.

Pneumonia

Pneumonia is an infection of the lung. It is usually caused by a bacterium or virus. However, aspiration pneumonia may also develop as a result of difficulty swallowing.

Pneumonia is a serious disease for the elderly. It is the seventh-leading cause of death in people age 65 and older. Its incidence increases with age at a rate of 10 percent for each decade beyond age 20. It is found in up to 60 percent of the

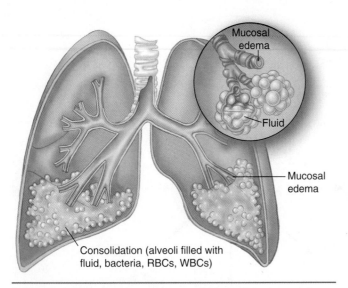

Consolidation (alveoli filled with fluid, bacteria, RBCs, WBCs)

● **Figure 5-15** Pneumonia is an infection of the lung or lungs usually caused by bacteria. It is a common cause of death in the elderly.

autopsies performed on the elderly. Reasons the elderly develop pneumonia more frequently than younger patients include:

● Decreased immune response

● Reduced pulmonary function

● Increased colonization of the pharynx by Gram-negative bacteria

● Abnormal or ineffective cough reflex

● Decreased effectiveness of mucociliary cells of the upper respiratory system (Figure 5-15 ●)

The elderly who are at greatest risk for contracting pneumonia include frail adults and those with chronic, multiple diseases or compromised immunity. Institutionalized patients in hospitals or nursing homes are especially vulnerable because of increased exposure to microorganisms and limited mobility. A patient in an institutional setting is up to 50 times more likely to contract pneumonia than an elderly patient receiving home care.

Common signs and symptoms of pneumonia include increasing dyspnea, congestion, fever, chills, tachypnea, sputum production, and altered mental status. Occasionally, abdominal pain may be the only symptom. Because of thermoregulatory changes, a fever may be absent in an elderly patient.

Prevention strategies include immunization with the current pneumonia and influenza vaccines. Efforts should also be taken to reduce exposure to infectious patients and to promote patient mobility.

In treating an elderly patient with pneumonia, manage all life threats. Maintain adequate oxygenation. Transport the patient to the hospital for diagnosis, keeping in mind that patients with respiratory disease often have other underlying problems.

Chronic Obstructive Pulmonary Disease

Chronic obstructive pulmonary disease (COPD) is really a collection of diseases, characterized by chronic airflow obstruction with reversible and/or irreversible components. Although each COPD has its own distinct features, elderly patients commonly have two or more types at the same time. COPD usually refers to some combination of emphysema, chronic bronchitis, and, to a lesser degree, asthma. Pneumonia, as well as other respiratory disorders, can further complicate chronic obstructive pulmonary disease in the elderly.

In the United States, chronic obstructive pulmonary disease is the third leading cause of death. Its prevalence has been increasing during the past 20 years. Several factors combine to produce the damage of COPD:

● Genetic disposition

● Exposure to environmental pollutants

● Existence of a childhood respiratory disease

● Cigarette smoking, a contributing factor in up to 80 percent of all cases of COPD

The physiology of COPD varies, but may include inflammation of the air passages with increased mucus production or actual destruction of the alveoli. The outcome is decreased airflow in the alveoli, resulting in reduced oxygen exchange. Usual signs and symptoms include:

● Cough

● Increased sputum production

● Dyspnea

● Accessory muscle use

● Pursed-lip breathing

● Tripod positioning

● Exercise intolerance

● Wheezing

● Pleuritic chest pain

● Tachypnea

COPD is progressive and debilitating (Figure 5-16 ●). The patient can often keep the signs and symptoms under control

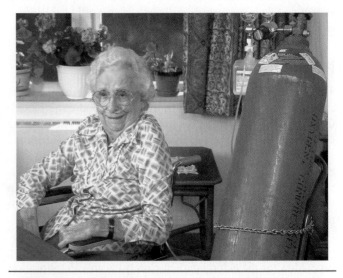

● **Figure 5-16** The COPD patient may use a nasal cannula with an oxygen unit.

until the body is stressed. When the condition becomes disabling, it is called *exacerbation of COPD*. This condition can lead rapidly to patient death because the accompanying hypoxia and hypercapnia alter the acid-base balance and deprive the tissues of the oxygen needed for efficient energy production.

The most effective prevention involves elimination of tobacco products and reduced exposure to cigarette smoke (in nonsmokers). Recent legislation has sought to keep public places smoke free and to discourage cigarette smoking in the young. Once the disease is present, patients are taught to identify stresses that exacerbate the condition. Appropriate self-care includes exercise, avoidance of infections, appropriate use of drugs, and, when necessary, calling EMS.

When confronted with an elderly patient with COPD, treatment is essentially the same as for all age groups. Supply supplemental oxygen to correct hypoxia and possibly drug therapy, usually for reducing dyspnea.

Pulmonary Embolism

Pulmonary embolism (PE) should always be considered as a possible cause of respiratory distress in the elderly. Although statistics for the elderly are unavailable, approximately 650,000 cases occur annually in the United States alone. Of this number, a pulmonary embolism is the primary cause of death in 100,000 people and a contributing factor in another 100,000 deaths. Nearly 11 percent of PE deaths take place in the first hour and 38 percent in the second hour after occurrence.

Blood clots are the most frequent cause of pulmonary embolism. However, the condition may also be caused by fat, air, bone marrow, tumor cells, or foreign bodies. Risk factors for developing pulmonary embolism include:

- Deep venous thrombosis
- Prolonged immobility, common among the elderly
- Malignancy (tumors)
- Paralysis
- Fractures of the pelvis, hip, or leg
- Obesity
- Trauma to the leg vessels
- Major surgery
- Presence of a venous catheter
- Use of hormones (estrogen and progestin) in women
- Atrial fibrillation

Pulmonary emboli usually originate in the deep veins of the thigh and calf. The condition should be suspected in any patient with the acute onset of dyspnea. Often, it is accompanied by pleuritic chest pain and right heart failure. If the pulmonary embolus is massive, you can often expect severe dyspnea, cardiac arrhythmias, and, ultimately, cardiovascular collapse (Figure 5-17 ●).

Definitive diagnosis of a pulmonary embolism takes place in a hospital setting. The goals of field treatment are to manage and minimize complications of the condition. General treatment considerations include delivery of supplemental oxygen via mask to maintain a SpO_2 of 92 to 94 percent. Establishment

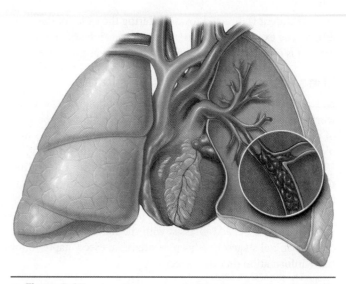

● **Figure 5-17** A pulmonary embolism is a blood clot lodged in a pulmonary artery, thus interrupting blood flow and adversely affecting the oxygenation of hemoglobin.

of an IV for possible administration of medications is appropriate, but vigorous fluid therapy should be avoided, if possible.

Prehospital pharmacological therapy for pulmonary embolism is limited. On advice from medical direction, you may administer small doses of morphine sulfate to reduce patient anxiety. After confirming the absence of GI bleeding, medical direction may also prescribe anticoagulants to prevent clot formation and/or to speed clot dissolution. If the administration of a vasopressor is indicated by low blood pressure, then dopamine may be prescribed. In such cases, remember to titrate the dopamine to a desirable blood pressure.

The risk of death from pulmonary embolism is greatest in the first few hours. As a result, rapid transport is essential. Position the patient in an upright position and avoid lifting the patient by the legs or knees, which may dislodge thrombi in the lower extremities. During transport, continue to monitor changes in skin color, pulse oximetry, and breathing rate and rhythm. Your field assessment and interventions can save the patient's life and guide the hospital physician in a direction that will result in an accurate diagnosis and rapid treatment.

Pulmonary Edema

Pulmonary edema is an effusion or escape of serous fluids into the alveoli and interstitial tissues of the lungs. Acute pulmonary edema can develop rapidly in the elderly. Although most commonly associated with acute myocardial infarction and congestive heart failure (acute on chronic congestive heart failure), it can also result from pulmonary infections, inhaled toxins, narcotic overdose, pulmonary embolism, and decreased atmospheric pressure.

Pulmonary edema causes severe dyspnea associated with congestion. Other signs and symptoms include rapid labored breathing, cough with blood-stained sputum, cyanosis, and cold extremities. Physical examination usually reveals the presence of moist crackles and accessory muscle use. Severe cases will exhibit rhonchi.

Treatment is directed toward altering the cause of the condition. The existence of pulmonary edema can be life threatening and is often the symptom of a fatal cardiovascular disease.

Lung Cancer

North America has the highest incidence of lung cancer in the world. The incidence increases with age, with about 65 percent of all lung cancer deaths occurring among people age 65 and older. The leading cause of lung cancer is cigarette smoking.

Often, progressive dyspnea will be the first presentation of a cancerous lesion. Hemoptysis (bloody sputum), chronic cough, and weight loss are also common symptoms.

Treatment of lung cancer occurs in a hospital setting. However, you may be called to assist with the follow-up home care or, in terminal stages, in a hospice situation. (See Chapter 8 for more information on this subject.)

Cardiovascular Disorders

The leading cause of death in the elderly is cardiovascular disease. Assessment and treatment of cardiovascular disease in the elderly patient is often complicated by non-age-related factors and disease processes in other organ systems. In conducting your history, determine the patient's level of cardiovascular fitness, changes in exercise tolerance, recent diet history, use of medications, and use of cigarettes and/or alcohol. Ask questions about breathing difficulty, especially at night, and evidence of palpitations, flutter, or skipped beats.

In performing the physical exam, look for hypertension and orthostatic hypotension (a decrease in blood pressure and an increase in heart rate when rising from a seated or supine position). Watch for dehydration or dependent edema. When taking an elderly patient's blood pressure, consider checking both arms. Routinely determine pulses in all the extremities. In auscultating the patient, remember that a bruit or noise in the neck, abdomen, or groin indicates a high probability of carotid, aortorenal, or peripheral vascular disease. Keep in mind, too, that heart sounds are generally softer in the elderly, probably because of a thickening of lung tissue between the heart and chest wall.

In evaluating the problem, recall the cardiovascular disorders commonly found in elderly patients. They include angina pectoris, myocardial infarction, heart failure, arrhythmias, aortic dissection, aneurysm, hypertension, and syncope.

Angina Pectoris

The likelihood of developing angina increases dramatically with age. This is especially true of women, who are protected by estrogen until after menopause. Angina is usually triggered by physical activity, especially after a meal, and by exposure to very cold weather. Attacks vary in frequency, from several a day to occasional episodes separated by weeks or months.

Angina pectoris literally means "pain in the chest." However, the pain of angina is actually felt in only about 10 to 20 percent of elderly patients. The changes in sensory nerves, combined with the myocardial changes of aging, make dyspnea a more likely symptom of angina than pain.

Angina develops when narrowing of coronary vessels as a result of plaque or vasospasm leads to an inability to meet the oxygen demands of the heart muscle. The heart muscle usually responds by sending out pain signals, which represent a buildup of lactic acid. In an elderly patient, exercise intolerance is a key symptom of angina. In obtaining a history, you should ask the patient about sudden changes in routine. In addition, inquire about any increased stresses on the heart, such as anemia, infection, arrhythmias, and thyroid changes.

General prevention strategies in the elderly are similar to those in young patients. Blood pressure control combined with diet, exercise, and smoking modifications reduces the risk in all groups.

Myocardial Infarction

A myocardial infarction (MI) involves actual death of muscle tissue owing to a partial or complete occlusion of one or more of the coronary arteries. The greatest number of patients hospitalized for acute myocardial infarction are older than 65. The elderly patient with myocardial infarction is less likely to present with classic symptoms, such as chest pain, than a younger counterpart. Atypical presentations that may be seen in the elderly include:

- Absence of pain
- Exercise intolerance
- Confusion/dizziness
- Syncope
- Dyspnea—common in patients over age 85
- Neck, dental, and/or epigastric pain
- Fatigue/weakness

The mortality rate associated with myocardial infarction and/or resulting complications doubles after age 70. Unlike younger patients, the elderly are more likely to suffer a **silent myocardial infarction**. They also tend to have larger myocardial infarctions. The majority of deaths that occur in the first few hours following a myocardial infarction are caused by arrhythmias.

A myocardial infarction is most commonly triggered by some form of physical exertion or a preexisting heart disease. Because of the high mortality associated with myocardial infarctions in the elderly, early detection and emergency management are critical.

Heart Failure

Heart failure takes place when cardiac output cannot meet the body's metabolic demands. The incidence rises exponentially after age 60. The condition is widespread among the elderly and is the most common diagnosis in hospitalized patients over age 65. The causes of heart failure fall into one of four categories: impairment to flow, inadequate cardiac filling, volume overload, and myocardial failure.

Typical age-related factors, such as prolonged myocardial contractions, make the elderly vulnerable to heart failure. Other factors that place them at risk include:

- Noncompliance with drug therapy
- Anemia
- Ischemia
- Thermoregulatory disorders (hypothermia/hyperthermia)

- Hypoxia
- Infection
- Use of nonsteroidal anti-inflammatory drugs (excluding low-dose aspirin)
- Arrhythmias (e.g., atrial fibrillation)

Signs and symptoms of heart failure vary. In most patients, regardless of age, some form of edema exists. However, edema in the elderly can indicate a range of problems, including musculoskeletal injury. Assessment findings specific to the elderly include:

- Fatigue (left failure)
- **Two-pillow orthopnea**
- Dyspnea on exertion
- Paroxysmal nocturnal dyspnea
- Dry, hacking cough progressing to productive cough
- Dependent edema (right failure)
- **Nocturia**
- Anorexia, **hepatomegaly**, ascites

Nonpharmacological management of heart failure includes modifications in diet (e.g., less fat and cholesterol), exercise, and reduction in weight, if necessary. Pharmacological management may include treatment with diuretics, vasodilators, antihypertensive agents, or inotropic agents. Check to see whether the patient is already on any of these medications and if the patient is compliant with scheduled doses.

Arrhythmias

Many cardiac arrhythmias develop with age. Atrial fibrillation is the most common arrhythmia encountered and can be a predictor of long-term mortality in elderly patients.[5]

Arrhythmias occur primarily as a result of degeneration of the patient's conductive system. Anything that decreases myocardial blood flow can produce an arrhythmia. They may also be caused by electrolyte abnormalities.

To complicate matters further, the elderly do not tolerate extremes in heart rate as well as a younger person would. For example, a heart rate of 140 in an older patient may cause syncope, whereas a younger patient can often tolerate a heart rate greater than 180. In addition, arrhythmias can lead to falls from cerebral hypoperfusion. They can also result in congestive heart failure (CHF) or a transient ischemic attack.

Treatment considerations depend on the type of arrhythmia. Patients may already have a pacemaker in place. In such cases, keep in mind that pacemakers have a low but significant rate of complications such as a failed battery, fibrosis around the catheter site, lead fracture, or electrode dislodgment. In a number of situations, drug therapy may be indicated. Whenever you discover an arrhythmia, remember that an abnormal or disordered heart rhythm may be the only clinical finding in an elderly patient suffering acute myocardial infarction.

Aortic Dissection/Aneurysms

Aortic dissection is a degeneration of the wall of the aorta, either in the thoracic or abdominal cavity. It can result in an **aneurysm** or in a rupture of the vessel. Generally speaking, dissections are more common in the thoracic aorta, whereas aneurysms are more common in the abdominal aorta—although both can occur in either location.

Approximately 80 percent of thoracic aneurysms are the result of atherosclerosis combined with hypertension. The remaining cases occur secondary to other factors, including blunt trauma to the chest. Patients with dissections will often present with tearing chest pain radiating through to the back or, if rupture occurs, cardiac arrest. **Marfan syndrome** is a connective system disorder resulting in abnormal growth of distal tissues and a dilation of the root of the aorta. It can cause aortic aneurysm and dissection; these should be considered in elderly patients with this condition.

The distal portion of the aorta is the most common site for abdominal aneurysms. Approximately 1 in 250 people over age 50 die from a ruptured abdominal aneurysm. The aneurysm may appear as a pulsatile mass in a patient with a normal girth, but lack of an identifiable mass does not eliminate this condition. Patients may present with tearing abdominal pain or unexplained low back pain. Pulses in the legs are diminished or absent and the lower extremities feel cold to the touch. The patient may experience sensory abnormalities such as numbness, tingling, or pain in the legs. The patient may fall when attempting to stand.

Treatment of an aneurysm depends on its size, location, and the severity of the condition. In the case of thoracic aortic dissection, continuous IV infusion and/or administration of drug therapy to lower the arterial pressure and to diminish the velocity of left ventricle contraction may be indicated. Rapid transport is essential, especially for the older patient who most commonly requires care and observation in an intensive care unit.

Hypertension

Hypertension appears to be a product of industrial society. In developed nations, such as the United States, the systolic and diastolic pressures have a tendency to rise until age 60. Systolic pressure may continue to rise after that time, but diastolic pressure stabilizes. Because this rise in blood pressure is not seen in less developed nations, experts believe that hypertension is not a normal age-related change.

Today more than 50 percent of Americans over age 65 have clinically diagnosed hypertension, which is defined as blood pressure greater than 140/90 mmHg. Prolonged elevated blood pressure will eventually damage the heart, brain, or kidneys. As a result of hypertension, elderly patients are at greater risk for heart failure, stroke, blindness, renal failure, coronary heart disease, and peripheral vascular disease. In men with blood pressure greater than 160/95 mmHg, the risk of mortality nearly doubles.

Hypertension increases with atherosclerosis, which is more common with the elderly than other age groups. Other contributing factors include obesity and diabetes. The condition can

CONTENT REVIEW

▶ Hypertension Prevention
Strategies

• Modified diet (low sodium)
• Exercise
• Smoking cessation
• Compliance with
  medications

be prevented or controlled through diet (sodium reduction), exercise, cessation of smoking, and compliance with medications.

Hypertension is often a silent disease that produces no clinically obvious signs or symptoms. It may be associated with nonspecific complaints such as headache, tinnitus, **epistaxis**, slow tremors, or nausea and vomiting. An acute onset of high blood pressure without any kidney involvement is often a telltale indicator of thyroid disease.

Treatment of hypertension for those between 60 and 80 years of age has been shown to increase their life span, whereas treatment of those above 80 years of age has not shown to increase life span. The management of hypertension depends on its severity and the existence of other conditions. For example, hypertension is often treated with angiotensin-converting enzyme (ACE) inhibitors or angiotensin II receptor blockers. Other medications, such as beta-blockers (medications that are contraindicated in patients with chronic obstructive lung disease, asthma, or heart block greater than first degree) and calcium-channel blockers can be effective. Diuretics, another common drug used in treating hypertension, should be prescribed with care for patients on digitalis. Keep in mind that centrally acting agents are more likely to produce negative side effects in the elderly. Unlike younger patients, the elderly may experience depression, forgetfulness, sleep problems, or vivid dreams and/or hallucinations.

Syncope

Syncope is a common presenting complaint among the elderly. The condition results when blood flow to the brain is temporarily interrupted or decreased. It is most often caused by problems with either the nervous system or the cardiovascular system. In general, syncope has a higher incidence of death in elderly patients than in younger individuals.[6] The following are some of the common presentations that you may encounter:

● *Vasodepressor syncope.* Vasodepressor syncope is commonly termed "fainting." It may occur following emotional distress; pain; prolonged bed rest; mild blood loss; prolonged standing in warm, crowded rooms; anemia; or fever.

● *Orthostatic syncope.* Orthostatic syncope occurs when a person rises from a seated or supine position. There are several possible causes. First, the person may have a disproportion between blood volume and vascular capacity. That is, there is a pooling of blood in the legs, reducing blood flow to the brain. Causes of this include hypovolemia, venous **varicosities**, prolonged bed rest, and **autonomic dysfunction**. Many drugs, especially blood pressure medicines, can cause drug-induced orthostatic syncope due to the effects of the medications on the capacitance vessels.

● *Vasovagal syncope.* Vasovagal syncope occurs as a result of a **Valsalva maneuver**, which happens during defecation,

coughing, or similar maneuvers. This effectively slows the heart rate and cardiac output, thus decreasing blood flow to the brain.

● *Cardiac syncope.* Cardiac syncope results from transient reduction in cerebral blood flow due to a sudden decrease in cardiac output. It can result from several mechanisms. Syncope can be the primary symptom of silent myocardial infarction. In addition, many arrhythmias can cause syncope. Arrhythmias that have been shown to cause syncope include bradycardias, **Stokes-Adams syndrome**, Brugada syndrome, heart block, tachyarrhythmia, and **sick sinus syndrome**.

● *Seizures.* Syncope may result from a seizure disorder or prolonged syncope may cause seizure activity. Syncope due to seizures tends to occur without warning. It is associated with muscular jerking or convulsions, incontinence, and tongue biting. Postictal confusion may follow.

● *Transient ischemic attacks.* Transient ischemic attacks occur more frequently in the elderly and they may cause syncope.

Neurologic Disorders

Elderly patients are at risk for several neurologic emergencies. Often, the exact cause is not initially known and may require probing at the hospital.

Many of the neurologic disorders that you will encounter in the field will exhibit an alteration in mental status. You may discover a range of underlying causes from stroke to degenerative brain disease. Some of the most common causes of altered mental status include:

● Cerebrovascular disease (stroke or transient ischemic attack)

● Myocardial infarction

● Seizures

● Medication-related problems (drug interactions, drug underdose, and drug overdose)

● Infection

● Fluid and electrolyte abnormalities (dehydration)

● Lack of nutrients (hypoglycemia)

● Temperature changes (hypothermia, hyperthermia)

● Structural changes (dementia, subdural hematoma)

As mentioned, it is often impossible to distinguish in the field the cause of an altered mental status. Even so, you should carry out a thorough assessment. Administer supplemental oxygen if the patient is hypoxic. As soon as practical, obtain a blood glucose level to exclude hypoglycemia as a possible cause. Overall, the approach to the elderly patient with altered mental status is the same as that for any other patient presenting with similar symptoms.

Cerebrovascular Disease (Stroke/TIAs)

Stroke is the fourth-leading cause of death in the United States. Annually, about 795,000 people suffer strokes and about 130,000 die. Incidence of stroke and the likelihood of dying from a stroke increase with age. Occlusive stroke is statistically more

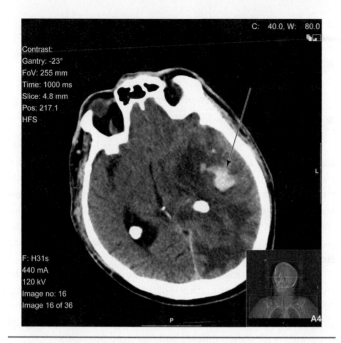

C: 40.0, W: 80.0

Contrast:
Gantry: -23°
FoV: 255 mm
Time: 1000 ms
Slice: 4.8 mm
Pos: 217.1
HFS

F: H31s
440 mA
120 kV
Image no: 16
Image 16 of 36

• **Figure 5-18** Large intracerebral hemorrhage with resultant midline shift. (© Dr. Bryan E. Bledsoe)

common in the elderly and relatively uncommon in younger individuals. Older patients are at higher risk of stroke because of atherosclerosis, hypertension, immobility, limb paralysis, congestive heart failure, and atrial fibrillation. Transient ischemic attacks are also more common in older patients. More than one-third of patients suffering TIAs will develop a major, permanent stroke. As previously mentioned, TIAs are a frequent cause of syncope in the elderly.

Strokes usually fall into one of two major categories. **Brain ischemia**—injury to brain tissue caused by an inadequate supply of oxygen and nutrients—accounts for about 80 percent of all strokes. Brain hemorrhage, the second major category, may be either **subarachnoid hemorrhage** or **intracerebral hemorrhage**. These different patterns of bleeding have different presentations, causes, and treatments. However, together they account for a high percentage of all stroke deaths (Figure 5-18 •).

Because of the various kinds of strokes, signs and symptoms can present in many ways: altered mental status, coma, paralysis, slurred speech, a change in mood, and seizures. Stroke should be highly suspect in any elderly patient with a sudden change in mental status.

Whenever you suspect a stroke, it is essential that you complete the Los Angeles Prehospital Stroke Screen or Cincinnati Prehospital Stroke Scale for later comparison in the emergency department. Fibrinolytic agents administered to a patient suffering an occlusive (ischemic) stroke can decrease the severity of damage if administered within 4.5 hours of onset. Rapid transport is essential for avoiding brain damage or limiting its extent. In the case of stroke, "time is brain tissue."

By far, the most preferred treatment is prevention of strokes in the first place. Strategies include:

- Control of hypertension
- Treatment of cardiac disorders, including arrhythmias and coronary artery disease

- Treatment of blood disorders, such as anemia and **polycythemia**
- Cessation of smoking
- Cessation of recreational drugs
- Moderate use of alcohol
- Regular exercise
- Good eating habits

Seizures

Seizures can be easily mistaken for strokes in the elderly. In addition, a first-time seizure may occur as a result of damage from a previous stroke. Not all seizures experienced by the elderly are of the major motor type. Some are more subtle. Many causes of seizure activity in the elderly have been identified. Common causes include:

- Seizure disorder (epilepsy)
- Syncope
- Recent or past head trauma
- Mass lesion (tumor or bleed)
- Alcohol withdrawal
- Hypoglycemia
- Stroke

Often the cause of the seizure cannot be determined in the field. Examination of the patient's home medications may give an indication as to whether the patient has a seizure disorder. Common antiseizure medications include:

- Phenytoin (Dilantin)
- Phenobarbital (Luminal)
- Carbamazepine (Tegretol)
- Ethosuximide (Zarontin)
- Levetiracetam (Keppra)
- Gabapentin (Neurontin)
- Valproic acid (Depakote)

Because the cause of a seizure cannot always be determined, treat the condition as a life-threatening emergency and transport as quickly as possible to eliminate the possibility of stroke. If the patient has fallen during a seizure, check for evidence of trauma and treat accordingly.

Dizziness/Vertigo

Dizziness is a frightening experience and a frequent complaint of the elderly. The complaint of dizziness may actually mean that the patient has suffered syncope, presyncope, light-headedness, or true **vertigo**. Vertigo is a specific sensation of motion perceived by the patient as spinning or whirling. Many patients will report that they feel as though they are spinning. Vertigo is often accompanied by sweating, pallor, nausea, and vomiting. Ménière's disease can cause severe, **intractable** vertigo. It is often, however, associated with a constant "roaring" sound in the ears, as well as ear "pressure."

Vertigo results from so many factors that it is often hard, even for the physician, to determine the actual cause. Any factor that impairs visual input, inner-ear function, peripheral sensory input, or the central nervous system can cause dizziness. In addition, alcohol and many prescription drugs can cause dizziness. So can hypoglycemia in its early stages. It is virtually impossible to distinguish dizziness, syncope, and presyncope in the prehospital setting.

Delirium, Dementia, and Alzheimer's Disease

Approximately 15 percent of all Americans over age 65 have some degree of dementia or delirium. **Dementia** is a chronic global cognitive impairment, often progressive or irreversible. The best known form of dementia is **Alzheimer's disease**, a condition that affects 5.5 million Americans. **Delirium** is a global mental impairment of sudden onset and self-limited duration. (For differences between dementia and delirium, see Table 5–6.)

Delirium Many conditions can cause delirium. The cause may be either organic brain disease or disorders that occur elsewhere in the body. Delirium in the elderly is a serious condition. According to some estimates, about 18 percent of hospitalized elderly patients with delirium die. Possible etiologies or causes include:

- Subdural hematoma
- Tumors and other mass lesions
- Drug-induced changes or alcohol intoxication
- CNS infections
- Electrolyte abnormalities

- Heart failure
- Fever
- Metabolic disorders, including hypoglycemia
- Chronic endocrine abnormalities, including hypothyroidism and hyperthyroidism
- Postconcussion syndrome

The presentation of delirium varies greatly and can change rapidly during assessment. Common signs and symptoms include the acute onset of anxiety, an inability to focus, disordered thinking, irritability, inappropriate behavior, fearfulness, excessive energy, or psychotic behavior such as hallucinations or paranoia. Aphasia or other speech disorders and/or prominent slurring of speech may be present. Normal patterns of eating and sleeping are almost always disrupted.

In distinguishing between delirium and dementia, err on the side of delirium. The condition is often caused by life-threatening, but reversible, conditions. Causes of delirium, such as infections, drug toxicity, and electrolyte imbalances, generally have a good prognosis if identified quickly and managed promptly.

Dementia Dementia is more prevalent in the elderly than delirium. More than 50 percent of all nursing home patients have some form of dementia. It is usually caused by an underlying neurologic disease. This mental deterioration is often called organic brain syndrome, **senile dementia**, or senility. It is important to find out whether an alteration in mental status is acute or chronic. Causes of dementia include:

- Small strokes
- Atherosclerosis
- Age-related neurologic changes
- Neurologic diseases
- Certain hereditary diseases (e.g., Huntington's disease)
- Alzheimer's disease

Signs and symptoms of dementia include progressive disorientation, shortened attention span, **aphasia** or nonsense talking, and hallucinations. Dementia often hampers treatment through the patient's inability to communicate, and it can exhaust caregivers. In moderate to severe cases, you will need to rely on the caregiver for information. (Remain alert to signs of abuse or neglect, which occurs in a disproportionate number of elderly suffering from dementia.)

Alzheimer's Disease Alzheimer's disease, a particular type of dementia, is a chronic degenerative disorder that attacks the brain and results in impaired memory, thinking, and behavior.[7] It accounts for more than half of all forms of dementia in the elderly (Figure 5-19 ●).

Alzheimer's disease generally occurs in stages, each with different signs and symptoms. These stages are:

- *Early stage.* Characterized by loss of recent memory, inability to learn new material, mood swings, and personality changes. Patients may believe someone is plotting against them when they lose items or forget things.

TABLE 5–6 | Distinguishing Dementia and Delirium*	
Dementia	**Delirium**
Chronic, slowly progressive development	Rapid in onset, fluctuating course
Irreversible disorder	May be reversed, especially if treated early
Greatly impairs memory	Greatly impairs attention
Global cognitive deficits	Focal cognitive deficits
Most commonly caused by Alzheimer's disease	Most commonly caused by systemic disease, drug toxicity, or metabolic changes
Does not require immediate treatment	Requires immediate treatment
*These are general characteristics that apply to most, but not all, cases.	

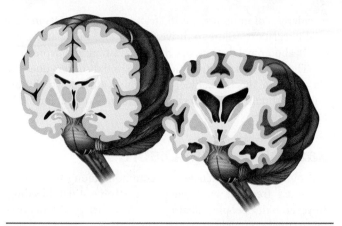

● **Figure 5-19** Illustration of normal human brain (left) and the brain of an Alzheimer's patient (right). Note the pronounced atrophy and ventricular enlargement. (© *J. Cavallini/Custom Medical Stock Photo*)

Aggression or hostility is common. Poor judgment is evident.

● *Intermediate stage.* Characterized by a complete inability to learn new material; wandering, particularly at night; increased falls; and loss of ability for self-care, including bathing and use of the toilet.

● *Terminal stage.* Characterized by an inability to walk and regression to infant stage, including the loss of bowel and bladder function. Eventually the patient loses the ability to eat and swallow.

Families caring for an Alzheimer's patient at home also present signs of stress. Remember to treat both the Alzheimer's patient and the family and/or caregivers with respect and compassion. Evaluate the needs of the family and make an appropriate report at your facility. Support groups are available to assist families.

Parkinson's Disease

Parkinson's disease is a degenerative disorder characterized by changes in muscle response, including tremors, loss of facial expression, and gait disturbances. It mainly appears in people over age 50 and peaks at age 70. The disease affects about 1 million Americans, with 50,000 new cases diagnosed each year. It is the fourth most common neurodegenerative disease among the elderly.

The cause of primary Parkinson's disease remains unknown.[8] However, it affects the basal ganglia in the brain, an area that deciphers messages going to muscles (Figure 5-20 ●). Secondary Parkinson's disease is distinguished from primary Parkinson's disease by having a known cause. Some of the most common causes include:

● Viral encephalitis

● Atherosclerosis of cerebral vessels

● Reaction to certain drugs or toxins, such as antipsychotics or carbon monoxide

● Metabolic disorders, such as anoxia

● Tumors

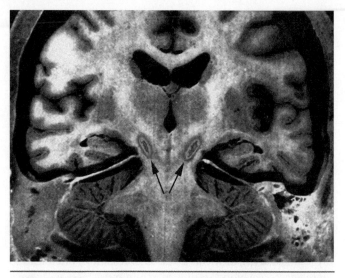

● **Figure 5-20** Degenerative disease of the extrapyramidal system (substantia nigra, arrows) in a 50-year-old man with Parkinson's disease. (*Custom Medical Stock Photo*)

● Head trauma

● Degenerative disorders, such as **Shy-Drager syndrome**

It is impossible in a field setting to distinguish primary and secondary Parkinson's disease. The most common initial sign of a Parkinson's disorder is a resting tremor combined with a **pill-rolling motion**. As the disease progresses, muscles become more rigid and movements become slower and/or more jerky. In some cases, patients may find their movements halted while carrying out some routine task. Their feet may feel "frozen to the ground." Gait becomes shuffled with short steps and unexpected bursts of speed, often to avoid falling. Kyphotic deformity is a hallmark of the disease.

Patients with Parkinson's disease commonly develop mask-like faces devoid of all expression. They speak in slow, monotone voices. Difficulties in communication, coupled with a loss of mobility, often lead to anxiety and depression.

There is no known cure for Parkinson's disease, with the exception of drug-induced secondary Parkinson's disorders. Exercise may help maintain physical activity or teach the patient adaptive strategies. In calls involving a Parkinson's patient, observe for the conditions that involved the EMS system, such as a fall or the inability to move. Manage treatable conditions and transport as needed.

Metabolic and Endocrine Disorders

As previously mentioned, the endocrine system undergoes a number of age-related changes that affect hormone levels. The most common endocrine disorders include diabetes mellitus and problems related to the thyroid gland. Of the two, you will more often treat diabetic-related emergencies, particularly hypoglycemia.

Diabetes Mellitus

An estimated 20 percent of older adults have diabetes mellitus, primarily type II diabetes. Almost 40 percent have some type of glucose intolerance. The elderly develop these disorders for these reasons:

- Poor diet
- Decreased physical activity
- Loss of lean body mass
- Impaired insulin production
- Resistance by body cells to the actions of insulin

Diagnosis of type II diabetes usually occurs during routine screening in a physical exam. In some cases, urine tests may register negative because of an increased renal glucose threshold in the elderly. The condition may present, in its early stages, with vague constitutional symptoms such as fatigue or weakness. Allowed to progress, diabetes can result in neuropathy and visual impairment. These manifestations often lead to more aggressive blood testing, which in most cases will reveal elevated glucose levels.

The treatment of diabetes involves diet, exercise, the use of sulfonylurea agents, and/or insulin. Many diabetics use self-monitoring devices to test glucose levels. Unfortunately, the cost of these devices and the accompanying test strips sometimes discourages the elderly from using them. Elderly patients on insulin also risk hypoglycemia, especially if they accidentally take too much insulin or do not eat enough food following injection. The lack of good nutrition can be particularly troublesome to elderly diabetics. They often find it difficult to prepare meals, fail to enjoy food because of altered taste perceptions, have trouble chewing food, or are unable to purchase adequate and/or the correct food because of limited income.

Management of diabetic and hypoglycemic emergencies for the elderly is generally the same as for any other patient. *Do not* rule out alcohol as a complicating factor, especially in cases of hypoglycemia. In addition, remember that diabetes places the elderly at increased risk of other complications, including atherosclerosis, delayed healing, **retinopathy**, blindness, altered renal function, and severe peripheral vascular disease, leading to foot ulcers and even amputations.

Thyroid Disorders

With normal aging, the thyroid gland undergoes moderate atrophy and changes in hormone production. An estimated 2 to 5 percent of people over age 65 experience hypothyroidism, a condition resulting from inadequate levels of thyroid hormones. It affects women in greater numbers than men, and the prevalence rises with age.

Less than 33 percent of the elderly present with typical signs and symptoms of hypothyroidism. When they do, their complaints are often attributed to aging. Common nonspecific complaints in the elderly include mental confusion, anorexia, falls, incontinence, and decreased mobility. Some patients also experience an increase in muscle or joint pain. Treatment involves thyroid hormone replacement.

Hyperthyroidism is less common among the elderly but may result from medication errors such as an overdose of thyroid hormone replacement. The typical symptom of heat intolerance is often present. Otherwise, hyperthyroidism presents atypically in the elderly. Common nonspecific features or complaints include atrial fibrillation, failure to thrive (weight loss and apathy combined), abdominal distress, diarrhea, exhaustion, and depression.

The diagnosis and treatment of thyroid disorders does not take place in the field. Elderly patients with known thyroid problems should be encouraged to go to the hospital for medical evaluation.

Gastrointestinal Disorders

Gastrointestinal emergencies are common among the elderly. The most frequent emergency is gastrointestinal bleeding. However, older people will also describe a variety of other gastrointestinal complaints: nausea, poor appetite, diarrhea, and constipation, to name a few. Remember that, like other presenting complaints, these conditions may be symptomatic of more serious diseases. Bowel problems, for example, may point to cancer of the colon or other abdominal organs.

Regardless of the complaint, remember that prompt management of a GI emergency is essential for young and old alike. For the elderly, there is a significant risk of hemorrhage and shock. There is a tendency to take GI patients less seriously than those suffering moderate or severe external hemorrhage. This is a serious mistake. Patients with gastrointestinal complaints, especially the elderly, should be managed aggressively. Keep in mind that older patients are far more intolerant of hypotension and anoxia than younger patients are. Treatment should include:

- Airway management
- Support of breathing and circulation
- Supplemental oxygen therapy if the patient is hypoxic
- IV fluid replacement with a crystalloid solution
- Rapid transport

Some of the most critical GI problems that you may encounter in the field will involve internal hemorrhage and bowel obstruction. You may also be called on to treat **mesenteric ischemia or infarct**, a serious and life-threatening condition in an elderly patient. The following descriptions will help you to recognize each of these gastrointestinal disorders.

GI Hemorrhage

Gastrointestinal bleeding falls into two general categories: upper GI bleed and lower GI bleed.

Upper GI Bleed   This form of gastrointestinal bleeding includes:

- *Peptic ulcer disease:* injury to the mucous lining of the upper part of the gastrointestinal tract due to stomach acids, digestive enzymes, and other agents, such as anti-inflammatory drugs
- *Gastritis:* an inflammation of the lining of the stomach
- *Esophageal varices:* an abnormal dilation of veins in the lower esophagus; a common complication of cirrhosis of the liver
- *Mallory-Weiss tear:* a tear in the lower esophagus that is often caused by severe and prolonged retching

Lower GI Bleed Conditions categorized as lower gastrointestinal bleeding include:

- *Diverticulosis:* the presence of small pouches on the colon that tend to develop with age; causes 70 percent of life-threatening lower GI bleeds
- *Tumors:* tumors of the colon can cause bleeding when the tumor erodes into blood vessels within the intestine or surrounding organs
- *Ischemic colitis:* an inflammation of the colon resulting from impaired or decreased blood supply
- *Arteriovenous malformations:* an abnormal link between an artery and a vein

Signs of significant gastrointestinal blood loss include the presence of "coffee-grounds" emesis; black, tarlike stools (**melena**); obvious blood in the emesis or stool; orthostatic hypotension; pulse greater than 100 (unless the patient is on beta-blockers); and confusion. Gastrointestinal bleeding in the elderly may result in such complications as a recent increase in angina symptoms, congestive heart failure, weakness, or dyspnea.

Bowel Obstruction

Bowel obstruction in the elderly typically involves the small bowel. Causes include tumors, prior abdominal surgery, use of certain medications, and occasionally the presence of vertebral compression fractures. The patient will typically complain of diffuse abdominal pain, bloating, nausea, and vomiting. The abdomen may feel distended when palpated. Bowel sounds may be hypoactive or absent, or hyperactive and "tinkling." If the obstruction has been present for a prolonged period of time, the patient may have fever, weakness, shock, and various electrolyte disturbances.

Mesenteric Ischemia/Infarct

Vessels arising from the superior or inferior mesenteric arteries generally serve the bowel. An infarct occurs when a portion of the bowel does not receive enough blood to survive. Certain age-related changes make the elderly more vulnerable to this condition. First, as a person ages, changes in the heart (such as atrial fibrillation) or the vessels (atherosclerosis) predispose the patient to a clot lodging in one of the branches serving the bowel. Second, changes in the bowel itself can promote swelling that effectively cuts off blood flow.

The primary symptom of a bowel infarct is pain out of proportion to the physical exam. Signs include:

- Bloody diarrhea, but usually not a massive hemorrhage
- Some tachycardia, although there may be a vagal effect masking the sign
- Abdominal distention

The patient is at great risk for shock because the dead bowel attracts interstitial and intravascular fluids, thus removing them from use. Necrotic products are released to the peritoneal cavity, leading to a massive infection. The prognosis is poor due, in part, to decreased physiologic reserves on the part of the older patient.

Skin Disorders

Younger and older adults experience common skin disorders at about the same rates. However, age-related changes in the immune system make the elderly more prone to certain chronic skin diseases and infections. They are also more likely to develop **pressure ulcers** (bedsores) than any other age group.

Skin Diseases

Elderly patients commonly complain about **pruritus**, or itching. This condition can be caused by dermatitis (eczema) or environmental conditions, especially during winter (i.e., from hot dry air in the home and cold windy air outside). Keep in mind that generalized itching can also be a sign of systemic diseases, particularly liver and renal disorders. When itching is strong and unrelenting, suspect an underlying disease and encourage the patient to seek medical evaluation.

Slower healing and compromised tissue perfusion in the elderly make them more susceptible to bacterial infection of wounds, appearing as cellulitis, impetigo, and, in the case of immunocompromised adults, staphylococcal scalded skin. The elderly also experience a higher incidence of fungal infections, partly because of decreases in the cutaneous immunologic response. In addition, they suffer higher rates of **herpes zoster** (shingles), which peaks between ages 50 and 70. Although these skin disorders also occur in the young, their duration and severity increases markedly with age.

In treating skin disorders, remember that many conditions may be drug induced. Beta-blockers, for example, can worsen psoriasis, which occurs in about 3 percent of elderly patients. Question patients about their medications, keeping in mind that certain prescription drugs (e.g., penicillins and sulfonamides) and some OTC drugs can cause skin eruptions. Also ask about topical home remedies, such as alcohol or soaps that may cause or worsen the disorder. Find out whether the patient is compliant with prescribed topical treatments. Finally, remember that some drugs and topical medications commonly used to treat skin disorders in the young can worsen or cause other problems for the elderly. Antihistamines and corticosteroids are two to three times more likely to provoke adverse reactions in the elderly than in younger adults.

Pressure Ulcers (Decubitus Ulcers)

Most pressure ulcers occur in people over age 70. As many as 20 percent of patients enter the hospital with a pressure ulcer or develop one while hospitalized. The highest incidence occurs in nursing homes, where up to 25 percent of patients may develop this condition.[9]

Pressure ulcers typically develop from the waist down, usually over bony prominences, in bedridden patients. However, they can occur anywhere on the body and with the

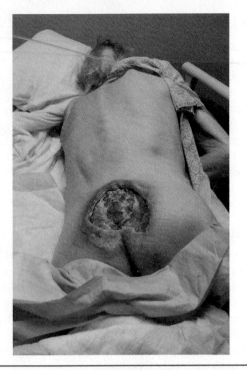

● **Figure 5-21** Multiple decubitus ulcers ("bedsores" or "pressure sores"). These often become infected, leading to the patient's death. They can be prevented with good nursing care.

patient in any position. Pressure ulcers usually result from tissue hypoxia and affect the skin, subcutaneous tissues, and muscle (Figure 5-21 ●). Factors that can increase the risk of this condition include:

● External compression of tissues (i.e., pressure)
● Altered sensory perception
● **Maceration**, caused by excessive moisture
● Decreased activity
● Decreased mobility
● Poor nutrition
● Friction or shear

To reduce the development of pressure ulcers or to alleviate their condition, you can take these steps:

● Assist the patient in changing position frequently, especially during extended transport, to reduce the length of time pressure is placed on any one point.
● Use a pull sheet to move the patient, reducing the likelihood of friction.
● Reduce the possibility of shearing by padding areas of skin prior to movement.
● Unless a life-threatening condition is present, take time to clean and dry areas of excessive moisture, such as urinary or fecal incontinence and excessive perspiration.
● Clean ulcers with normal saline solution and cover with hydrocolloid or hydrogel dressings, if available. With severe ulcers, pack with loosely woven gauze moistened with normal saline.

Musculoskeletal Disorders

The skeleton, as you know, is a metabolically active organ. Its metabolic processes are influenced by a number of factors, including age, diet, exercise, and hormone levels. The musculoskeletal system is also subject to disease. In fact, musculoskeletal diseases are the leading cause of functional impairment in the elderly. Although usually not fatal, musculoskeletal disorders often produce chronic disability, which in turn creates a context for illness. Two of the most widespread musculoskeletal disorders are osteoarthritis and osteoporosis.

Osteoarthritis

Osteoarthritis is the leading cause of disability among people age 65 and older. Many experts think the condition may not be one disease but several with similar presentations. Although wear and tear, as well as age-related changes such as loss of muscle mass, predispose the elderly to osteoarthritis, other factors may play a role as well. Presumed contributing causes include:

● Obesity
● Primary disorders of the joint, such as inflammatory arthritis
● Trauma
● Congenital abnormalities, such as hip dysplasia

Osteoarthritis in the elderly presents initially as joint pain, worsened by exercise and improved by rest. As the disease progresses, pain may be accompanied by diminished mobility, joint deformity, and crepitus or grating sensations. Late signs include tenderness on palpation or during passive motion.

The most effective treatment involves management before the disability develops or worsens. Prevention strategies include stretching exercises and activities that strengthen stress-absorbing ligaments (Figure 5-22 ●). Immobilization, even for short periods, can accelerate the condition. Drug therapy is usually aimed at lessening pain and/or inflammation. Surgery

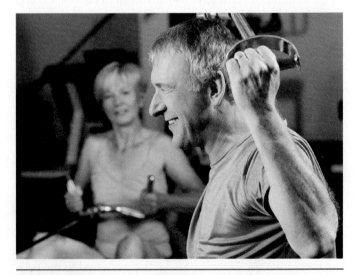

● **Figure 5-22** Regular stretching and weight-bearing exercises help prevent the development of osteoarthritis. (*Fotolia.com*)

(i.e., total joint replacement) is usually the last resort after more conservative methods have failed.

Osteoporosis

Osteoporosis affects an estimated 20 million Americans and is largely responsible for fractures of the hip, wrist, and vertebral bones following a fall or other injury. Risk factors include:

- *Age.* Peak bone mass for men and women occurs in their third and fourth decades of life and declines at varying rates thereafter. Decreased bone density generally becomes a treatment consideration at about age 50.
- *Gender.* The decline of estrogen production places women at a higher risk of developing osteoporosis than men. Women are more than twice as likely to have brittle bones, especially if they experience early menopause (before age 45) and do not take estrogen replacement therapy.
- *Race.* Whites and Asians are more likely to develop osteoporosis than African Americans and Latinos, who have higher bone mass at skeletal peak.
- *Body weight.* Thin people, or people with low body weight, are at greater risk of osteoporosis than obese people. Increased skeletal weight is thought to promote bone density. However, weight-bearing exercise can have the same effect.
- *Family history.* Genetic factors (i.e., peak bone mass attainment) and a family history of fractures may predispose a person to osteoporosis.
- *Miscellaneous.* Late menarche, nulliparity, and use of caffeine, alcohol, and cigarettes are all thought to be important determinants of bone mass.

Unless a bone density test is conducted, persons with osteoporosis are usually asymptomatic until a fracture occurs. The precipitating event can be as slight as turning over in bed, carrying a package, or even a forceful sneeze (Figure 5-23 ●). Management includes prevention of fractures through exercise and drug therapy, such as the administration of calcium, vitamin D, estrogen, and other medications or minerals. Once the condition occurs, pain management also becomes a consideration.

Ankylosing Spondylitis

Ankylosing spondylitis (AS) is a form of inflammatory arthritis that primarily affects the spine. It is estimated that approximately 500,000 people in the United States have the disease. AS primarily causes inflammation of the joints between the vertebrae of the spine and the sacroiliac joints in the pelvis (Figure 5-24 ●). It can also cause inflammation and pain in other parts of the body. As the condition worsens and the inflammation persists, new bone forms as a part of the healing process. The bone may grow from the edge of the vertebra across the disk space between two vertebrae, resulting in a bony bridge; this may occur throughout the spine so that the spine becomes stiff and inflexible—effectively fusing the spine. On spinal X-rays, this phenomenon is referred to as "bamboo spine." This fusion can also affect the rib cage, restricting lung capacity and function.

As the disease progresses, the spine becomes fused into a single unit incapable of flexion, extension, or lateral movement.

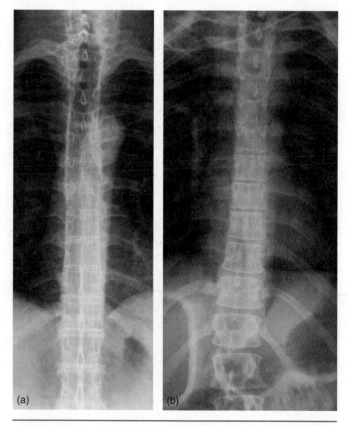

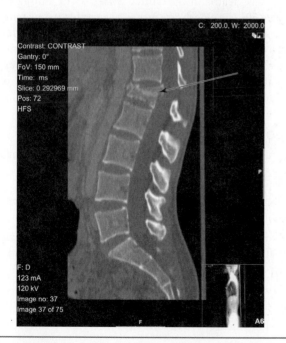

● **Figure 5-23**   Sagittal CT image of a traumatic L1 compression fracture with retropulsion of bone fragments into the spinal canal. (© *Dr. Bryan E. Bledsoe*)

● **Figure 5-24**   Typical "bamboo spine" as seen in ankylosing spondylitis (a) compared with a normal spine (b). (*Spondylitis Association of America*)

Usually the fusion progresses with the spine assuming a flexed position and the patient is forced to walk bent over.

EMS providers called to care for a victim of AS must remember that the patient's spine is inflexible and cannot be moved. Furthermore, the fused spine can be extremely fragile and subject to fracture, with resultant spinal cord injury. Numerous EMS techniques must be modified to accommodate patients with AS. These include airway management techniques, splinting techniques, and transport considerations. Because most AS patients have spinal flexion, it is important to adequately pad underneath the patient's head, neck, and upper back with pillow or pillows.[10] Likewise, airway management techniques must be applied without extending the neck. Airway devices that do not require visualization (e.g., extraglottic airways) should be considered instead of endotracheal intubation, with cricothyrotomy used as a last resort.

Although patients with AS are not common, improper EMS care of them can be devastating. Learn to identify the signs and symptoms of AS and be careful to protect the patient's spine accordingly.

Renal Disorders

The most common renal diseases in the elderly include renal failure, **glomerulonephritis**, and renal blood clots. These problems may be traced to two age-related factors: (1) loss in kidney size and (2) changes in the walls of the renal arteries and in the arterioles serving the glomeruli. In general, a person's kidney loses approximately one-third of its weight between the ages of 30 and 80. Most of this loss occurs in the tissues that filter blood. When filtering tissue is gone, blood is shunted from the precapillary side directly to venules on the postcapillary side, thus bypassing any tissue still capable of filtering. The result is a reduction in kidney efficiency. This condition is complicated by changes in renal arteries, which promote the development of renal emboli and thrombi.

With renal changes, elderly patients are more likely to accumulate toxins and medications within the bloodstream. Occasionally, this will be obvious to the patient because he will experience a substantial decrease in urine output. More often, however, the elderly are prone to a type of renal failure in which urine output remains normal to high while the kidney remains ineffective in clearing wastes.

Processes that precipitate acute renal failure include hypotension, heart failure, major surgery, sepsis, angiographic procedures (the dye is nephrotoxic), and use of nephrotoxic antibiotics (e.g., gentamycin, tobramycin). Ongoing hypertension also figures in the development of chronic renal failure.

Urinary Disorders

Urinary tract infections (UTIs) affect as much as 10 percent of the elderly population each year. Younger women generally suffer more UTIs than young men, but in the elderly the distribution is almost even. Most of these infections result from bacteria and easily lead to **urosepsis** owing to reduced immune system function among the elderly.

A number of factors contribute to the high rate of UTIs among the elderly:

- Bladder outlet obstruction from benign prostatic hyperplasia (in men)
- Atrophic vaginitis (in women)
- Stroke
- Immobilization
- Use of indwelling bladder catheters
- Diabetes
- Upper urinary tract stone
- Dementia, with resulting poor hygiene

Signs or symptoms of a UTI range from cloudy, foul-smelling urine to the typical complaints of bladder pain and frequent urination. Urosepsis presents as an acute process, including fever, chills, abdominal discomfort, and other signs of septic shock. The septicemia generally begins within 24 to 72 hours after catheterization or cystoscopy.

Treatment of urosepsis commonly includes placement of a large-bore IV catheter for administration of fluids and parenteral antibiotics. Diagnosis of urosepsis is based on history and other physical findings. Prompt transport is critical. The prognosis for elderly patients with urosepsis is poor, with a mortality rate of approximately 30 percent. Maintenance of fluid balance, as well as adequate blood pressure, is essential.

Environmental Emergencies

As previously mentioned, environmental extremes represent a great health risk for the elderly. Nearly 50 percent of all **heatstroke** deaths in the United States occur among people over age 50. The elderly are just as susceptible to low temperatures, suffering numerous winter deaths annually, primarily from hypothermia and "winter risks" such as pneumonia and influenza. As you may already know from your EMT experience, thermoregulatory emergencies represent some of the most common EMS calls involving the elderly.

Hypothermia

A number of factors predispose the elderly to hypothermia:

- Accidental exposure to cold
- CNS disorders, including head trauma, stroke, tumors, or subdural hematomas
- Endocrine disorders, including hypoglycemia and diabetes (patients with diabetes are six times as likely to develop hypothermia as other patients)
- Drugs that interfere with heat production, including alcohol, antidepressants, and tranquilizers
- Malnutrition or starvation
- Chronic illness
- Forced inactivity as a result of arthritis, dementia, falls, paralysis, or Parkinson's disease

- Low or fixed income, which discourages the use of home heating
- Inflammatory dermatitis
- AV shunts, which increase heat loss

Signs and symptoms of hypothermia can be slow to develop. Many times, elderly patients with hypothermia lose their sensitivity to cold and fail to complain. As a result, hypothermia may be missed. Nonspecific complaints may suggest a metabolic disorder or stroke. Hypothermic patients may exhibit slow speech, confusion, and sleepiness. In the early stages, patients will exhibit hypertension and an increased heart rate. As hypothermia progresses, however, blood pressure drops and the heart rate slows, sometimes to a barely detectable level.

Remember that the elderly patient with hypothermia often does not shiver. Check the abdomen and back to see if the skin is cool to the touch. Expect subcutaneous tissues to be firm. If your unit has a low-temperature thermometer, check the patient's core temperature. (Regular thermometers often do not "shake down" far enough for an accurate reading.)

As with other medical disorders, prevention is the preferred treatment. However, once elderly patients develop hypothermia, they become progressively impaired. Treat even mild cases of hypothermia, or suspected hypothermia, as a medical emergency. Focus on the rewarming techniques used with other patients and rapid transport. Maintain reassessment to ensure that the hypothermia does not complicate existing medical problems or heretofore untreated disorders. Death most commonly results from cardiac arrest or ventricular fibrillation.

Hyperthermia (Heatstroke)

Age-related changes in sweat glands and increased incidence of heart disease place the elderly at risk of heat stress. They may develop heat cramps, heat exhaustion, or heatstroke. Although the first two disorders rarely result in death, heatstroke is a serious medical emergency. Risk factors for severe hyperthermia include:

- Altered sensory output, which would normally warn a person of overheating
- Inadequate liquid intake
- Decreased functioning of the thermoregulatory center
- Commonly prescribed medications that inhibit sweating such as antihistamines and tricyclic antidepressants
- Low or fixed income, which may result in a lack of air conditioning or adequate ventilation
- Alcoholism
- Concomitant medical disorders
- Use of diuretics, which increase fluid loss

Like hypothermia, early heatstroke may present with non-specific signs and symptoms, such as nausea, light-headedness, dizziness, or headache. High temperature is the most reliable indicator, but consider even a slight temperature elevation as symptomatic if coupled with an absence of sweating

and neurologic impairment. Severe hypotension also exists in many critical patients.

Prevention strategies include adequate fluid intake, reduced activity, shelter in an air-conditioned environment, and use of light clothing. If hyperthermia develops, however, rapid treatment and transport are necessary.

Toxicologic Emergencies

As previously mentioned, aging alters pharmacokinetics and pharmacodynamics in the elderly. Functional changes in the kidneys, liver, and gastrointestinal system slow the absorption and elimination of many medications. In addition, the various compensatory mechanisms that help buffer against medication side effects are less effective in the elderly than in younger patients.

A significant number of all hospital admissions are a result of drug-related illnesses. Many of these result in drug-related deaths in people over age 60. Accidental overdoses may occur more frequently in the aged as a result of confusion, vision impairment, self-selection of medications, forgetfulness, and concurrent drug use. Intentional drug overdose also occurs in attempts at self-destruction. Another complicating factor is the abuse of alcohol among the elderly.

The paramedic must be familiar with the range of side effects that can be caused by the polypharmacy of medications taken by geriatric patients. The usage of multiple doctors and polypharmacy in the aging patient increase the chances of receiving multiple medications for the same medical conditions. This problem is further compounded as a result of the usage of both trade and generic medication names.

In assessing the geriatric patient, always take these steps:

- Obtain a full list of medications currently taken by the patient.
- Elicit any medications that are newly prescribed. (Some side effects appear within a few days of taking a new medication.)
- Obtain a good past medical history. Find out if your patient has a history of renal or hepatic depression.
- Know your medications, their routes of elimination, and their potential side effects.
- If possible, always take all medications to the hospital along with the patient.

A knowledge of pharmacology is important in all patients; however, it is critical in recognizing potential toxicologic emergencies in the geriatric patient. Some of the drugs or substances that have been identified as commonly causing toxicity in the elderly are described in the following sections.

Beta-Blockers

Beta-blockers are widely used to treat hypertension, angina pectoris, and cardiac arrhythmias. Commonly prescribed beta-blockers include propranolol hydrochloride (Inderal), nadolol, atenolol, sotalol, timolol, esmolol, metoprolol, penbutolol, and labetalol.

Although fairly well tolerated in younger adults, elderly patients tend to be more susceptible to the side effects of these agents. In particular, central nervous system side effects—depression, lethargy, and sleep disorders—are more common in the elderly.

Because geriatric patients often have preexisting cardiovascular problems that can cause decreased cardiac function and output, beta-blockers will limit the heart's ability to respond to postural changes, causing orthostatic hypotension. Beta-blockers also limit the heart's ability to increase contractile force and cardiac output whenever a sympathetic response is necessary in situations such as exercise or hypovolemia. This can be detrimental to the trauma patient who is hemorrhaging and cannot mount the sympathetic response necessary to maintain perfusion of vital organs. Also remember that all beta-blockers can worsen heart failure in patients with poor left ventricular function. Beta-blockers decrease intraocular pressure and are often used to treat glaucoma in the elderly. Remember, even beta-blocker eyedrops can cause systemic effects.

Treatment of beta-blocker overdose includes general supportive measures, the removal of gastric contents, cardiorespiratory support, fluids, and administration of nonadrenergic inotropic agents, such as glucagon, for hypotension. Excessive bradycardia can be treated with atropine.

Antihypertensives/Diuretics

Diuretics act on the kidneys to increase urine flow and the excretion of water and sodium. They are used primarily in the treatment of hypertension and congestive heart failure.

This group of medications includes hydrochlorothiazide (HCTZ), furosemide, bumetanide, and torsemide. Of these drugs, furosemide is the most widely used diuretic in the elderly. The elimination half-life of furosemide is markedly prolonged in the patient with acute pulmonary edema and renal and hepatic failure. As a result, the geriatric patient is at risk for a drug buildup.

Because the elderly may be sensitive to adult dosages, a smaller dose is often prescribed and the patient usually takes a daily potassium supplement. Excessive urination caused by the drug may put the elderly at risk for postural hypotension, circulatory collapse, potassium depletion, and renal function impairment.

Angiotensin-Converting Enzyme Inhibitors

Angiotensin-converting enzyme (ACE) inhibitors are a relatively recent addition to the group of medications used in the treatment of hypertension and congestive heart failure. They are used either as a first-line treatment or when other, more established, drugs are contraindicated, are poorly tolerated, or fail to produce the desired effect. Specific examples of ACE inhibitors include captopril, enalapril, lisinopril, fosinopril, benazepril, quinapril, and ramipril.

For the treatment of congestive heart failure, ACE inhibitors reduce renin–angiotensin-mediated vasoconstriction, which reduces the pressure against which the heart has to pump (afterload). Geriatric patients generally respond well to treatment with ACE inhibitors. However, these drugs can cause chronic hypotension in patients with severe heart failure if they are also taking high-dose loop diuretics. ACE inhibitors can also cause plasma volume reduction and hypotension with prolonged vomiting and diarrhea, especially in the elderly. Some hemodialysis patients can experience anaphylactic reactions if treated with ACE inhibitors.

Other side effects of ACE inhibitors include dizziness or light-headedness upon standing; presence of a rash; muscle cramps; swelling of the hands, face, or eyes; cough (especially in women); headache; stomach upset; and fatigue. Captopril, in particular, can cause a loss of taste.

Digitalis (Digoxin, Lanoxin)

Digoxin is the most widely used cardiac glycoside for the management of congestive heart failure, atrial fibrillation, atrial flutter, paroxysmal atrial tachycardia, and cardiogenic shock. The drug is unique in that it has a positive inotropic effect, but a negative chronotropic effect. In congestive heart failure, digoxin increases the strength of myocardial contractions (positive inotropic effect) with a resulting increase in cardiac output. Digoxin also slows conduction and increases the refractory period in cardiac conducting tissue, resulting in a reduced ventricular rate (negative chronotropic effect). This allows the ventricle to adequately fill with blood, also improving cardiac output.

In the patient with moderate to severe heart failure, digitalis is often combined with ACE inhibitors and diuretics. Remember that digoxin has a low therapeutic index. As a result, the dose must be adjusted for each patient.

Digoxin serum levels should be monitored carefully during therapy. The drug is excreted in the urine, with 50 to 70 percent of the dose as unchanged drug. The half-life ranges from 32 to 48 hours in patients with normal renal function. Because the elderly have a reduced volume of distribution for digoxin and may have impaired renal or hepatic function, the dose should be reduced and individualized to minimize the risk of toxicity. Digitalis-induced appetite loss is also a danger in frail elderly patients.

The most common adverse drug effect that occurs in elderly patients is digoxin toxicity. The primary reason is that digoxin has a low margin of safety and a narrow therapeutic index. The amount of the drug needed to produce beneficial or therapeutic effects is close to the toxic amount.

Digoxin toxicity in the elderly can result from accidental or intentional ingestion. For the renal-impaired elderly patient, any change in kidney function usually warrants an alteration in the dosing of digoxin. Failure to adjust the dose can lead to toxicity. Diuretics, which are often given to patients with congestive heart failure, cause the loss of large amounts of potassium in the urine. If potassium is not adequately replenished in the patient taking digoxin, toxicity will develop. Therefore, elderly patients on digoxin should be taking a daily potassium supplement such as potassium chloride (Micro-K, K-Tabs, Slow-K).

Signs and symptoms of digoxin toxicity include visual disturbances, fatigue, weakness, nausea, loss of appetite, abdominal discomfort, dizziness, abnormal dreams, headache, and vomiting. Patients who are taking digoxin for the first time are instructed to call their physician if any of these symptoms occur.

Low potassium (hypokalemia) is also common with chronic digoxin toxicity due to concurrent diuretic therapy. Arrhythmias commonly associated with digoxin toxicity include sinoatrial (SA) exit block, SA arrest, second- or third-degree AV block, atrial fibrillation with a slow ventricular response, accelerated AV junctional rhythms, patterns of premature ventricular contractions (bigeminy and trigeminy), ventricular tachycardia, and atrial tachycardia with AV block.

Management of digoxin toxicity includes gastric lavage with activated charcoal, correction of confirmed hypokalemia with K^+ supplements, treatment of bradycardias with atropine or pacing, and treatment of rapid ventricular rhythms with an antiarrhythmic. A digoxin-specific FAB fragment antibodies treatment (Digibind), an antidote for digoxin toxicity, is used in the treatment of potentially life-threatening situations.

Anticoagulants

The use of anticoagulant medications by the elderly is common. Low-dose aspirin is commonly used as an antiplatelet inhibitor for the prophylaxis of cardiovascular and cerebrovascular disease. A commonly encountered anticoagulant is warfarin (Coumadin). It is used to prevent blood clots from forming or enlarging. It is commonly used in patients with atrial fibrillation, those who have prosthetic (artificial) heart valves, and in selected patients following cardiac events (STEMI). It is also used to prevent pulmonary emboli and deep venous thrombosis.

Warfarin can be difficult to dose and requires routine monitoring of the patient's prothrombin time (PT) or the derivative value called the International Normalized Ratio (INR). The goal is to keep the INR within a target range—not too high or the patient will bleed, or too low where it is ineffective. Warfarin toxicity can be reversed with vitamin K if required.

A newer anticoagulant is dabigatran (Pradaxa). It is effective and does not require PT or INR monitoring. However, there is no reversal agent. Patients on anticoagulants (besides aspirin) are at an increased risk for hemorrhage following trauma—especially head trauma.

Antipsychotics/Antidepressants

Psychotropic medications comprise a variety of agents that affect mood, behavior, and other aspects of mental function. The elderly often experience a high incidence of psychiatric disorders and may take any number of medications, including antidepressants, antianxiety agents, sedative-hypnotic agents, and antipsychotics.

Depression is the most common mental disorder in the elderly. Drug therapy may be prescribed to help resolve the feelings of sadness or hopelessness that result from the death of a spouse, divorce, declining health, and/or loss of independence. Commonly prescribed antidepressants include serotonin reuptake inhibitors (SSRIs) such as fluoxetine (Prozac) and bupropion (Wellbutrin). Tricyclic antidepressants (amitriptyline [Elavil] and imipramine [Tofranil]) are less popular. Monoamine oxidase inhibitors (isocarboxazid [Marplan] and phenelzine [Nardil]) are rarely used.

Antidepressant use in the elderly may result in side effects such as sedation, lethargy, and muscle weakness. Some antidepressants tend to produce anticholinergic effects, including dry mouth, constipation, urinary retention, and confusion. Newly prescribed tricyclic antidepressants can also cause orthostatic hypotension, which can be compounded if the geriatric patient is taking diuretics or other antihypertensive medications. Side effects such as sedation and confusion may also impair the patient's cognitive abilities and possibly endanger the elderly patient who lives alone.

Elderly patients with a history of bipolar disorder may be treated with lithium carbonate. This drug stabilizes the mood swings associated with bipolar disorder. Because lithium cannot be degraded by the body into an inactive form, the kidneys are the sole routes of elimination for this drug. If renal function is impaired, the drug may quickly accumulate to toxic levels, causing lithium toxicity. Symptoms include a metallic taste in the mouth, hand tremors, nausea, muscle weakness, and fatigue. As the levels of toxicity increase, blurred vision, lack of coordination, coma, and even death may occur.

Antipsychotic medications produce a number of minor side effects such as sedation and anticholinergic effects. Extrapyramidal side effects can also occur, including restlessness and involuntary muscle movements, particularly in the face, jaw, and extremities. Examples of these medications include chlorpromazine (Thorazine), thioridazine (Mellaril), chlorprothixene (Taractan), thiothixene (Navane), and haloperidol (Haldol).

Sedative-hypnotic drugs are prescribed to relax the patient, allay anxiety, and promote sleep. Antianxiety medications, chemically similar to the sedative-hypnotics, are intended to decrease anxiety without producing sedation. These drugs are helpful in geriatric patients who suffer from insomnia and feelings of fear or apprehension.

Benzodiazepines are the most commonly prescribed sedative-hypnotic and anxiolytic drugs. These medications can produce drowsiness, sluggishness, and addiction if used over a long period of time. Examples of benzodiazepines include flurazepam (Dalmane), temazepam (Restoril), and triazolam (Halcion). Specific antianxiety agents include diazepam (Valium), lorazepam (Ativan), and chlordiazepoxide (Librium).

Field treatment for overdoses of these medications are aimed primarily at the ABCs, with special emphasis on airway management.

Medications for Parkinson's Disease

Parkinson's disease is a common disorder of the elderly and is caused by a breakdown of dopamine-secreting neurons located in the basal ganglia. This leads to an imbalance in other neurotransmitters, which eventually results in the parkinsonian motor symptoms of rigidity, bradykinesia, resting tremor, and postural instability. Drug treatment is aimed at restoring the balance of neurotransmitters in the basal ganglia. The most commonly prescribed medications include carbidopa/levadopa (Sinemet), bromocriptine (Parlodel), benztropine mesylate (Cogentin), and amantadine (Symmetrel).

Toxicity of these drugs commonly presents as dyskinesia (the inability to execute voluntary movements) and psychological disturbances such as visual hallucinations and nightmares. When these medications are first taken, orthostatic hypotension may also occur.

Tolcapone (Tasmar) is a Parkinson's drug that is given in combination with Sinemet. It potentiates the effects of Sinemet and can cause liver failure. Toxicity in a patient on Tasmar will present as acute jaundice.

The goal of field management is aimed at decreasing the patient's anxiety and providing a supportive environment. Remember that patients with gross involuntary motor movements are at risk for aspiration and choking. Continued assessment of this patient is necessary.

Antiseizure Medications

Seizure disorders are not uncommon in elderly patients. In most cases, the cause of seizures is related to a previous central nervous system injury such as stroke or trauma, tumor, or degenerative brain disease. The selection of a specific antiseizure medication depends on the type of seizure present in the patient.

The most common side effect of antiseizure medications is sedation. Other side effects include GI distress, headache, dizziness, lack of coordination, and dermatologic reactions (rashes). Recommended treatment involves airway management and supportive therapy.

Analgesics and Anti-Inflammatory Agents

Treatment of pain and inflammation for chronic conditions such as rheumatoid arthritis and osteoarthritis includes narcotics and nonnarcotic analgesics and corticosteroids. The narcotic analgesics used to reduce pain in the elderly include codeine, meperidine (Demerol), morphine, hydrocodone (Vicodin), oxycodone (Percodan, Percocet), and hydromorphone (Dilaudid). Remember that these agents alter pain perception, rather than eliminating the condition. As they wear off, pain reappears, encouraging a patient to increase the frequency of dosage.

Adverse side effects of these drugs include sedation, mood changes, nausea, vomiting, and constipation. Orthostatic hypotension and respiratory depression may also occur. Over long periods of time, patients may develop drug tolerance and physical dependence on narcotic agents.

The nonsteroidal anti-inflammatory drugs (NSAIDs) and acetaminophen (Tylenol) are prescribed for mild to moderate pain. They are also the principal therapeutic agents for osteoarthritis and other inflammatory musculoskeletal considerations. The most common side effect of these agents is gastric irritation. Higher doses can cause renal and hepatic toxicity. Acetaminophen is particularly toxic to the liver when taken in high doses. Confusion and hearing problems (ringing or buzzing in the ears) and gastrointestinal hemorrhaging may occur with aspirin use.

Corticosteroids

Corticosteroids are powerful anti-inflammatory agents used to treat rheumatoid arthritis and other inflammatory conditions. Side effects from these agents include hypertension, peptic ulcer, aggravation of diabetes mellitus, glaucoma, increased risk of infection, and suppression of normally produced corticosteroids. Commonly prescribed corticosteroids include cortisone (Cortone), hydrocortisone (Hydrocortone), and prednisone (Deltasone).

Substance Abuse

Substance abuse is a widespread problem in the United States. It affects nearly all age groups, including the elderly. Many Americans over age 60 are addicted to substances. That number is expected to rise as the baby boomer generation swells to the size of the elderly population.

In general, the factors that contribute to substance abuse among the elderly are different from those of younger people. They include:

- Age-related changes
- Loss of employment
- Loss of spouse or partner
- Multiple prescriptions
- Malnutrition
- Loneliness
- Moving from a long-loved house to an apartment

Like people in other age groups, the elderly may intentionally abuse substances to escape pain or life itself. Other times, particularly in the case of prescription drugs, the abuse is accidental. Substance abuse in the elderly may involve drugs, alcohol, or both drugs and alcohol.

Drug Abuse

As previously mentioned, people age 65 and older have more illnesses, consume more drugs, and are more sensitive to adverse drug reactions than younger adults. The sheer number of medications taken by the elderly makes them vulnerable to drug abuse. Of the 1.5 billion prescriptions written each year in the United States, more than one-third go to the elderly. People age 65 and older fill an average of 13 prescriptions per year. The elderly also use a disproportionate percentage of OTC drugs.

Polypharmacy, coupled with impaired vision and/or memory, increases the likelihood of complications. The elderly might experience drug–drug interactions, drug–disease interactions, and drug–food interactions.

The elderly who become physically and/or psychologically dependent on drugs (or alcohol) are more likely to hide their dependence and less likely to seek help than other age groups. Common signs and symptoms of drug abuse include:

- Memory changes
- Drowsiness
- Decreased vision/hearing
- Orthostatic hypotension
- Poor dexterity
- Mood changes
- Falling
- Restlessness
- Weight loss

In cases of suspected drug abuse, carefully document your findings. Collect medications for identification at the hospital, where the patient can be evaluated and, if necessary, referred for substance abuse treatment.

Alcohol Abuse

In a national survey, nearly 50 percent of the elderly reported abstinence from alcohol. However, the same survey found that 15 percent of the men and 12 percent of the women interviewed regularly drank in excess of the one-drink-a-day limit suggested by the National Institute on Alcohol Abuse and Alcoholism. Those percentages are expected to rise with the aging of the baby boomer generation, which has generally used alcohol more frequently than their predecessors.

The use or abuse of alcohol places the elderly at high risk of toxicity. Physiologic changes, such as organ dysfunction, makes older adults more susceptible to the effects of alcohol. Consumption of even moderate amounts of alcohol can interfere with drug therapy, often leading to dangerous consequences. Severe stress and a history of heavy and/or regular drinking predisposes a person to alcohol dependence or abuse in later life.

Unless a patient is openly intoxicated, discovery of alcohol abuse depends on a thorough history. Signs and symptoms of alcohol abuse in the elderly may be very subtle or confused with other conditions. Remember that even small amounts of alcohol can cause intoxication in an older person. If possible, question family, friends, or caregivers about the patient's drinking patterns. Pertinent findings include:

- Mood swings, denial, and hostility (especially when questioned about drinking)
- Confusion
- History of falls
- Anorexia
- Insomnia
- Visible anxiety
- Nausea

Treatment follows many of the same steps as for any other patient with a pattern of abusive drinking. (See Volume 4, Chapter 8.) *Do not* judge the patient. Evaluate the need for fluid therapy, and keep in mind the possibility of withdrawal. Transport the patient to the hospital for evaluation and referral for treatment. Ideally, these patients will seek support from community organizations such as Alcoholics Anonymous (AA). Many communities have AA groups specifically for senior citizens.

Behavioral/Psychological Disorders

When behavioral or psychological problems develop later in life, they are often dismissed as normal age-related changes. This attitude denies an elderly person the opportunity to correct a treatable condition and/or overlooks an underlying physical disorder. Studies have shown that the elderly retain their basic personalities and their adaptive cognitive abilities. In other words, intellectual decline and/or regressive behavior are not normal age-related changes. Unless an organic brain disorder

is involved, alterations in behavior should be considered symptomatic of a possible psychological problem.

It is important to keep in mind the emotionally stressful situations facing many elderly people: isolation, loneliness, loss of self-dependence, loss of strength, fear of the future, and more. The elderly also face a higher incidence of secondary depression as a result of neuroleptic medications such as Haldol and Thorazine. Some of the common classifications of psychological disorders related to age include:

- Organic brain syndrome
- Affective disorders (depression)
- Personality disorders (dependent personality)
- Dissociative disorders (paranoid schizophrenia)

As with other people, the emotional well-being of the elderly affects their overall physical health. Therefore, it is important that you note evidence of altered behavior in any elderly patient you assess and examine. Common signs and symptoms of a psychological disorder include lapses in memory, cognitive difficulty, changes in sleep patterns, fear of death, changes in sexual interest, thoughts of suicide, or withdrawal from society.

In general, management of psychological disorders in the elderly is the same as that for other age groups. Two of the most common emotional disturbances that you may encounter in the elderly are depression and suicide.

Depression

Up to 15 percent of the noninstitutionalized elderly experience depression. Within institutions, that figure rises to about 30 percent. The incidence of depression among the elderly is expected to rise in the early twenty-first century as the baby boomers—with their larger numbers and more prevalent depression at an earlier age—enter their 60s.

Some of the general signs and symptoms noted previously may indicate depression. Ask the patient about feelings of sadness or despair. Determine whether he has suffered episodes of crying. Inquire about past psychological treatment and current stressful events, particularly the death of a loved one. Keep in mind that sensory changes, especially deafness and blindness, may make the patient vulnerable to depression. Serious acute diseases can have the same effect. If the patient recognizes the depression, ask about the duration and any prior bouts. Find out whether the patient has been given any medications to treat the depression. If so, check compliance.

Some depressed patients may exhibit **hypochondriasis** (hypochondria). If this condition is a side effect of the depression, the patient will still show some degree of emotional pain and/or **dysphoria**. Although you may not be able to identify hypochondria in the field, remember that the condition is an illness and requires treatment by trained medical personnel.

In general, depressed patients should receive supportive care. Encourage them to talk, delicately raising questions about suicidal thoughts. The seriously depressed patient should be transported to the hospital. Treatment of depression usually entails psychotherapy and/or antidepressants.

Suicide

The highest suicide rates in the United States are among people over age 65, especially men. The elderly account for 20 percent of all suicides, but represent only 12 percent of the total population. Someone over age 65 commits suicide about every 90 minutes. Suicide is the third-leading cause of death among the elderly, following falls and car accidents.

Depression is the leading cause of suicide among the elderly. As a group, the elderly are less likely to seek help than the young. They are also less likely to express their anger or sorrow, turning their feelings inward instead. Other stressors that put the elderly at risk of suicide include:

- Chronic illness
- Physical impairment
- Unrelieved pain
- Living in a youth-oriented society
- Family issues
- Financial problems
- Isolation and loneliness
- Substance abuse
- Low serotonin levels (serotonin declines with age)
- Bereavement
- Family history of suicide

Suicidal behavior is related to stress. As a paramedic, you should try to evaluate the stress from an elderly patient's point of view, keeping the preceding factors in mind. In cases of a seriously depressed patient, elicit behavior patterns from family, friends, or caregivers. Warning signs may include:

- Loss of interest in activities that were once enjoyable
- Curtailing social interaction, grooming, and self-care
- Breaking from medical or exercise regimens
- Grieving a personal loss ("I don't want to live without him/her")
- Feeling useless ("nobody would miss me")
- Putting affairs in order, giving away things, finalizing a will
- Stockpiling medications or other lethal means of self-destruction, including firearms

Be particularly alert to suicide among the acutely ill. With more patients being returned home to care for themselves, there is a higher incidence of suicide among the terminally ill, especially cancer victims. A lack of postacute hospital care can be interpreted as a lack of caring in general.

Prevention of suicide among the elderly involves intervention by all levels of society, from family to EMS to hospital workers. It is important to dispel the common myths about aging and age-related diseases. Recognition of warning signs and involvement of appropriate individuals and agencies is critical.

Your first priorities in the management of a suicidal elderly patient are to protect yourself and then to protect the patient from self-harm. To do this, you must gain access to the patient. This may require breaking into a house or room, particularly if the patient is unconscious or can be readily seen. Remember to summon law enforcement personnel as necessary. *Do not* rule out firearm use among the elderly.

If you reach the patient, emergency care has the highest priority secondary to crew safety. Conduct a brief interview with the patient, if possible, to determine the need for further action. *Do not* leave the suicidal patient alone. Administer medications with caution, keeping in mind polypharmacy and drug interactions in the elderly. (Consult with medical direction.) *All* suicidal elderly patients should be transported to the hospital.

TRAUMA IN THE ELDERLY PATIENT

Trauma is the leading cause of death among the elderly. Older patients who sustain moderate to severe injuries are more likely to die than their younger counterparts. Postinjury disability is also more common in the elderly than in the young.

Contributing Factors

A number of factors contribute to the high incidence and severity of trauma among the elderly. Slower reflexes, arthritis, and diminished eyesight and hearing predispose the elderly to accidents, especially falls. The elderly, because of their physical state and vulnerability, are also at high risk from trauma caused by criminal assault. Purse snatching, armed robbery, and assault occur all too frequently in the elderly population, especially among those living in urban areas. Fall and trauma prevention programs can be effective in reducing elderly trauma—especially falls.[11]

Age-related factors that place the elderly at risk of severe injury and complications include:

- *Osteoporosis and muscle weakness*—increased likelihood of fractures
- *Reduced cardiac reserve*—decreased ability to compensate for blood loss
- *Decreased respiratory function*—increased likelihood of **acute respiratory distress syndrome (ARDS)**
- *Impaired renal function*—decreased ability to adapt to fluid shifts
- *Decreased elasticity in the peripheral blood vessels*—greater susceptibility to tearing

General Assessment

As with any other trauma patient, determine the mechanism of injury. Leading causes of trauma in the elderly include falls, motor vehicle crashes, burns, assault or abuse, and underlying medical problems such as syncope.

In assessing elderly trauma patients, remember that blood pressure readings may be deceptive. Older patients typically have higher blood pressures than younger patients. Although a blood pressure of 110/70 may be normal for a 30-year-old, it could represent a low blood pressure, and possibly shock, for an older patient. Elderly trauma patients also may not exhibit an elevated pulse, a common early sign of hypoperfusion. This may be because of a chronic heart disease or the use of medications to treat hypertension or a myocardial infarction. Fractures may also be obscured or concealed because of a diminished sense of pain among the elderly. One of the best indicators of shock in the elderly is an altered mental status or changes in consciousness during assessment. Elderly trauma patients who exhibit confusion or agitation are candidates for rapid transport.

Observing for Abuse/Neglect

Make sure you observe the scene for signs of abuse and neglect. Abuse of the elderly is as big a problem in our society as child abuse and neglect. **Geriatric abuse** is defined as a syndrome in which an elderly person has received serious physical or psychological injury from family members or other caregivers. Abuse of the elderly knows no socioeconomic bounds. It often occurs when an older person is no longer able to be totally independent, and the family members have difficulty upholding their commitment to care for the patient. It can also occur in nursing homes and other health care facilities. The profile for the potential geriatric abuser may often show a great deal of life stress. In many cases, there is sleep deprivation, marital discord, financial problems, and work-related problems. As the abuser's life falls into further disarray, and as the patient further deteriorates, abuse may be the outcome.

Signs and symptoms of geriatric abuse and neglect are often obvious. Unexplained trauma is usually the primary presentation. The average abused patient is older than 80 and has multiple medical problems, such as cancer, congestive heart failure, heart disease, and incontinence. Senile dementia is often present. In these cases, it can be hard to determine whether the dementia is chronic or acute, especially if there is an increased likelihood of head trauma from abuse.[12]

Whenever you suspect geriatric abuse, obtain a complete patient and family history. Pay particular attention to inconsistencies. *Do not* confront the family. Instead, report your suspicions to the emergency department and the appropriate governmental authority. Many states have very strong laws protecting the elderly from abuse or neglect. In fact, many states consider it a criminal offense *not* to report suspected geriatric abuse. These states also offer legal immunity to those who report geriatric abuse, as long as the report is made in good faith.

General Management

The priorities of care for the elderly trauma patient are similar to those for any trauma patient. However, you must keep in mind age-related systemic changes and the presence of chronic diseases. This is especially true of the cardiovascular, respiratory, and renal systems.

Cardiovascular Considerations

Recent or past myocardial infarctions may contribute to the risk of arrhythmia or congestive heart failure in the trauma patient. In addition, there may be a decreased response of the heart, in adjusting heart rate and stroke volume, to hypovolemia. An elderly trauma patient may require higher than usual arterial pressures for perfusion of vital organs, owing to increased peripheral vascular resistance and hypertension. Care must be taken in intravenous fluid administration because of decreased myocardial reserves. Hypotension, hypovolemia, and hypervolemia are poorly tolerated in the elderly patient.

Respiratory Considerations

In managing the airway and ventilation in an elderly trauma patient, you must consider the physical changes that may affect treatment. Check for dentures and determine whether they should be removed. Keep in mind that age-related changes can decrease chest wall movement and vital capacity. Age also reduces the tolerance of all organs for anoxia. Remember, too, that chronic obstructive pulmonary disease is widespread among the elderly.

Make necessary adjustments in treatment to provide adequate oxygenation and appropriate CO_2 removal. Monitor with oximetry and capnography.

Renal Considerations

The decreased ability of the kidneys to maintain a normal acid-base balance and to compensate for fluid changes can further complicate the management of the elderly trauma patient. Any preexisting renal disease can decrease the kidney's ability to compensate. The decrease in renal function, along with a decreased cardiac reserve, places the elderly injured patient at risk for fluid overload and pulmonary edema. Remember, too, that renal changes allow toxins and medications to accumulate more readily in the elderly.

Transport Considerations

You may have to modify the positioning, immobilization, and packaging of the elderly trauma patient before transport. Be attentive to physical deformities such as arthritis, spinal abnormalities, or frozen limbs that may cause pain or require special care (Figure 5-25 ●). Recall the frailty of an elderly person's skin and avoid creating skin tears or pressure sores. Keep in mind that trauma places an elderly person at increased risk of hypothermia. Ensure that the patient is kept warm at all times.

Specific Injuries

The elderly can be subject to a variety of injuries, just like any other age group. The three most common categories of injuries among the elderly are orthopedic injuries, burns, and injuries of the head and spine.

Orthopedic Injuries

As previously mentioned, the elderly suffer the greatest mortality and greatest incidence of disability from falls. Some falls in the elderly result in at least one fractured bone (Figure 5-26 ●). The most common fall-related fracture is a fracture of the hip or pelvis. Osteoporosis and general frailty contribute to this. The older patient who has fallen should be assumed to have a hip fracture until proven otherwise. Signs and symptoms of a hip fracture include tenderness over the affected joint and

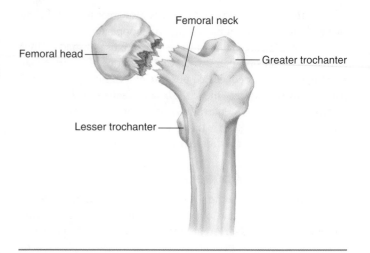

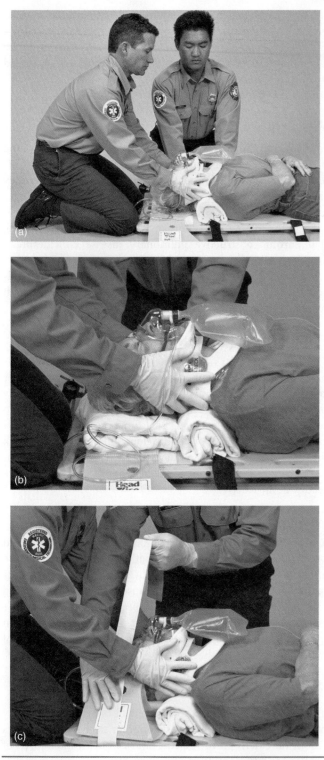

● **Figure 5-26** Subcapital femoral neck fracture. Patients with a displaced femoral neck fracture present with groin pain and a shortened externally rotated leg.

of this, they may remain on the floor for a prolonged period of time. This can lead to hypothermia, hyperthermia, and/or dehydration.

Falls also result in a variety of other stress fractures in the elderly, including fractures of the proximal humerus, distal radius, proximal tibia, and thoracic and lumbar bodies. Falls may also lead to soft-tissue injuries and hot-water burns if the incident occurred in a tub or hot shower.

In treating orthopedic injuries, remember to ask questions aimed at detecting an underlying medical condition. Ask whether the patient recalls "blacking out." Remain alert for evidence of potential cardiac emergencies. Package and transport the patient according to the general guidelines mentioned earlier.

Burns

People age 60 and older are more likely to suffer death from burns than any other age group except neonates and infants. Several factors help explain the high mortality rate among elderly burn victims:

● Reaction time slows as people age, so the elderly often stay in contact with thermal sources longer than their younger counterparts.

● Preexisting diseases place the elderly being treated for burns at risk of medical complications, particularly pulmonary and cardiac problems.

● Age-related skin changes (thinning) result in deeper burns and slower healing time.

● Immunologic and metabolic changes increase the risk of infection.

● Reductions in physiologic function and the reduced reserve of several organ systems make the elderly more vulnerable to major systemic stress.

Management of elderly burn patients follows the same general procedures as other patients. However, remember that the elderly are at increased risk of shock. Administration of fluids is important to prevent renal tubular damage. Assess hydration in

● **Figure 5-25** (a) In an elderly patient with curvature of the spine, place padding behind the neck when immobilizing a patient to a long spine board. (b) Additional padding, such as rolled blankets or towels behind the head, may be needed to keep the head in a neutral, in-line position. (c) Secure the patient's head with a head immobilizer device. To prevent spinal damage, maintain manual stabilization until the head is secured.

shortening and external rotation of the leg. The patient is unable to bear weight on the affected leg. Patients who live alone may not be able to get to a phone to summon help. Because

the initial hours after a burn injury by blood pressure, pulse, and urine output (at least 1 to 2 mL/kg per hour).

In the case of the elderly, complications from a burn may manifest themselves in the days and weeks following the incident. For serious burns to heal, the body may use up to 20,000 calories a day. Elderly patients, with altered metabolism and complications such as diabetes, may not be able to meet this demand, increasing the chances for infection and systemic failure. Part of your job may be to prepare the family for such a delayed response and to provide necessary psychological support.

Head and Spinal Injuries

As a group, the elderly experience more head injuries, even from relatively minor trauma, than their younger counterparts. Elderly patients with a seemingly less severe head injury often have increased mortality and decreased functional outcomes compared with non-elderly patients. A major factor is the difference in proportion between the brain and the skull. As mentioned earlier, the brain decreases in size and weight with age. The skull, however, remains constant in size, allowing the brain more room to move, thus increasing the likelihood of brain injury. Because of this, signs of brain injury may develop more slowly in the elderly, sometimes over days and weeks. In fact, the patient may often have forgotten the offending injury.

The cervical spine is also more susceptible to injury due to osteoporosis and spondylosis. **Spondylosis** is a degeneration of the vertebral body. The elderly often have a significant degree of this disease. In addition, arthritic changes can gradually compress the nerve rootlets or spinal cord. Thus, injury to the spine in the elderly makes the patient much more susceptible to spinal cord injury. In fact, sudden neck movement, even without fracture, may cause spinal cord injury. This can occur with less than normal pain, owing to the absence of fracture. Therefore, it is important to provide older patients with suspected spinal injuries, especially those involved in motor vehicle collisions, with immediate manual cervical spinal stabilization at the time of primary assessment.

CONTENT REVIEW

▶ Common Fractures among the Elderly

- Hip or pelvis fractures
- Proximal humerus
- Distal radius
- Proximal tibia
- Thoracic and lumbar bodies

SUMMARY

Providing EMS in the twenty-first century means treating a growing elderly population. The "graying of America" has resulted in a greater number of people age 65 and older, many of whom are in home settings. When treating elderly patients, keep in mind the anatomic, physiologic, and emotional changes that occur with age. However, never jump to conclusions based solely on age. Weigh normal age-related changes against abnormal changes—that is, those resulting from a medical condition or trauma. Recall that elderly patients are much more susceptible to medication side effects and toxicity than younger patients. They also are more susceptible to trauma and environmental stressors. Abuse of the elderly occurs; you should bear this in mind whenever injuries do not match the history. Any suspected abuse or neglect of an elderly patient should be reported to the emergency department and/or the appropriate governmental authorities.

Just as in pediatric calls, the call for an elderly patient can present with a variety of scenarios that are unique to the population or related to the normal physiology. Maintaining a current knowledge and understanding of these two unique populations will help you make quicker, more accurate assessments and treatment plans.

YOU MAKE THE CALL

Just after 3 A.M., a call comes in to the station to assist an elderly man who has fallen. His wife requests lifting assistance because she has a disability. She reports: "I have arthritis and cannot possibly help him back into bed."

You arrive at a small, one-family home just off a major thoroughfare. A small, severely arthritic woman in a wheelchair greets you: "He's inside. The nerve of him. He won't even answer me—just makes fun of me by repeating everything I say and slurring his words. I'll bet he's been drinking and didn't want me to know. As if I couldn't tell by his behavior! We've been married for 47 years, and he still takes care of me. But not tonight!"

The home is clean and well cared for—not a speck of dust or a single cobweb to be seen. The woman's husband is lying on his side on the carpeted floor next to the bed. He is awake, drooling, and repeating words in a thick speech.

1. What general impression do you have of this patient?

2. Do you suspect that this is an acute or chronic problem? Explain.

During the primary assessment, the patient is at V on the AVPU scale. Pupils are deviated left. You ensure that all spinal precautions are taken. Then you check hand grasp; the left is strong, the right absent. The airway is open, but needs suctioning of saliva. Respirations are present and unlabored. You note strong, but irregular, distal pulses.

You apply oxygen to correct mild hypoxia and determine that the patient, Mr. Jones, is a high priority due to the field diagnosis of a stroke. His airway will need close management and definitive treatment.

3. Aside from the patient's presentation and response to your interventions, what other information should be included in your hospital report?

4. What support do you provide for Mrs. Jones?

See Suggested Responses at the back of this book.

REVIEW QUESTIONS

1. _____ is defined as discrimination against aged or elderly people.
   a. Ageism   c. Congregate
   b. Polypharmacy   d. Comorbidity

2. The most common cause of injury in the elderly is _____.
   a. falls
   b. motor vehicle collisions
   c. skydiving
   d. gunshot wounds

3. Multiple drug therapy in which there is a concurrent use of a number of drugs is termed _____.
   a. multipharmacy
   b. polypharmacy
   c. hyperpharmacy
   d. comorbidity

4. _____ injuries represent the leading cause of accidental death among the elderly.
   a. Burn   c. Abuse-related
   b. Fall-related   d. Vehicle collision

5. By-products of malnutrition may include all of the following *except* _____.
   a. vitamin deficiencies
   b. dehydration
   c. hypoglycemia
   d. hyperthermia

6. A pathophysiologic change may cause a reduction in brain size, leaving room for increased bleeding following a blow to the head, making the elderly more prone to _____.
   a. dissecting aneurysm
   b. cardiac arrhythmias
   c. epidural hematomas
   d. subdural hematomas

7. A common drug toxicity problem seen in the elderly is _____.
   a. aspirin   c. vitamin E
   b. digitalis   d. acetaminophen

8. The leading cause of death in the elderly is _____ disease.
   a. renal   c. cardiovascular
   b. respiratory   d. immune system

9. In elderly patients, the changes in sensory nerves, combined with the myocardial changes of aging, make _____ a more likely symptom of angina than pain.
   a. anoxia   c. weakness
   b. dyspnea   d. diaphoresis

10. Toxicity in a patient on tolcapone (Tasmar) will present as acute _____.
    a. hypoxia   c. anxiety
    b. jaundice   d. anemia

See Answers to Review Questions at the back of this book.

REFERENCES

1. Administration on Aging, Department of Health and Human Services. *Aging into the 21st Century*. [Available at http://www.aoa.gov/AoARoot/Aging_Statistics/future_growth/aging21/program.aspx]

2. Grudzen, C. R., J. R. Hoffman, W. J. Koenig, et al. "The LA Story: What Happened after a New Policy Allowing Paramedics to Forgo Resuscitation Attempts in Prehospital Cardiac Arrest." *Resuscitation* 81 (2010): 685–690.

3. Byrd, L. "More Drugs Equal More Problems: Polypharmacy in Elders—More Problems than Benefits?" *Geriatr Nurs* 31 (2010): 389–390.

4. Xu, W., S. Parera, D. Medich, et al. "Height Loss, Vertebral Fractures, and the Misclassification of Osteoporosis." *Bone* 48 (2011): 301–311.

5. Testa, G., F. Cacciatore, D. Della-Morte, et al. "Role of Permanent Atrial Fibrillation (AF) on Long-Term Mortality in Community-Dwelling Elderly People with and without Chronic Heart Failure (CHF)." *Arch Gerontol Geriatr* 54 (2011): 121–126.

6. Kessler, C., J. M. Tristano, and R. DeLorenzo. "The Emergency Department Approach to Syncope: Evidence-Based Guidelines and Prediction Rules." *Emerg Med Clin N Am* 28 (2010): 487–500.

7. Querfurth, H. W. and F. M. LaFeria. "Alzheimer's Disease." *N Engl J Med* 362 (2010): 329–344.

8. Lees, A. "The Bare Essentials: Parkinson's Disease." *Pract Neurol* 10 (2010): 240–246.

9. Naccarato, M. K. and T. Kelechi. "Pressure Ulcer Prevention in the Emergency Department." *Adv Emerg Nurs J* 33 (2011): 155–162.

10. Carnell, J., J. Fahimi, and C. P. Wills. "Cervical Spine Fracture in Ankylosing Spondylitis." *West J Emerg Med* 10 (2009): 267.

11. Weiss, S. J., R. Chong, M. Ong, A. A. Ernst, and M. Balash. "Emergency Medical Services Screening of Elderly Falls in the Home." *Prehosp Emerg Care* 7 (2003): 79–84.

12. Rinker, A. G., Jr. "Recognition and Perception of Elder Abuse by Prehospital and Hospital-Based Care Providers." *Arch Gerontol Geriatr* 48 (2009): 110–115.

FURTHER READING

Abrams, W. B., et al., eds. *The Merck Manual of Geriatrics.* 3rd ed. Whitehouse Station, NJ: Merck Research Laboratories, 2000.

American Geriatrics Society, National Council of State EMS Coordinators. *Geriatric Education for Emergency Medical Services.* Sudbury, MA: Jones and Bartlett Publishers, 2003.

Bledsoe, B. and D. Clayden. *Prehospital Emergency Pharmacology.* 7th ed. Upper Saddle River, NJ: Pearson/Prentice Hall, 2012.

"Drug Therapy in the Elderly," in Beers M. H., et al., eds. *The Merck Manual of Diagnosis and Therapy.* 18th ed. Whitehouse Station, NJ: Merck Research Laboratories, 2006.

"Geriatric Trauma" and "Abuse in the Elderly and Impaired," in Tintinalli J. E., et al., eds. *Emergency Medicine: A Comprehensive Study Guide.* 7th ed. New York: McGraw-Hill, 2010.

6

Abuse, Neglect, and Assault

Bryan Bledsoe, DO, FACEP, FAAEM, EMT-P

STANDARD
Special Patient Populations (Patients with Special Needs)

COMPETENCY
Integrates assessment findings with principles of epidemiology and pathophysiology and knowledge of psychosocial needs to formulate a field impression and implement a comprehensive treatment/disposition plan for patients with special needs.

OBJECTIVES

Terminal Performance Objective
After reading this chapter, you should be able to integrate patient assessment findings, patient history, and knowledge of therapeutic communication and medical/legal considerations to recognize and manage patients suffering from abuse, neglect, and assault.

Enabling Objectives
To accomplish the terminal performance objective, you should be able to:

1. Define key terms introduced in this chapter.
2. Describe the epidemiology and demographics of abuse, assault, and neglect.
3. Describe the characteristics of abusers and abused and neglected patients, including partner abuse, elder abuse, and child abuse.
4. Adapt your approach to history and assessment to interact effectively with abused or neglected patients.
5. Explain the importance of communicating the availability of resources to patients in suspected partner abuse situations.
6. Explain the ethical and legal obligations to report suspected abuse and neglect.
7. Identify patterns of injuries and behavior suspicious for abuse and neglect.
8. Describe special considerations in interacting with victims of sexual assault.
9. Recognize the effects of date rape drugs.
10. Describe the epidemiology of hate crimes.
11. Document relevant observations and information regarding suspected abuse, neglect, hate crimes, and sexual assault.

KEY TERMS

You are awakened during the middle of the night to respond to an unknown emergency. You arrive to find a police officer on the scene with a 36-year-old woman who was found at the side of the road, partially clothed. She is crying and nearly incoherent. You learn from scattered comments and from remarks by the police officer that a male assailant abducted the patient at gunpoint and sexually assaulted her. He then threw the patient from a moving vehicle and fled the scene. A passing motorist spotted the woman curled up along the roadside and used a cell phone to summon police.

Because you have a female partner, you decide that she might be a more appropriate choice than you to maintain contact with this patient. As you return to the ambulance to retrieve equipment, your partner begins the primary assessment. She looks for immediate life threats, while exhibiting a compassionate and consoling attitude just as any EMS professional should do. During the secondary assessment, she uses a blanket to protect the patient's privacy. All clothing removed during the assessment is placed in a paper bag and given to the police officer as evidence.

Because of the mechanism of injury, you and your partner decide to apply spinal immobilization. You find extensive abrasions when you logroll the patient, but do not detect any life-threatening injuries. Because your partner has noted blood around the patient's perineum, she places a dressing over the patient's genitals.

Vital signs are good, so you begin transport to a hospital designated as a rape crisis center. En route, you notify the receiving hospital so the staff can prepare for your arrival. The staff readies a private room for the patient and summons a social worker, a nurse with specialized training as a sexual assault nurse examiner (SANE), and a detective.

After you transfer the patient, you complete your patient report, giving special attention to the narrative. Both you and your partner realize that you might be called to testify in court sometime in the future.

INTRODUCTION

Because of underreporting, it is difficult to provide accurate statistics on the incidence of abuse and assault in the United States today. That makes available figures even more overwhelming in their seriousness. To grasp the magnitude of the problem, consider these facts:

- Nearly three million children suffer abuse each year and almost five children a day die as a result of child abuse.[1]

- Between 2 and 4 million women each year are battered by their partners or spouses.

- Elder abuse occurs at an incidence of 700,000 to 1.1 million annually.[2]

Abuse and assaults transcend gender, race, age, and socioeconomic status. The effects are serious and long-lasting. Victims may die as a result of their injuries or have long-term health care problems. No victim ever forgets his or her pain. Even after the physical wounds have healed, the emotional injuries never fade completely.

Unfortunately, the pattern of abuse and assault forms a cycle that is difficult to break. Parents who harm each other are more likely to abuse their children. Children who suffer abuse have a greater likelihood of becoming abusers themselves. At some point in their lives, they may abuse their dates, their partners, their children, their elders, or others.

The EMS system is involved with many cases of abuse. Although law enforcement is not always present, you have a responsibility to identify victims of abuse and initiate some kind of action. In many areas, laws require health care personnel to report actual or suspected incidences of abuse. Early detection is critical to breaking the cycle of abuse through social services support and alterations in behavior.

PARTNER ABUSE

The potential for **partner abuse** has existed for as long as couples have interacted. It results when a man or woman subjects a domestic partner to some form of physical or psychological violence. The victim may be a husband or wife, someone who shares a residence, or simply a boyfriend or girlfriend.

The most widespread and best known form of abuse involves the abuse of women by men. However, battery is not limited to women. Men can be—and are—abused by women. They suffer the same feelings of guilt, humiliation, and loss of control. A battered man feels trapped, just like a battered woman,

CONTENT REVIEW

▶ Reasons for Not Reporting Abuse

- Fear of reprisal
- Fear of humiliation
- Denial
- Lack of knowledge
- Lack of financial resources

but is often even less likely to report the abuse, out of either a sense of shame, a lack of resources for support, or both.

Battery also affects same-sex couples. Abusive relationships between men or between women follow the same patterns and the same conditioning as those seen in heterosexual relationships. What can be said of women battered by men can generally be said of most battery situations, regardless of the gender of the victim or the abuser.

Reasons for Not Reporting Abuse

Victims of partner abuse hesitate or fail to report the problem for a number of reasons. Fear is one of the biggest obstacles to taking action. Most battered partners fear reprisals, either to themselves or to their children. They also fear being humiliated for their powerlessness or inability to stop the violence, especially if the battered partner is a male.

Reporting abuse is usually the last resort. Many partners hope the abusive behavior will simply just end. This hope is fueled when the abuser promises to change—a common reaction after a violent episode. The abused partner may also be in denial, claiming that the situation is less serious than it is or rationalizing that the violence was somehow justified. Some abused women, for example, believe that they are the cause of the abusive behavior or that the abuse is part of the marriage and should be endured to preserve the family.

Finally, many victims of abuse lack the knowledge or financial means to seek help. They may not know where to turn or whom to trust. They may also lack the money to seek counseling, intervention, or a safe place to live. A partner who lacks job training and/or who must support dependent children may find the prospect of starting life anew more frightening than the abuse. Unfortunately, an abusive situation rarely ceases without some kind of separation or intervention. Escalation of violence is common, with injuries becoming more severe. Over time, abuse becomes more frequent, often occurring without provocation, and more inclusive. If children were not initially involved, they may become victims as the episodes escalate. All too often, victims of abuse are eventually killed by their abuser.

Identification of Partner Abuse

Partner abuse can fall into several categories. The most obvious form is physical abuse, which involves the application of force in ways too numerous to list here. In addition to direct personal injury, physical abuse may exacerbate existing medical conditions, such as hypertension, diabetes, or asthma. These conditions can also be affected by verbal abuse, which consists of words chosen to control or harm a person. Verbal abuse may leave no physical mark, but it damages a person's self-esteem and can lead to depression, substance abuse, or other self-destructive behavior.

Sexual abuse, which is a form of physical abuse, can also occur between partners. It involves forced sexual contact and includes marital or date rape. (For more on sexual abuse and assault, see material later in this chapter.)

In identifying an abusive family situation, keep in mind the 10 generic risk factors identified in *Domestic Violence: Cracking the Code of Silence*, a source often cited.[3] These 10 factors, based on research on battered women, are as follows:

1. Male is unemployed.
2. Male uses illegal drugs at least once a year.
3. Partners have different religious backgrounds.
4. Family income is below the poverty level.
5. Partners are unmarried.
6. Either partner is violent toward children at home.
7. Male did not graduate from high school.
8. Male is unemployed or has a blue-collar job.
9. Male is between 18 and 30 years old.
10. Male saw his father hit his mother.

Characteristics of Partner Abusers

As already indicated, partner abuse occurs in all demographic groups. However, abuse is more common in lower socioeconomic levels in which wage earners have trouble paying bills, holding down jobs, or keeping pace with technological changes that make their job skills outdated or obsolete.

A history of family violence makes a person more likely to repeat the pattern as an adult. Typically, the abuser does not like being out of control but at the same time feels powerless to change. The situation is made worse if both parties do not know how to back down from a conflict. Lacking any alternative, one or both of the partners may turn to physical and/or verbal violence (Figure 6-1 ●). In some cases, abusers will think they are demonstrating discipline rather than violent behavior.

Abusers usually exhibit overly aggressive personalities—an outgrowth of low self-esteem. They often feel insecure and jealous, flying into sudden and unpredictable rages. Use of alcohol or drugs increases the likelihood that the abuser will lose control and may not even clearly remember his or her actions.

In the aftermath of an abusive incident, the abuser often feels a sense of remorse and shame. The person may seek to relieve his or her guilt by promising to change or even seeking help. For a time, the abuser may appear charming or loving, convincing an abused partner to think that perhaps the pattern has finally been broken. All too often, however, the cycle of violence repeats itself in just a few days, weeks, or months.[4]

Characteristics of Abused Partners

It may be difficult to identify an abused partner. As mentioned, the primary risk factor for abuse is a history of violence between parents, a factor that will not be immediately known to you or other EMS providers. However, studies have revealed that abused partners share certain common characteristics. They include:

- *Pregnancy:* Many women suffer some form of battery during pregnancy.

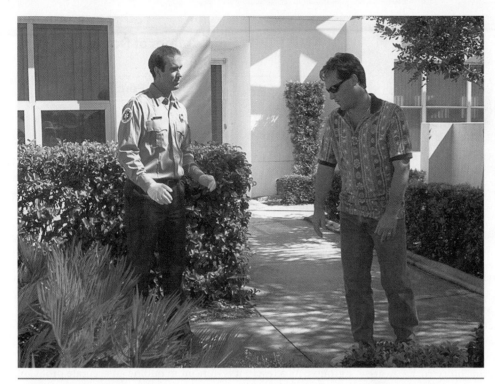

● **Figure 6-1**   When called to the scene of domestic violence, you may encounter hostility from the person responsible for the abuse. Remain calm when you speak to the person and do not enter his personal space. Remain alert to changes in emotional status, and be prepared to summon law enforcement officials as necessary.

- *Substance abuse.* Abused partners often seek the numbing effect of alcohol and/or drugs.
- *Emotional disorders.* Abused partners frequently exhibit depression, evasiveness, anxiety, or suicidal behavior.

As mentioned earlier, the victim may seek to protect the attacker, either by delaying care and/or by providing alternative explanations for injuries. Remain alert to subtle signs

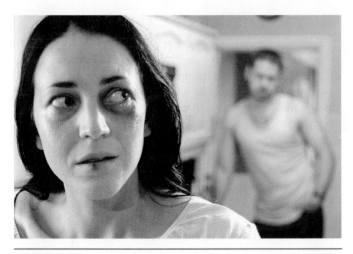

● **Figure 6-2**   A domestic abuse situation is among the most dangerous of situations an EMS crew can encounter. While the abuser is often aggressive, it is not uncommon to have the abused person become aggressive as well. Alcohol and drugs of abuse are often confounding factors in these situations. *(Ian Thraves/Alamy Images)*

that the patient is being less than honest. Many victims, for example, avoid eye contact, exhibit nervous behavior, and/or watch the abuser, if present (Figure 6-2 ●). The victim may also provide verbal clues, saying such things as "We've been having some problems lately" or "I always seem to be causing some kind of trouble."

Approaching the Battered Patient

In assessing the battered patient, direct questioning usually works best. Convey an awareness that the person's partner may have caused the harm or created conditions that led to the injury and/or the emotional trauma. Once the subject of abuse has been introduced, exhibit a willingness to discuss it. Remember to avoid both judgmental questions such as "Why don't you leave?" or judgmental statements such as "How awful!"

Throughout the assessment, listen carefully to the patient. Indicate your attention by saying, "I hear what you are telling me." Often victims of abuse feel a sense of relief when someone else knows about the situation. This can be the first step toward seeking help.

Keep in mind that in cases of partner abuse, the abuser may be reported and taken into custody by the police. However, the person may soon be released on his own recognizance, sometimes within a matter of hours. The patient may already know this and be reluctant to take any action. If the patient does not know this, it is your duty to inform the patient of this possibility and to provide information about available protection programs.

ELDER ABUSE

As noted in Chapter 5, elder abuse is a widespread medical and social problem caused by many factors, including:

- Increased life expectancies
- Increased dependency on others, as a result of longevity
- Decreased productivity in later years
- Physical and mental impairments, especially among the old-old
- Limited resources for long-term care of the elderly
- Economic factors, such as strained family finances
- Stress on middle-aged caretakers responsible for two generations—children and parents

The problem of elder abuse is expected to grow along with the size of the elderly population, which will increase

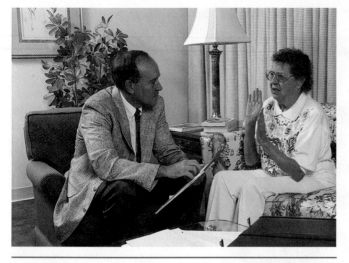

● **Figure 6-3** You are obligated to report suspected elder abuse to the appropriate authorities. In the case of institutional elder abuse, your actions may result in an investigation by an outside agency who will question the patient more closely.

dramatically within the next 20 to 30 years as baby boomers turn age 65 and older. It is your responsibility to be aware of this situation and to remain alert to signs of elder abuse (Figure 6-3 ●).

Identification of Elder Abuse

The two basic types of elder abuse are domestic and institutional. **Domestic elder abuse** takes place when an elder is being cared for in a home-based setting, usually by relatives. **Institutional elder abuse** occurs when an elder is being cared for by a person with a legal or contractual responsibility to provide care, such as paid caregivers, nursing home staff, or other professionals. Both types of abuse can be either acts of commission (acts of physical, sexual, or emotional violence) or acts of omission (neglect).[5]

In some cases, signs of elder abuse are subtle, such as theft of the victim's belongings or loss of freedom. Other signs, such as wounds, untreated decubitus ulcers, or poor hygiene, are more obvious. For additional information on the signs of elder abuse, see Chapter 5.

Theories about Domestic Elder Abuse

There are four main theories about causes of domestic elder abuse. Commonly, caregivers feel stressed and overburdened. They are ill equipped to provide care or simply lack the knowledge to do the job correctly. Another cause of elder abuse is the patients' physical and/or mental impairment. Elders in poor health are more likely to be abused than elders in good health. This situation results, in part, from their inability to report the abuse. Yet another cause of elder abuse is family history, or the cycle of violence mentioned earlier. Finally, elder abuse increases proportionately with the personal problems of the caregivers. Abusers of the elderly tend to have more difficulties, either financial or emotional, than nonabusers.

TABLE 6–1 | Perpetrators of Domestic Elder Abuse	
Group	Percentage
Adult children	32.5
Grandchildren	4.2
Spouse	14.4
Sibling	2.5
Other relatives	12.5
Friend/neighbor	6.5
All others	18.2
Unknown	8.2

Characteristics of Abused Elders

Like partner abuse, elder abuse cuts across all demographic groups. As a result, it is difficult to outline an accurate profile of the abused elder. The most common cases involve elderly women abused by their sons. However, this pattern is skewed by the fact that women live longer than men. Elder abuse most frequently occurs among people who are dependent on others for their care, especially among those elders who are mentally or physically challenged. In such cases, elders may be repeatedly abused by relatives who believe the elder will not or cannot ask for help.

In cases of neglect, abused elders most commonly live alone. They may be mentally competent, but fear asking for help because relatives have complained about providing care or have threatened to place them in a nursing home. Like abused partners, they may be reluctant to give information about their abusers for fear of retaliation.

Characteristics of Elder Abusers

It is also difficult to profile the people who are most likely to abuse elders. According to the National Aging Resource Center on Elder Abuse, the percentages in Table 6–1 reflect the reported perpetrators of elder abuse in domestic settings. As you can see, the most typical abusers are adult children who are either overstressed by care of the elder or who were abused themselves.

As with partner abusers, several characteristics in common are found in abusers of the elderly. Often, the perpetrators exhibit alcoholic behavior, drug addiction, or some mental impairment. The abuser may also be dependent on the income or assistance of the elder, a situation that can cause resentment, anger, and, in some cases, violence.

For more on the management of elder abuse, see Chapter 5.

CHILD ABUSE

As pointed out in Chapters 3 and 4, child abuse is one of the most difficult circumstances that you will face as a paramedic. **Child abuse** may range from physical or emotional impairment

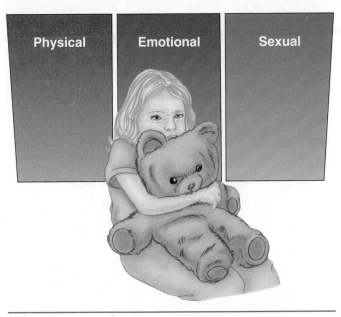

Physical **Emotional** **Sexual**

● **Figure 6-4**   Child abuse comes in many forms. Be alert and report any concerns you may have regarding abuse or neglect.

to neglect of a child's most basic needs (Figure 6-4 ●). It can occur from infancy to age 18 and can be inflicted by any number of caregivers: parents, foster parents, stepparents, babysitters, siblings, stepsiblings, or other relatives or friends charged with a child's care.

Although you may be familiar with some of the following information from your training or from earlier chapters in this book, it bears repeating. The damage done to a child can last a lifetime and, as stressed earlier, can perpetuate a cycle of violence in generations to come.

Characteristics of Child Abusers

As with other types of abusers, you cannot relate child abuse to social class, income, or education. However, certain patterns do emerge, most notably a history of abuse within their own families. Most child abusers were physically or emotionally abused as children. They often would prefer to use other forms of discipline, but under stress they regress to their earliest and most familiar patterns. Once they resort to physical discipline, the punishments become more severe and more frequent.

In cases of reported physical abuse, perpetrators tend to be men. However, the statistics for men and women even out when neglect is taken into account. As indicated earlier, potential child abusers can include a wide variety of caregivers. In most cases, however, one or both parents are the most likely abusers. Frequent behavioral traits include:

● Use or abuse of drugs and/or alcohol

● Immaturity and preoccupation with self

● Lack of obvious feeling for the child, rarely looking at or touching the child

● Apparent lack of concern about the child's injury, treatment, or prognosis

● Open criticism of the child, with little indication of guilt or remorse for involvement in the child's condition

● Little identification with the child's pain, whether it is physical or emotional

CONTENT REVIEW

▶ Conditions Commonly Mistaken for Abuse

• Car seat burns
• Staphylococcal scalded skin syndrome
• Chickenpox (cigarette burns)
• Hematologic disorders that cause easy bruising

Any one of these signs should raise suspicion in your mind of possible child abuse. The infant or child will provide other clues, even before you begin your physical examination.

Characteristics of Abused Children

A child's behavior is one of the most important indicators of abuse. Some behavior is age related. For example, abused children under age six usually appear excessively passive, whereas abused children over age six seem aggressive. Other behavioral clues include:

● Crying, often hopelessly, during treatment—or not crying at all

● Avoiding the parents or showing little concern for their absence

● Unusual wariness or fear of physical contact

● Apprehension and/or constant alertness for danger

● Being prone to sudden behavioral changes

● Absence of nearly all emotions

● Neediness, constantly requesting favors, food, or things

In general, use your instincts and knowledge of age-appropriate behavior (see Chapters 3 and 4) to guide your first impression of the child. If the child's behavior is atypical, maintain an index of suspicion throughout your assessment.[6]

Identification of the Abused Child

As you know, children very commonly get injured, and not all injured children are abused. If a child volunteers the story of his injury without hesitation and if it matches the story told by the parent and the symptoms of injury, child abuse is very unlikely. However, in cases in which the behavior of a caregiver and/or child has raised an index of suspicion, you may face a challenge in distinguishing between an intentional injury and an authentic accident. Conditions commonly mistaken for abuse are car seat burns, staphylococcal scalded skin syndrome, chickenpox (cigarette burns), and hematologic disorders that can cause bruising. In assessing a child, look for common patterns of physical abuse, evidence of emotional abuse, and/or environmental clues of neglect.

Physical Examination

In most cases, signs of physical mistreatment of a child should be the easiest type of abuse for you to recognize. Soft-tissue injuries are the most common indicators, especially multiple bruises

Medicinal Practices of the Hmong

Some cultural folk medicine practices can be easily mistaken for child abuse. An Asian population, referred to as the Hmong or "Hill People," is among the oldest populations in Asia. Many Hmong were recruited by the Central Intelligence Agency and were allied with the United States in the secret war in Laos that was fought contemporaneously with the war in Vietnam. When these countries fell, more than 100,000 Hmong were killed by the Communist insurgents. Numerous Hmong families immigrated to the United States—usually with the help of various church groups—and settled primarily in southern California and the Midwest.

In their folk medicine belief system, coining, cupping, and pinching are common practices. With coining, a utensil with a rounded edge (such as a coin or spoon) is used to rub the skin until bruising appears. This procedure leaves an oval ecchymotic area with an irregular border. Cupping treatment creates a vacuum effect that is thought to draw out pain. It is done by burning cotton in a small jar and placing the jar over the affected area after the flame is out. The sign of this is a round ecchymotic area. Pinching is commonly used to alleviate headaches. It is performed by pinching the skin until bruising appears. The result is a narrow bruise, often found between the eyes. As noted, all these folk remedies result in bruising. It is also common to puncture and bleed these ecchymotic areas in an effort to release toxins thought to cause the illness. The puncture usually is done with a sewing needle.

Soon after their settlement in the United States, numerous Hmong children were referred to child protection authorities for investigation of suspected child abuse—usually by well-meaning health care professionals. Some of the bruising secondary to coining, cupping, or pinching seemed symptomatic of child abuse to those unfamiliar with Hmong culture. However, following investigation, it was learned that these were loving actions designed to make the child or adult well.

In areas where Hmong are present, cultural diversity education programs are available to provide information on the folk medicine and cultural practices of this interesting group of people.[7]

TABLE 6–2 | Determining the Age of a Bruise by Its Color

Color of Bruise	Age of Bruise
Red (swollen, tender)	0–2 days
Blue, purple	2–5 days
Green	5–7 days
Yellow	7–10 days
Brown	10–14 days
No further evidence of bruising	2–4 weeks

From Portable Guides to Investigating Child Abuse, *Office of Juvenile Justice and Delinquency Prevention, Office of Justice Programs, U.S. Department of Justice. https://www .ncjrs.gov/html/ojjdp/portable_guides/abuse/bruises.html (accessed May 30, 2012)*

is too hot, you can expect to see "splash" burns—marks created by spattering water as children try to escape. Intentional scalding, however, is characterized by the conspicuous lack of splash burns. Such "dipping injuries" are a common form of child abuse.

Fractures   Fractures constitute the second most common form of child abuse. Sites of fractures include the skull, nose, facial structures, and upper extremities (Figure 6-5 ●). Twisting

in different places of the body, in different stages of healing, and with distinctive shapes (Table 6–2). Other common warning signs include defensive wounds on the hands and forearms and symmetrical injuries such as bites or burns. Any of these conditions carries a high index of suspicion of abuse.

Burns and Scalds   Some injuries often have distinctive patterns that indicate the implement or source used to injure the child. The burns tend to be in certain common locations: the soles of the feet, palms of the hands, back, or buttocks. They may or may not be found in conjunction with other injuries.

Because children have thinner skin than adults (other than elders), they also tend to scald more easily. The temperature of hot water in most residences is about 140°F, which can scald an adult in only about 5 seconds. (Bathwater for children should be kept below 120°F.) When children accidentally get into water that

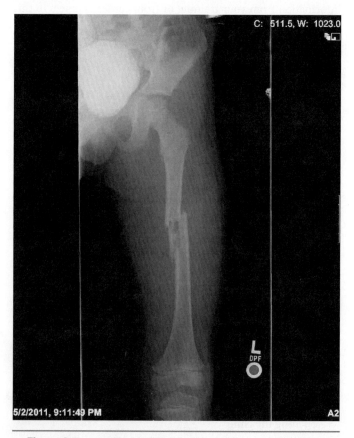

● **Figure 6-5**   Evidence of child abuse—X-ray of a femur fracture in a six-year-old girl. *(© Dr. Bryan E. Bledsoe)*

and jerking fractures result from grabbing a child by an extremity, and neck injuries occur from shaking a child. Because children have soft, pliable ribs, they rarely experience accidental fractures to this region. As a result, you should maintain a high index of suspicion of abuse whenever you encounter a child with fractured ribs.

Head Injuries   Over time, injuries from abuse tend to progress from the extremities and trunk to the head. Head injuries commonly found in abused children include scalp wounds, skull fractures, subdural hematomas, and repeated contusions.

Injuries to the head claim the largest number of lives among abused children. They also account for most of the long-term disability associated with child abuse.

Shaken Baby Syndrome   Shaken baby syndrome frequently occurs when a parent or caregiver becomes frustrated with a crying infant and all other attempts to quiet the baby have failed. It happens when a person picks up the infant and shakes the baby vigorously. The movement can cause permanent brain damage, such as subdural hematomas or diffuse swelling. It may also result in injuries to the neck and spine or retinal hemorrhages, which in turn can lead to blindness. If the infant is shaken hard enough or repeatedly, the baby may die from the injuries.

Abdominal Injuries   Although abdominal injuries represent a small proportion of the injuries suffered by abused children, they are usually very serious. Blunt force can result in trauma to the liver, spleen, or mesentery. You should look for pain, swelling, and vomiting, as well as hemodynamic compromise from these injuries.

Maternal Drug Abuse

Drug abuse by the mother during pregnancy is a subtle, but devastating, form of child abuse. Certain drugs, particularly cocaine and alcohol, are associated with long-term problems

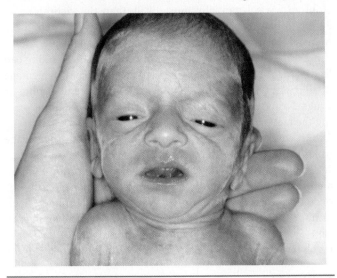

● **Figure 6-6**   Face of a premature cocaine baby. The mother of this child was a cocaine addict. Developmental abnormalities are common. The infant may develop acute cocaine withdrawal signs and symptoms. (© *Stevie Grand/ Photo Researchers, Inc.*)

for the fetus. Fetal alcohol syndrome (FAS) can occur following repeated exposure to alcohol during the first trimester of pregnancy. In addition, maternal use of cocaine can result in a specific pattern. Children of mothers addicted to cocaine, most commonly "crack cocaine," are a particular problem. Premature birth and numerous complications are often seen in cocaine babies or "crack babies" (Figure 6-6 ●).

Signs of Neglect

Some forms of child abuse are less obvious than physical injuries. Abuse may result from neglect. Caregivers simply do not provide children with adequate food, clothing, shelter, or medical care.

As a paramedic, you may be in a unique position to observe and report neglect. Unlike many other health care or public safety workers, EMS personnel get an opportunity to see the child's home environment for themselves. Unhealthy or unclean conditions are clear evidence of a caregiver's inability to provide for a child's safety or well-being.

In examining a child, keep in mind the following common signs of neglect:

- Malnutrition (neglected children are often underweight, sometimes by up to 30 percent)
- Severe diaper rash
- Diarrhea and/or dehydration
- Hair loss
- Untreated medical conditions
- Inappropriate, dirty, torn clothing or lack of clothing
- Tired and listless attitudes
- Near constant demands for physical contact or attention

Signs of Emotional Abuse

Emotional abuse is often the hardest form of abuse to identify. It may take any one of the following six forms:

1. Parents or caregivers simply ignore the child, showing indifference to the child's needs and failing to provide any stimulation.
2. Parents or caregivers reject, humiliate, or criticize the child.
3. The child may be isolated and deprived of normal human contact or nurturing.
4. A child may be terrorized or bullied through verbal assaults and threats, creating feelings of fear and anxiety.
5. A parent or caregiver may encourage destructive or antisocial behavior.
6. The child may be overpressured by unrealistic expectations of success.

Recording and Reporting Child Abuse

As with all other forms of abuse, you have a responsibility to report suspected cases of child abuse. In some instances, you might have a chance to provide early intervention. An abusive adult may actively seek help or may send out signals for help. For example, a potential abuser may make several calls within a 24-hour period. The person may also summon help for inconsequential symptoms or demonstrate an inability to handle an impeding crisis. These are warning signs and should be duly noted.

When confronted with an actual case of child abuse, try to conduct the examination with another colleague present. You must keep your personal reactions to yourself and record only your objective observations. Assumptions must not be included in your report. The final document should be objective, legible, and written with the knowledge that it may be used in a future court or child custody case. At all times, put the child's interest first, treating him with the utmost kindness and gentleness. (For more on your EMS and legal responsibilities, see material later in this chapter.)

SEXUAL ASSAULT

Anyone can be a victim of sexual violence. Statistics from the National Victims Center and the U.S. Department of Justice reveal that males and females of all backgrounds, from infancy to old age, have reported crimes involving forced or unwanted sexual contact. According to the Bureau of Justice Statistics, more than 260,000 rapes and nearly 100,000 sexual assaults are reported each year. However, these figures reflect only a small percentage of cases, with an estimated 63 to 74 percent of all incidents going unreported.[8]

Although the legal definitions vary from state to state, courts generally interpret **sexual assault** as unwanted sexual contact, whether it is genital, oral, rectal, or manual. **Rape** is usually defined as penile penetration of the genitalia or rectum (however slight) without the consent of the victim. Both forms of sexual violence are prosecuted as crimes, with rape constituting a felony offense. As a result, your actions at the scene and the report that you file will, in all likelihood, affect the outcome of a trial.

Characteristics of Victims of Sexual Assault/Rape

It is difficult to profile a victim of sexual assault or rape because of the variety of victims. However, statistics reveal certain patterns. The group most likely to be victimized is made up of adolescent females younger than age 18. Nearly two-thirds of all rapes and sexual assaults take place between the hours of 6 P.M. and 6 A.M. at the victim's home or at the home of a friend, relative, or acquaintance. A woman is raped, on average, every 2 minutes in the United States; a woman is four times as likely to be raped by someone she knows than by a stranger.

Particularly alarming is the number of children who suffer some form of sexual abuse. According to the Department of Justice, one in two rape victims is under age 18; one in six is under age 12. Other government figures show that approximately one-third of all juvenile victims of sexual abuse are children younger than six years of age. Typically, contact involves a male assailant and a female victim, but not always. The contact can range from exposure to fondling to penetration. Although sexual abuse can occur in families of all descriptions, children

raised in families in which there is domestic violence are eight times more likely to be sexually molested within that family.

Sexual assault and rape carry serious consequences. Victims may be physically injured, or even killed, during the assault. They commonly suffer internal injuries, particularly if multiple assailants are involved in the attack. Rape can result in infections, sexually transmitted diseases, and unwanted pregnancies. The psychological damage is deep and long lasting. Shame, anger, and a lack of trust can persist for years—or even for a lifetime.

Children, in particular, find it difficult to speak about molestation. It is likely that they know the person and fear reprisal or, in some instances, even seek to protect the individual. In many cases, the assailants physically explore the child without intercourse or force the child to touch or fondle them. Victims, especially very young children, may be confused about the situation or, lacking physical evidence of abuse, fear that nobody will believe them. Symptoms of sexual abuse, regardless of its form, may include:

- Nightmares
- Restlessness
- Withdrawal tendencies
- Hostility
- Phobias related to the offender
- Regressive behavior, such as bed wetting
- Truancy
- Promiscuity, in older children and teens
- Drug and alcohol abuse

Characteristics of Sexual Assailants

Like the victims of sexual assaults, the assailants can come from almost any background. However, the violent victimizers of children are substantially more likely than the victimizers of adults to have been physically or sexually abused as children. Many assailants, particularly adolescents and abusive adults, think domination is part of any relationship. Such thinking can lead to date rape or marital rape. In a significant percentage of all cases, the assailants are under the influence of alcohol or drugs. Nearly 30 percent of all rapists use weapons, underscoring the fact that sexual assaults are violent crimes.

In cases of date rape, the assailant may have drugged the unknowing victim with one of the drugs described in the next section. The victim may exhibit extreme intoxication without a corresponding strong smell of alcohol or may have drug-induced amnesia (a common effect), making questioning difficult or impossible. More often than not, the alleged assailant in such cases lives on a college campus, the location of most EMS calls involving what is known as a "date rape drug."

Date Rape Drugs

The use of drugs to facilitate a sexual assault is occurring with increasing frequency.[9] These medications will generally render a person unresponsive or weaken the person to the point of being unable to resist an attacker. Some of these medications cause amnesia, thus eliminating or distorting the victim's recall of the assault. Because these drugs have become more commonplace in society, it is important for EMS personnel to be aware of these agents and their effects. Date rape drugs have a rapid onset of action with a varying duration of effect. Drugs that have been associated with rape, which are also known as *predator drugs*, include the following:

- *Rohypnol.* Rohypnol is a potent benzodiazepine that produces a sedative effect, amnesia, muscle relaxation, and slowing of the psychomotor response. It is widely prescribed outside the United States as a sleeping pill. It is colorless, odorless, and tasteless and can be dissolved in a drink without being detected. Rohypnol can be potentiated by the concomitant effects of alcohol. Street names for rohypnol include *Roofies, Rope, Ruffies, R2, Ruffles, Roche, Forget-Pill,* and *Mexican Valium.*

- *GHB.* Gamma-hydroxybutyrate, commonly called GHB, is an odorless, colorless liquid depressant with anesthetic-type qualities. It is also used as an amino acid supplement by body builders. The drug causes relaxation, tranquility, sensuality, and loss of inhibitions. Street names for GHB include *Liquid Ecstasy, Liquid X, Scoop, Easy Lay,* and *Grievous Bodily Harm.*

- *Ketamine.* Ketamine is a potent anesthetic agent. Widely used in veterinary practice, ketamine is also used in human anesthesia. It is chemically similar to the hallucinogenic LSD. It causes hallucinations, amnesia, and dissociation. Street names for ketamine include *K, Special K, Vitamin K, Jet,* and *Super Acid.*

- *MDMA.* 3,4-Methylenedioxymethamphetamine (MDMA) is most commonly known as *Ecstasy.* It is known to cause psychological difficulties including confusion, depression, sleep problems, drug craving, severe anxiety, and paranoia (both during and sometimes weeks after taking the drug). It can also cause physical symptoms such as muscle tension, involuntary teeth clenching, nausea, blurred vision, rapid eye movement, faintness, and chills or sweating. Street names for MDMA, in addition to *Ecstasy,* include *Beans, Adam, XTC, Roll, E,* and *M.*

Persons attending parties and other events should be cautious with regard to predator drugs. It is best not to drink from a punch bowl or a bottle that is being passed around. Notice the behavior of others at the party. If a person seems more intoxicated than the amount of alcohol consumed would warrant, then consider the possibility of predator drugs. If a rape victim thinks she has been drugged, a drug screen should be requested on arrival at the emergency department. EMS personnel should note any suspicions or observations that may point to the use of a predator drug.

EMS Responsibilities

Your response to a call involving a sexual assault is similar in many ways to your response to any abusive situation. In both instances, your primary responsibility is safety—both your own and that of the patient. You should never enter a scene if your safety is compromised, and you should leave the scene as soon as you feel unsafe.

You can expect victims of assault or abuse to feel unsafe as a result of the violence they have suffered. One of your primary responsibilities is to provide a safe environment for an already traumatized patient. Sometimes you can provide safety merely by your official presence. Other times, you may have to move the patient to the ambulance, where you can lock the doors, or move to a different location entirely. In still other instances, you may have to summon additional personnel. (For more on crime scene management, see Volume 7, Chapter 6.)

LEGAL CONSIDERATIONS

As noted throughout this chapter, abuse and assault constitute crimes. Although the nature and extent to which an assault is considered a crime often depends on local laws, you have a responsibility to report suspected cases to the appropriate law enforcement officials. Because the assailants may be detained only a short time, you also have an obligation to find out about the victim and witness protection programs available in your area.

Specialized resources include both private and state or federally funded programs. Make a point of learning about hospital units for the victims of sexual assault, public and private shelters for battered persons, and state agencies responsible for youths and their families. Also acquaint yourself with nurses trained as sexual assault nurse examiners (SANEs). They have completed programs allowing them to perform the physical exam for sexual assaults. They have detailed information on the protection of evidence, something that you must keep in mind throughout the call.

As you have read, your actions can affect the prosecution of a crime. Clothing should be removed from a patient only when necessary for assessment and treatment. All items should then be turned over to the proper authorities.

In the case of rape, patients should not urinate, defecate, douche, bathe, eat, drink, or smoke. Some jurisdictions have specific rules for evidence protection, such as using paper bags to collect evidence or placing bags over the patient's hands to preserve trace evidence. Remember that any evidence that you collect must remain in your custody until you can give it directly to a law enforcement official to preserve the **chain of evidence.**

As indicated, it is important that you carefully and objectively document all your findings. You may end up defending your words in a court of law. Regardless of the emotions evoked by the call, you must remain a professional at all times.

Finally, you should study the local laws and protocols regarding cases of abuse and assault. All 50 states require health care workers to report suspected cases of child abuse. Some states require EMS personnel to report even a suspicion of abuse or assault. Some states allow minors to seek medical care for sexual assault without parental consent. The Joint Commission mandates that hospital personnel screen incoming patients for abuse. Regardless of where you live, take time to learn the rules and regulations that affect your practice, both for your sake and for the sake of your patients.

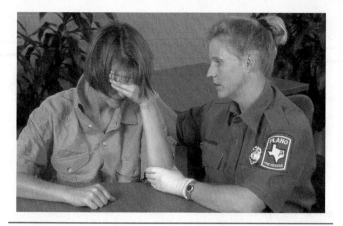

● **Figure 6-7** If possible, a paramedic or EMT of the same sex as the victim of rape or an alleged sexual assault should maintain contact with the victim, accompanying the patient to the hospital.

You are also responsible for providing proper psychosocial care for the victims of abuse and assault. Privacy is a major consideration. In many cases, a paramedic of the same sex as the victim should maintain contact with the victim (Figure 6-7 ●). Although you may need to expose the victim during assessment, you should cover the patient and remove him or her from public view as soon as possible.

When talking with the patient, use open-ended questions to reestablish a sense of control. You might say, for example, "Would you like to sit on a seat or ride on the stretcher?" Or you might ask, "Is there someone you would like us to call?" As mentioned in earlier sections, remain nonjudgmental throughout treatment, avoiding subjective comments about both the patient and the assailant. In a reassuring voice, encourage the patient to report the rape, explaining the importance of preserving evidence.

Medical treatment of victims of abuse and assault is essentially the same as with other patients. However, you should always remember the origins of the patient's injuries and provide appropriate emotional support. Keep in mind that the patient has been harmed by another human being, in many cases a person that the patient knows intimately.

HATE CRIMES

A **hate crime** is a crime of hatred or prejudice in which the perpetrator targets a particular victim or victims because of the victim's perceived membership in a certain social group. These groups can include racial, religious, sexual orientation, political, disability, and other social groups. The crime is based on bias and sometimes referred to as **bias-motivated crime**. Most hate crimes result from racial bias. This is followed by religious bias, sexual orientation bias, ethnicity/national origin bias, and disability bias. The vast majority of racial hate crimes are against blacks. Most religious hate crimes are directed at Jews. In terms of sexual orientation bias, most hate crimes are motivated by anti-male homosexual bias. Anti-female homosexual hate crimes are much less common. Most ethnicity/national origin hate crimes are directed at Hispanics.

Most hate crimes involve vandalism. Intimidation is also common. Approximately one in three hate crimes involves assault. Certain hate crimes, especially those that are racially motivated, can result in widespread violence. EMS can become involved in any aspect of hate crimes, from simple intimidation to full-fledged riots. Paramedics must recognize that hate crimes and their aftermath are emotionally charged events and paramedics, because of their race, gender, or sexual orientation, can be drawn into the fray. Always treat hate crimes as particularly dangerous situations. Involve law enforcement early and always ensure the safety of you and your partner first.

◤ SUMMARY

The incidence of assault and abuse is more widespread today than ever before. You will encounter more cases during your paramedic career than you can imagine. For the sake of your patients, it is imperative that you learn the hallmarks of partner abuse, elder abuse, child abuse, and sexual assaults. Remember that you have a duty to report these situations, whether you transport the patients or not. By learning to recognize significant physical and emotional assessment findings, as well as characteristics of the victims and assailants, you will be able to provide better treatment of victims of abuse and assault. This includes knowing the legal requirements of your area, protecting evidence, and properly documenting your findings and actions. You may be the only chance a victim has of being saved from further abuse. Be vigilant in your observations and document objectively.

◤ YOU MAKE THE CALL

You and your partner respond to a police request to evaluate an injured child. You find several police officers on the scene of a domestic disturbance. The patient is a three-year-old boy found sitting quietly on the couch. The boy's parents are present and being questioned by the police officers.

You find the patient dressed in underwear with no other clothing, although it is wintertime. He has obvious and different-colored bruises to both his upper arms and his back. During your exam, the boy is silent, not answering your questions or looking toward either of his parents.

1. What do you suspect is taking place?

2. What physical evidence do you have to support this suspicion?

3. What emotional evidence do you have to support this suspicion?

4. What other clues lead you to believe that abuse might be taking place?

5. What are your priorities in this case?

See Suggested Responses at the back of this book.

REVIEW QUESTIONS

1. Physical or emotional violence from a man or woman toward a domestic partner is termed _____.
  a. child abuse
  b. spousal abuse
  c. partner abuse
  d. transient abuse

2. The form of partner abuse most obvious to an observer is _____ abuse.
  a. sexual
  b. physical
  c. emotional
  d. psychological

3. Child abuse can occur from infancy to age _____ and can be inflicted by any number of caregivers.
  a. 19
  b. 18
  c. 20
  d. 21

4. Bath water for children should be kept below _____ degrees Fahrenheit.
  a. 125
  b. 130
  c. 120
  d. 140

5. Fractures constitute the second most common form of child abuse. Common sites of fractures include all of the following *except* the _____.
  a. ribs   c. nose
  b. skull   d. face

6. Injuries to the _____ claim the largest number of lives among abused children.
  a. chest
  b. head
  c. femur
  d. pelvis

7. _____ abuse is often the hardest form of abuse to identify.
  a. Verbal
  b. Sexual
  c. Physical
  d. Emotional

8. Soft-tissue injuries are common indicators of abuse, especially multiple bruises _____.
  a. with distinctive shapes
  b. in different stages of healing
  c. in different planes of the body
  d. all of the above

See Answers to Review Questions at the back of this book.

REFERENCES

1. Childhelp. *National Child Abuse Statistics*. [Available at http://www.childhelp.org/pages/statistics]

2. Bureau of Justice Statistics, Office of Justice Programs. *Violent Crime*. [Available at http://bjs.ojp.usdoj.gov/]

3. Pixley, C. *Domestic Violence: Cracking the Code of Silence*. Los Angeles: Do It Now Foundation, 1995.

4. Weiss, S. J., A. A. Ernst, D. Blanton, et al. "EMT Domestic Violence Knowledge and Results of an Educational Intervention." *Am J Emerg Med* 18 (2000): 168–171.

5. Rinker, A. G., Jr. "Recognition and Perception of Elder Abuse by Prehospital and Hospital-Based Providers." *Arch Gerontol Geriatr* 48 (2009): 110–115.

6. American Academy of Pediatrics, Stirling, J., Committee on Child Abuse and Neglect and Section on Adoption and Foster Care, American Academy of Child and Adolescent Psychiatry, Amaya-Jackson, L., National Center for Child Traumatic Stress. "Understanding the Behavioral and Emotional Consequences of Child Abuse." *Pediatrics* 122 (2008): 667–673.

7. Her, C. and K. A. Culhane-Pera. "Culturally Responsive Care in Hmong Patients: Collaboration Is a Key Treatment Component." *Postgrad Med* 116 (2004): 39–42.

8. Center for National Victims of Crime. "Statistics." [Available at http://www.ncvc.org/ncvc/main.aspx?dbID=DB_Statistics584]

9. Meehan, T. J, S. M. Bryant, and S. E. Aks. "Drugs of Abuse: The Highs and Lows of Altered Mental Status in the Emergency Department." *Emerg Med Clin North Am* 28 (2010): 663–682.

10. Federal Bureau of Investigation, Department of Justice. *Hate Crime Statistics*. [Available at http://www2.fbi.gov/ucr/hc2009/incidents.html]

FURTHER READING

American Nurses Association. *Culturally Competent Assessment for Family Violence*. Washington, DC: American Nurses Publishing, 1998.

Federal Bureau of Investigation. *Uniform Crime Statistics*. Washington, DC: FBI, 2009.

Giardino, A. P. and E. R. Giardino. *Recognition of Child Abuse for the Mandated Reporter*. 3rd ed. St. Louis: G. W. Medical Publishers, 2003.

Hamberger, L. K. and C. Renzetti. *Domestic Partner Abuse*. New York: Springer Publishing, 1996.

Hobbs, C. J. and J. M. Wynne. *Physical Signs of Child Abuse: A Colour Atlas*. 2nd ed. London: W. B. Saunders, 2002.

Kehner, G. *Date Rape Drugs*. Broomall, PA: Chelsea House Publishers, 2004.

Reece, R. M. *Child Abuse: Medical Diagnosis and Management*. 3rd ed. Elk Grove, IL: American Academy of Pediatrics, 2008.

The Challenged Patient

Bryan Bledsoe, DO, FACEP, FAAEM, EMT-P

STANDARD
Special Patient Populations (Patients with Special Needs)

COMPETENCY
Integrates assessment findings with principles of epidemiology and pathophysiology and knowledge of psychosocial needs to formulate a field impression and implement a comprehensive treatment/disposition plan for patients with special needs.

OBJECTIVES

Terminal Performance Objective
After reading this chapter, you should be able to integrate patient assessment findings, patient history, and knowledge of therapeutic communication and medical/legal considerations to recognize and manage patients with a variety of special challenges.

Enabling Objectives
To accomplish the terminal performance objective, you should be able to:

1. Define key terms introduced in this chapter.

2. Describe the epidemiology and demographics of each of the following challenges:
   a. Vision impairment
   b. Hearing impairment
   c. Speech impairment
   d. Obesity
   e. Paralysis
   f. Mental illness
   g. Developmental disabilities
   h. Emotional disabilities
   i. Cognitive disabilities (such as those associated with past traumatic brain injury)
   j. Physical disabilities (such as arthritis and neuromuscular and movement disorders)
   k. Chronic and terminal illnesses (such as cancer, cystic fibrosis, and communicable illnesses)

3. Adapt your approach to communication, history taking, assessment, and management to interact effectively with patients with a variety of pathologic problems and sensory, physical, mental, emotional, cognitive, and developmental disabilities.

4. Adapt your approach to communication, history taking, assessment, and management to interact effectively with patients from a variety of cultural backgrounds.

5. Anticipate the special needs and concerns of patients with financial challenges.

6. Document relevant observations and information regarding patients with special challenges.

CASE STUDY

You sit down for the first meal on your shift at Medic 211, but just as you take out something to eat, you are dispatched to a private residence to aid the victim of a fall. You and your partner look at each other, throw your food back into your lunch bags, and hit the road.

En route to the call, you learn that a 72-year-old woman has fallen out of her wheelchair and is unable to get back up. Dispatch tells you that the door is locked, but the woman has hidden a spare key under a fake rock in the garden near the front door.

Fifteen minutes later, you and your partner gain access to the house. You find a woman lying on her side on the bedroom floor, her wheelchair off to the side behind her. You notice what appears to be a brace on the woman's right leg.

When you introduce yourself, the patient tells you her name is Bonnie Wade. "I was trying to put a dress up in my closet," explains Mrs. Wade, "when I lost my balance and fell."

On further questioning, Mrs. Wade indicates that she is widowed and lives alone. Although she can ambulate for short periods of time, she is, for the most part, wheelchair bound. Mrs. Wade denies losing consciousness and says she feels no neck or back pain and no tingling in her extremities. When asked about pain, she replies, "My left hip and shoulder hurt real bad. I fell so hard that I almost dropped the cell phone. I carry it all the time just in case I ever need help."

During your neurologic exam, you find that the patient is unable to move her right leg. Mrs. Wade responds, "Oh that, I had polio when I was young—long before the vaccination they give to kids today." She also tells you that her left arm is weak from post-polio syndrome.

Your partner goes to the ambulance to get the scoop stretcher. Meanwhile, you put the patient's left arm in a cravat sling. You then explain how the scoop stretcher works and assure Mrs. Wade that it is the safest and most comfortable way to get her off the floor. When Mrs. Wade asks whether her leg brace will be in the way, you tell her that you'd like to keep it in place until a doctor evaluates her.

Once you have packaged the patient in the scoop stretcher, you carefully place her on the ambulance stretcher. Mrs. Wade tells you that the sling has relieved some of the pain in her arm, but asks you to take the bumps slowly because of the pain in her hip. You place her in the back of the ambulance and begin transport to Memorial Hospital.

INTRODUCTION

Throughout your EMS career, you can expect to encounter a number of patients who live with a variety of impairments or special challenges. Many will have met these challenges so successfully that you may not notice them right away. For example, people with hearing impairments might lip-read so well that you may not initially realize they cannot hear. People with more obvious challenges, such as paralysis, may have accepted their impairments and built active and rewarding lives. A patient with a history of polio, for example, may have lived with the problem so long that he neglects to tell you about it right away. Instead, the patient talks about a more immediate problem—the reason for summoning EMS.

The one thing that challenged patients share is their variety. They might have any number of physical, mental, or emotional impairments. They might have contracted a pathologic illness that necessitates a special living or working arrangement. They might be suffering from a terminal illness or a communicable disease. They may come from a cultural or financial situation that dictates medical practices contrary to those of the EMS community. The key to treating the "challenged" patient is to understand and recognize the special condition or situation and to make any accommodations that may be needed for proper patient care.

PHYSICAL CHALLENGES

A number of physical impairments—conditions that limit the use of one or more parts of the body—can affect patient assessment and/or treatment. These impairments may be the result of accidents, birth injuries, chronic illnesses, aging, and more. Impairments can limit the ability of a patient to hear, see, speak, or move. Patients will react to their impairments in different ways—from acceptance to denial, anger, or shame. It is important that you quickly recognize the impairment and exhibit knowledge and sensitivity to assure the patient that you understand his special needs.

Hearing Impairment

Hearing impairments involve a decrease or loss in the ability to distinguish or hear sounds, particularly those involving speech. An inability to hear is commonly described as **deafness**. A person may be completely deaf or partially deaf. A person may be deaf in one ear or both ears. The condition may be present at birth or may occur later in life as a result of an accident, illness, or aging.

Types of Hearing Impairment

The two basic types of deafness are **conductive deafness** and **sensorineural deafness**. Many forms of conductive deafness can be treated and cured, especially if caught early. Sensorineural deafness, on the other hand, is often incurable.

Conductive Deafness Conductive deafness results from any condition that prevents sound waves from being transmitted from the external ear to the middle or inner ear. The condition can be either temporary or permanent.

If an infant or child does not respond to verbal stimulation or questions, rule out the possibility of conductive deafness when performing your assessment of disability. Congenital malformation of the ear is a possible but rare cause of conductive deafness in the neonate. A more common cause of conductive deafness in children is **otitis media**, an infection of the middle ear. This condition often arises from various childhood illnesses, particularly those involving the upper respiratory tract. To prevent hearing loss, children under age six who experience recurrent otitis media may need to take daily prophylactic antibiotics or have tympanostomy (myringotomy) tubes placed.

In addition to infection, a number of other conditions can result in a temporary loss of hearing. Anyone can experience conductive deafness during an airline flight, where changes in air pressure can affect hearing. A deep-water dive can have a similar effect. Impacted cerumen, or earwax, is yet another common and easily treatable cause of conductive deafness.

Other causes might be the temporary blockage of the ear canal by various irritants, such as dust, hair spray, insects, or water ("swimmer's ear"). Patient attempts to clean the canal with cotton applicators may disrupt the ear's natural cleaning process and push the debris deeper into the ear, which sets the stage for bacterial infections and conductive deafness.

Obstructions can also be caused by hematomas, which may result from blunt trauma to the ear. Force to the mandible, such as a fractured jaw, can also produce a temporary loss of hearing and may in fact result in fragments of bone displaced to the ear canal. Although these conditions cannot be treated in the field, they should be taken into account when a trauma patient appears not to respond to, or "hear," your questions.

Sensorineural Deafness Sensorineural deafness arises from the inability of nerve impulses to reach the auditory center of the brain because of damage either to the inner ear or to the brain itself. It is usually a permanent condition.

In the case of infants and children, sensorineural deafness often results from congenital defects or birth injuries. Preterm infants are particularly at risk for sensorineural deafness, especially those with severe asphyxia or recurrent apnea in the neonatal period. Ototoxic drugs, such as furosemide (Lasix) and gentamycin, can also cause sensorineural deafness if administered to infants in neonatal intensive care units. Finally, many children who develop this type of hearing loss have mothers who contracted rubella (German measles) or cytomegalovirus (CMV) during the first three months of pregnancy.

Diseases such as bacterial meningitis or viral illnesses such as **labyrinthitis** (inner ear infection) can lead to sensorineural deafness at any age. Taking high doses of ototoxic drugs such as aspirin can also cause sensorineural deafness in both children and adults. A common symptom of aspirin toxicity is "ringing in the ears" (tinnitus). Other causes of sensorineural deafness include tumors of the brain or middle ear, concussion, severe blows to the ear, and repeated loud noises such as chain saws, heavy machinery, gunfire, rock music, or sudden blasts of sound.

Conditions associated with aging can also lead to permanent hearing loss. **Presbycusis** is a progressive sensorineural hearing loss that begins after age 20 but is usually significant only in people over age 65. More common in men than women, this type of hearing loss affects high-frequency sounds first, then low-frequency sounds. Eventually, human voices become harder to detect, especially if background noise is present. Elderly people with this condition will often tell others not to "mumble" or will ask them to speak louder.

Recognition of Deafness

As mentioned, it is important to detect deafness early in your assessment. A partially deaf person may ask questions repeatedly, misunderstand answers to questions, or respond inappropriately. Such reactions can easily be mistaken for head injury, leading to misdirected treatment.

The most obvious sign of deafness is a hearing aid. Unfortunately, hearing aids do not work for all types of deafness. Also, many people do not wear hearing aids, even when

CONTENT REVIEW

▶ Causes of Visual Impairment

- Injury
- Disease
- Congenital conditions
- Infection
- Degeneration of the retina, optic nerve, or nerve pathways

they have been prescribed. In addition, deaf people may have poor diction due to partial hearing loss or hearing loss later in life. They might use their hands to gesture or use sign language. As noted, deaf people may ask you to speak louder or they may speak excessively loudly themselves. Finally, deaf people will commonly face you so that they can read your lips.

Accommodations for Deaf Patients

When managing a patient with a hearing impairment, you can do several things to ease communication. Begin by identifying yourself and making sure the patient knows that you are speaking to him. Get the patient's attention by moving so you can be seen or by gently touching the person, if appropriate. By addressing deaf patients face to face, you give them the opportunity to read your lips and interpret your expression.

When talking with a deaf patient, speak slowly in a normal voice. Never yell or use exaggerated gestures. These techniques often distort your facial and body language, making you seem angry or threatening. Keep in mind that nearly 80 percent of hearing loss is related to high-pitched sounds. As a result, you might use a low-pitched voice to speak directly into the patient's ear. Whatever you do, make sure that background noise is reduced as much as possible by turning off the TV, radio, or other sources of sound.

If you are called to a deaf patient's home during the night, you may need to help find or adjust a hearing aid. If you cannot locate the device, you might put stethoscope earpieces into the patient's ears and try speaking into the mouthpiece. Alternatively, you might make use of an "amplified" listener (e.g., an ear microphone).

Don't forget one of the most simple and effective means of communication: use of pen and paper. As long as you do not need to move quickly, you can write out notes for the patient to read and wait for the person to respond by speaking or writing. You can also use a pen and paper to draw pictures to illustrate basic needs or procedures. This approach can ease a patient's anxiety, reducing the fear of miscommunication or lack of control over his treatment.

Finally, many people with hearing impairments know sign language, usually American Sign Language (ASL). If you do not know sign language, try to find an interpreter, such as a family member or even a neighbor. Make sure that you document the name of the person who did the interpreting and the information received. Also, notify the receiving hospital of the need to have an interpreter on hand if the interpreter you have used is unable to accompany you.

Visual Impairments

When caring for the patient with a visual impairment, it is important to note whether the impairment is a permanent disability or a new symptom as a result of the illness or injury for which you were called. It is necessary to understand the causes of blindness before this determination can be made.

Etiologies

Visual impairments can result from a number of causes. Possible etiologies include injury, disease, congenital conditions, infection (such as CMV), and degeneration of the retina, optic nerve, or nerve pathways. Descriptions of each of the etiologies follow.

Injury   A previous injury to the eye can cause a permanent vision loss. An injury to the orbit usually includes injury to the tissue around the orbit as well as to the eye itself. This can cause muscle and nerve damage that may lead to permanent loss of eyesight. Penetrating injuries can result in **enucleation**, which is removal of the eyeball. Chemical and thermal burns to the eye can result in damage to the cornea and can also lead to permanent vision loss if not treated quickly. A temporary loss of vision can result from an injury, such as the chemical burn that may occur with the deployment of an air bag, or from a corneal abrasion. Once treated, these injuries rarely lead to permanent loss of vision.

Disease   Visual impairments may also be caused by a disease of the eye, or as a secondary result of a primary disease process. **Glaucoma**, for example, is a group of eye diseases that results in increased intraocular pressure on the optic nerve. If not treated, glaucoma leads to loss of peripheral vision and to blindness. The incidence of glaucoma is higher in blacks than in whites. A black person between the ages of 45 and 65 is 15 times more likely to have glaucoma than a white person in the same age group.

Diabetic retinopathy is another disease-related visual impairment. It results from diabetes mellitus, which causes disorders in the blood vessels that lead to the retina. Small hemorrhages in these blood vessels lead to a slow loss of vision and possible blindness.

Congenital and Degenerative Disorders   A congenital disorder that causes visual disturbances is cerebral palsy. Premature birth can lead to blindness in the neonate. Degeneration of the eyeball, optic nerve, or nerve pathways is most commonly caused by aging and can slowly lead to loss of vision. Cytomegalovirus, an opportunistic infection often seen in AIDS patients, can lead to blindness by causing retinitis, an inflammation of the retina.

Recognizing and Accommodating Visual Impairments

Many people with visual impairments live independent, active lives (Figure 7-1 ●). Depending on the degree of impairment and a person's adjustment to the loss of vision, you may or may not recognize the condition right away. In cases of obvious blindness, identify yourself as you approach the patient so the person knows you are there. Also, describe everything you are doing as you do it.

Many people who are blind have tools to assist them in their activities of daily living. The most obvious is a service dog.

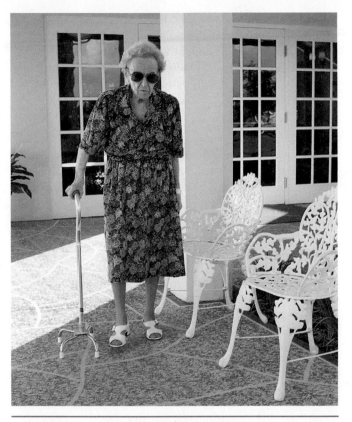

● **Figure 7-1** Individuals who are visually impaired can still maintain active, independent lives.

When approaching a person with a service dog, *do not* pet the dog or disturb it while the dog is in its harness. For the dog, the harness means that it is working. Ask permission from the patient to touch the dog. Never grab the leash, the harness, or the patient's arm without asking permission. Doing this may place you, the dog, or the owner in danger.[1]

Accommodation must be made for transporting the guide dog with the patient. Circumstances and local protocols will dictate whether you transport the dog in the ambulance with the patient or have the dog transported in another vehicle.

If your patient does not have a guide dog, inquire about other tools that the person may want brought to the hospital. If the patient is ambulatory, have the person take your arm for guidance rather than taking the patient's arm.

Speech Impairments

When performing an assessment, you may come across a patient who is awake, alert, and oriented, but cannot communicate with you because of a speech impairment. Possible miscommunication can hinder both the treatment you administer and the information that you provide to the receiving facility.

Types of Speech Impairment

You may encounter four types of speech impairment: language disorders, articulation disorders, voice production disorders, and fluency disorders.

Language Disorders A language disorder is an impaired ability to understand the spoken or written word. In children,

language disorders result from a number of causes, such as congenital learning disorders, cerebral palsy, or hearing impairments. A child who receives inadequate language stimulation in the first year of life may also experience delayed speaking ability.

In an adult patient, language disorders may result from a variety of illnesses or injuries. The person may have experienced a stroke, aneurysm, head injury, brain tumor, hearing loss, or some kind of emotional trauma. The loss of the ability to communicate in speech, writing, or signs is known as **aphasia**. Aphasia can manifest itself in the following ways:

- *Sensory aphasia*—a person can no longer understand the spoken word. Patients with sensory aphasia will not respond to your questions because they cannot understand what you are saying.

- *Motor aphasia*—a person can no longer use the symbols of speech. Patients with motor aphasia, also known as *expressive aphasia*, will understand what you say, but cannot clearly articulate a response. They may respond to your questions slowly, use the wrong words, or act out answers. It is important to allow such patients to express their responses in whatever way they can.

- *Global aphasia*—occurs when a person has both sensory and motor aphasia. These patients can neither understand nor respond to your questions. A brain tumor in Broca's region can cause this condition.

Articulation Disorders Articulation disorders, also known as *dysarthria*, affect the way a person's speech is heard by others. These disorders occur when sounds are produced or put together incorrectly or in a way that makes it difficult to understand the spoken word. Articulation disorders may start at an early age, when the child learns to say words incorrectly or when a hearing impairment is involved. This type of disorder can also occur in both children and adults when neural damage causes a disturbance in the nerve pathways leading from the brain to the larynx, mouth, or lips.

When speaking with people who have articulation disorders, you will notice that they pronounce their words incorrectly or that their speech is slurred. They may leave certain sounds out of a word because they are too difficult for them to pronounce. Again, it is important for you to listen carefully and let the person complete a response.

Voice Production Disorders When a patient has a voice production disorder, the quality of the person's voice is affected. This can be caused by trauma or may be due to overuse of the vocal cords or infection. Cancer of the larynx can also cause a speech failure by impeding air from passing through the vocal cords. A patient with a production disorder will exhibit hoarseness, harshness, an inappropriate pitch, or abnormal nasal resonance, or may have a total loss of voice.

CONTENT REVIEW

▶ Types of Speech Impairment

- Language disorders
- Articulation disorders
- Voice production disorders
- Fluency disorders

Fluency Disorders Fluency disorders present as stuttering. Although the cause of stuttering is not fully understood, the condition is found more often in men than in women. Stuttering occurs when sounds or syllables are repeated and the patient cannot put words together fluidly. When speaking with patients who stutter, do not interrupt or finish their answers out of frustration. Let patients complete what they have to say, and do not correct how they say it.

Accommodations for Speech Impairments

When speaking to a patient with a speech impairment, never assume that the person lacks intelligence (Figure 7-2 ●). It will be difficult, if not impossible, to complete a thorough interview if you have insulted the patient. Do not rush the patient or predict an answer. Try to form questions that require short, direct answers. Prepare to spend extra time during your interview.

When asking questions, look directly at the patient. If you cannot understand what the person has said, politely ask him to repeat it. Never pretend to understand when you don't. You might miss valuable information about the patient's chief complaint—the reason for the call. If all else fails, give the patient an opportunity to write responses to your questions.

Obesity

More than 40 percent of people in the United States are considered obese, and many more are heavier than their ideal body weight. An obese patient can make a difficult job even more

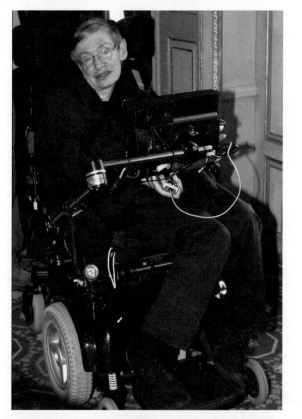

● **Figure 7-2** Physical disabilities do not often impact intellect. Stephen Hawking, the renowned British physicist and mathematician, has done important work despite the crippling effects of Lou Gehrig's disease and the loss of his voice as a result of a tracheostomy. (© *REUTERS/Tobias Schwarz*)

difficult for an EMS provider. Besides the obvious difficulty of lifting and moving the obese patient, excess weight can exacerbate the complaint for which you were called. Obesity can also lead to a number of serious medical conditions, including hypertension, heart disease, strokes, diabetes, and joint and muscle problems.

Etiologies

People require a certain amount of body fat to metabolize vitamins and minerals. Obesity occurs when a person has an abnormal amount of body fat and a weight 20 to 30 percent heavier than is normal for people of the same age, gender, and height.

Obesity occurs for a number of reasons. In many cases, it happens when a person's caloric intake is higher than the amount of calories required to meet his energy needs. In such cases, diet, exercise, and lifestyle choices play a role in the person's condition. Genetic factors may also predispose a patient toward obesity. In rare cases, an obese patient may have a low basal metabolic rate, which causes the body to burn calories at a slower rate. In such cases, the condition may be produced by an illness, particularly hypothyroidism.

Accommodations for Obese Patients

Regardless of the cause of your patient's obesity, your primary responsibility is to provide thorough and professional medical care. Conduct an extensive medical history, keeping in mind the chronic medical conditions commonly associated with obesity.

Obese patients often mistakenly blame signs and symptoms of an untreated illness on their weight. For example, they may quickly dismiss shortness of breath by saying: "When you're as heavy as me, you can't expect to walk up a flight of stairs without some extra breathing." Don't accept such an answer. The shortness of breath may be caused by congestive heart failure. Obtain a complete history of the symptoms and the activities the person was doing when they appeared. Although the patient usually experiences shortness of breath when climbing stairs, this time the condition may have started while he was sitting down or may have been more severe than usual.

When doing your patient assessment, you may also have to make accommodations for the person's weight. For example, if the patient's adipose tissue presents an obstruction, you may need to place ECG monitoring electrodes on the arms and thighs instead of on the chest. You may also need to auscultate lung sounds anteriorly on a patient who is too obese to lean forward. In assessing an obese patient, flexibility is the key. Keep in mind that no two patients and no two environments will be just alike.[2, 3]

Positioning an obese patient for transport may prove especially difficult, because many EMS transportation devices are not designed or rated for heavy weights. Always be sure you have enough lifting assistance for the circumstances. Never compromise your health or safety during the transport process. Another EMS crew or the fire department may be necessary to help move your patient safely. Finally, remember to let the emergency department know that extra lifting assistance and special stretchers will be needed on your arrival (Figure 7-3 ●).

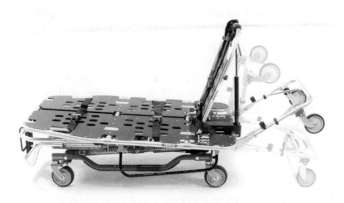

● **Figure 7-3a**   The Ferno LBS (large body surface) board converts a Ferno cot into a bariatric cot handling up to 1,000 pounds. (© *Ferno-Washington, Inc.*)

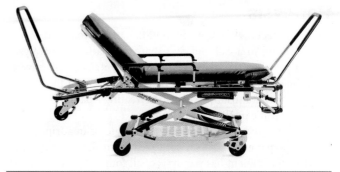

● **Figure 7-3b**   The Stryker MX-PRO® Bariatric Transport cot will handle patients up to 850 pounds, and will accommodate patient weights from 850 to 1,600 pounds at its lowest height position. This cot can be used with accessory winch and ramp-loading devices. (© *Stryker Medical Corporation*)

PATHO PEARLS

Dealing with the Morbidly Obese Patient

Obesity is one of the leading health care problems in the United States today. Several factors can be blamed for this. First, in the 20th century we made a change from a largely agrarian diet to one of processed foods. In the latter half of the 20th century we saw the advent of fast foods. These foods are tasty and readily available—but they contain a large number of calories and saturated fats. In addition, the American lifestyle has become more sedentary with nearly 200 television channels to watch and numerous video games to play. All these contribute to increasing obesity.

Obesity is often determined using the body mass index (BMI). The BMI incorporates the person's weight and height using the metric system. It is defined as:

$$Body\ Mass\ Index\ (BMI) = \frac{mass\ (kilograms)}{height\ (meters)^2}$$

The following definitions of obesity have been established by the World Health Organization based on the BMI:

- *Overweight: BMI of 25–29.9 kg/m²*
- *Obesity: BMI of 30–39.9 kg/m²*
- *Morbid obesity: BMI ≥ 40 kg/m²*

The BMI corresponds to the percentage of total body fat. Obesity can also be determined by measuring total body fat; a male with greater than 25 percent total body fat or a female with greater than 30 percent total body fat is considered obese.

Morbid obesity is defined as being 50 to 100 percent, or 100 pounds or more, above ideal body weight. Morbidly obese persons are at increased risk for diabetes, hypertension, heart disease, stroke, certain cancers (breast and colon), depression, and osteoarthritis. In addition, they tend to develop chronic hypoxemia from inadequate ventilation. This is often complicated by sleep apnea. Morbid obesity is a significant disability, and EMS personnel now encounter the morbidly obese more frequently. Some morbidly obese people can weigh more than 500 pounds and cannot typically be handled by standard ambulance stretchers and equipment. Because of this, several ambulance stretcher

manufacturers now manufacture equipment specifically for the morbidly obese. Many ambulance services have developed special ambulances for the obese that contain winches and ramps to ease patient loading.

Moving an obese patient can be a very trying event for all involved. For EMS personnel, it presents several logistical problems. For the patient, it can be a tremendous source of embarrassment. Many of these patients have not been out of their houses in years and now find themselves the center of attention, surrounded by emergency vehicles, often the media, and curious onlookers. Sometimes structural modifications must be made to the house before they can be removed.

Every EMS system must have a protocol and strategy for dealing with the morbidly obese. Many have added bariatric transport vehicles to their fleets (Figure 7-4 ●). They should be treated with the same compassion and care afforded all EMS patients.

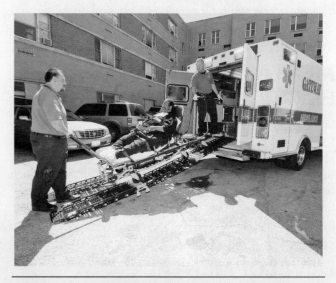

● **Figure 7-4**   With an increasing number of morbidly obese patients, many EMS systems have developed specialized bariatric transport units. (© *Ray Kemp/911 Imaging*)

Paralysis

Always expect the unexpected in EMS. During your career, you may respond to a call and find that your patient is paralyzed from a previous traumatic or medical event. You will have to treat the chief complaint while taking into account the accommodations that must be made when treating a patient who cannot move some or all of his extremities.

A paralyzed patient may be paraplegic or quadriplegic. A paraplegic patient has been paralyzed from the waist down; a quadriplegic patient has paralysis of all four extremities. In addition, spinal cord injuries in the area of C3 to C5 and above may also paralyze the patient's respiratory muscles and compromise the ability to breathe.

If your patient depends on a home ventilator, it is important to maintain a patent airway and to keep the ventilator functioning. Also, a paralyzed patient may have been breathing through a tracheostomy for some time. Therefore, you should keep suction nearby in case the person experiences an airway obstruction. You may also need to use a bag-valve-mask unit to transport the patient to the ambulance if the ventilator does not transport easily. If your ambulance is equipped, use the ventilator with an onboard power supply to save the ventilator's batteries. This is an already anxious time for your patient, so you may need to spend some extra time reassuring the person before making any changes in the life support system.

If the patient has suffered a recent spinal cord injury, halo traction may still be intact. Be sure to stabilize the traction before transport. The patient can probably tell you how to assist with the halo traction; if not, a call to the patient's physician may be necessary.

While performing your physical assessment, you may come across a **colostomy** appliance. This device is necessary when the patient does not have normal bowel function from paralysis of the muscles needed for proper elimination. Be sure to take any other assisting devices, such as canes or wheelchairs, so the patient can get around once out of your care. (For more on acute interventions for people with physical disabilities and other chronic care patients, see Chapter 8.)

MENTAL CHALLENGES AND EMOTIONAL IMPAIRMENTS

Mental and emotional illnesses present a special challenge to the EMS provider. They may range from psychoses such as schizophrenia to personality disorders to psychological conditions resulting from trauma. Emotional impairments can include such conditions as anxiety or depression. For a detailed discussion of the etiologies, assessment, management, and treatment of these patients, see Volume 4, Chapter 11.

DEVELOPMENTAL DISABILITIES

People with developmental disabilities are individuals with impaired or insufficient development of the brain who are unable to learn at the usual rate. In recent years, a large number of people with developmental disabilities have been mainstreamed into the day-to-day activities of life. They hold jobs and live in residential settings, either on their own, with their families, or in group homes.

Developmental disabilities can have a variety of causes. They can be genetic, such as in Down syndrome, or they can be the product of brain injury caused by some hypoxic or traumatic event. Such injuries can take place before birth, during birth, or anytime thereafter.

Accommodations for Developmental Disabilities

Unless a patient has Down syndrome or lives in a group home or other special residential setting, it may be difficult to recognize someone with a developmental disability. The disability may become obvious only when you start your interview, and even then the person may be able to provide adequate information (Figure 7-5 ●). Remember that persons with developmental disabilities can recognize body language, tone, and disrespect just like anyone else. Treat them as you would any other patient, listening to their answers, particularly if you suspect physical or emotional abuse. As mentioned in previous chapters, this group has a higher than average chance of being abused, particularly by someone they know.

If a patient has a severe cognitive disability, you may need to rely on others to obtain the chief complaint and history. In this case, plan to spend a little extra time on the physical assessment, because the patient may not be able to tell you what is wrong. Also, many children or young people with learning disabilities have been taught to be wary of strangers who may seek to touch them. You will have to establish a basis of trust with the patient, perhaps by making it clear that you are a member of the medical community or by asking for the support of a person the patient does trust. Also, some people with developmental disabilities have been judged "stupid" or "bad" for behavior that results in an accident and, therefore, they may try to cover up the events that led up to the call.

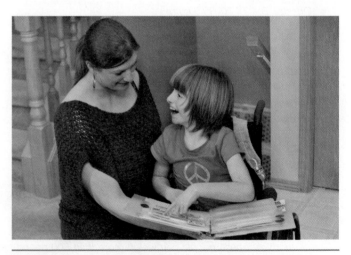

● **Figure 7-5** People with developmental disabilities may have trouble communicating but can often still understand what you say.

At all times, keep in mind that a person with a developmental disability may not understand what is happening. The ambulance, special equipment, and even your uniform may confuse or scare him. In cases of severe disabilities, it will be important to keep the primary caregiver with you at all times, even in the back of the ambulance. Talk to patients with disabilities in terms they will understand and demonstrate what you are doing, as much as possible, on yourself or your partner.

Down Syndrome

Until the mid-1900s, people with Down syndrome lived largely out of public view and tended to die at an early age. Today, people with Down syndrome attend special schools, hold paid jobs, and, because of improved medical care, can live long lives.

Down syndrome is named after J. Langdon Down, the British physician who studied and identified the condition. It results from an extra chromosome, usually on chromosome 21 or 22. Instead of 46 chromosomes, a person with Down syndrome has 47.

Although the cause is unknown, the incidence of this chromosomal abnormality increases with the age of the mother, especially after age 40. It also occurs at a higher rate in parents with a chromosomal abnormality such as the translocation of chromosome 21 to chromosome 14. In such cases, the parent, usually the mother, has only 45 chromosomes. Theoretically, the chance is one in three that this mother will have a child with Down syndrome.

Typically, Down syndrome presents with easily recognized physical features, including:

- Eyes sloped up at the outer corners
- Folds of skin on either side of the nose that cover the inner corner of the eye
- Small face and features
- Large and protruding tongue
- Flattening of the back of the head
- Short and broad hands

In addition to mild to moderate developmental disability, patients with Down syndrome may have other physical ailments, such as heart defects, intestinal defects, and chronic lung problems. People with Down syndrome are also at risk of developing cataracts, blindness, and Alzheimer's disease at an early age.

When assessing the patient with Down syndrome, consider the level of developmental delay and follow the general guidelines mentioned earlier for dealing with patients who have developmental disabilities (Figure 7-6 ●). Transport to the hospital should be uneventful, especially if the caregiver accompanies you.

Fetal Alcohol Syndrome

Fetal alcohol syndrome (FAS) is sometimes confused with Down syndrome because of similar facial characteristics. Unlike Down syndrome, however, FAS is a preventable disorder,

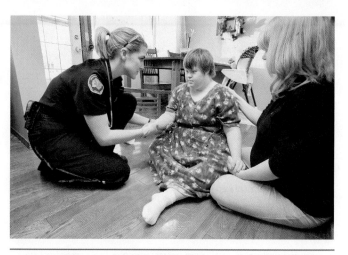

● **Figure 7-6** A patient with Down syndrome may have a mild to moderate developmental impairment.

caused by excessive alcohol consumption during pregnancy. Children who suffer FAS have characteristic features, including:

- Small head with multiple facial abnormalities
- Small eyes with short slits
- Wide, flat nose bridge
- Lack of a groove between the nose and lip
- Small jaw

FAS patients often exhibit delayed physical growth, mental disabilities, and hyperactivity. Again, follow the preceding general guidelines when treating children with FAS.

PATHOLOGICAL CHALLENGES

During your career in EMS, you will probably encounter a number of patients with chronic conditions. You should be aware of the most common of these conditions, because chronic care patients require a higher-than-average number of interventions and transports, as discussed in the following sections and in Chapter 8.

Arthritis

The three most common types of arthritis are:

- *Juvenile rheumatoid arthritis (JRA)*—a connective tissue disorder that strikes before age 16
- *Rheumatoid arthritis*—an autoimmune disorder
- *Osteoarthritis*—a degenerative joint disease, the most common arthritis seen in elderly patients

All forms of arthritis cause painful swelling and irritation of the joints, making everyday tasks sometimes impossible. Arthritis patients commonly have joint stiffness and limited range of motion. Sometimes the smaller joints of the hands and feet become deformed (Figure 7-7 ●). In addition, children with JRA may suffer complications involving the spleen or liver.

Treatment for arthritis includes aspirin, nonsteroidal anti-inflammatory drugs (NSAIDs), and/or corticosteroids. You

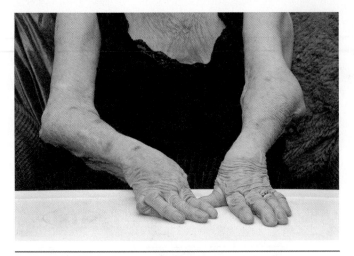

● **Figure 7-7** Rheumatoid arthritis causes joints to become painful and deformed.

should be able to recognize the side effects of these medications because you may be called on to treat a medication side effect rather than the disease. NSAIDs can cause stomach upset and vomiting, with or without bloody emesis. Corticosteroids, such as prednisone, can cause hyperglycemia, bloody emesis, and decreased immunity. You should also take note of all the patient's medications so you do not administer a medication that can interact with the ones already taken by the patient.

When transporting arthritis patients, keep in mind their high level of discomfort. Use pillows to elevate affected extremities. The most comfortable patient position might not be the best position to start an IV, but try to make the patient as comfortable as possible. Special padding techniques may be required because of the patient's arthritis.

Cancer

Entire books have been written about cancer. It is impossible to list here all that a health care provider could learn about this subject. However, some basic points follow that you should keep in mind when treating a patient with cancer.

Cancer is really a blanket term for many different diseases, each with its own characteristics but having in common the abnormal growth of cells in normal tissue. The primary site of origin of the cancer cells determines the type of cancer that the patient has. If the cancer starts in epithelial tissue, it is called a *carcinoma*. If the cancer forms in connective tissue, it is called a *sarcoma*.

It may be difficult for you to recognize a cancer patient, because the disease often has few obvious signs and symptoms. However, treatments for the disease do tend to produce telltale signs, such as alopecia (hair loss) or anorexia (loss of appetite) leading to weight loss. Tattoos may be left on the skin by radiation oncologists to mark positioning of radiation therapy equipment. In addition, physical changes, such as removal of a breast (mastectomy), may be obvious.

Management of the patient with cancer can present a special challenge to the paramedic. Many patients undergoing chemotherapy treatments become **neutropenic**. This is a

condition in which chemotherapy creates a dangerously low level of neutrophils, the white blood cells responsible for the destruction of bacteria and other infectious organisms. Frequently during chemotherapy the neutrophils are destroyed along with the cancer cells, severely increasing the patient's risk for infection.

If patients have recently undergone chemotherapy, assume that they are neutropenic. Reduce their exposure to infection as much as possible. Remember that, once infected, a neutropenic patient can quickly go into septic shock, sometimes in a matter of hours. For this reason, keep a mask on such patients during both transport and transfer at the emergency department (Figure 7-8 ●).

Also keep in mind that cancer patients' veins may have become scarred and difficult to access as a result of frequent IV starts, blood draws, and caustic chemotherapy transfusions. A patient with cancer may also have an implanted infusion port, found just below the skin, with the catheter inserted into the subclavian vein or brachial artery. This port is accessed for infusion of chemotherapy drugs or IV fluids using sterile technique.

You need special training to use these implanted ports and should not attempt to access them unless you have such training. Local protocols usually dictate whether an EMS provider may access one of these devices. Patients may request that you do not start a peripheral IV if their port can be accessed at the hospital. In such cases, you need to consider if your IV is a lifesaving necessity that cannot wait or if the patient can indeed wait for access at the emergency department.

Patients with cancer may also have a peripheral access device, such as a Groshong catheter or Hickman catheter, that has access ports that extend outside the skin. In this situation, it may simply be a matter of flushing the line and then hooking up your IV fluids to this external catheter. Whatever you decide to do, involve the patient in the decision-making process whenever possible. Patients with cancer lose much control over their lives during treatment, so it is important for them to maintain as much control over their EMS care as possible.

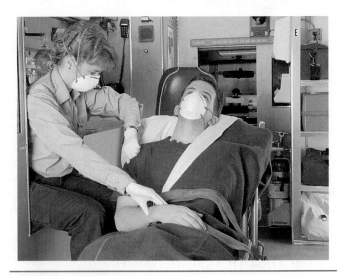

● **Figure 7-8** Make every effort to protect cancer patients from infection. Keep a mask on yourself and the patient during transport and during transfer at the hospital.

Cerebral Palsy

Cerebral palsy is a group of disorders caused by damage to the cerebrum *in utero* or by trauma during birth. Prenatal exposure of the mother to German measles can cause cerebral palsy, along with any event that leads to hypoxia in the fetus. Premature birth or brain damage from a difficult delivery can also lead to cerebral palsy. Other causes include encephalitis, meningitis, or head injury from a fall or the abuse of an infant.

Patients with cerebral palsy have difficulty controlling motor functions, causing spasticity of the muscles. This condition may affect a single limb or the entire body. About two-thirds of cerebral palsy patients have a below-normal intellectual capacity, and about half experience seizures. Conversely, a full third of patients with cerebral palsy have normal intelligence and a few are highly gifted.

The three main types of cerebral palsy are spastic paralysis, athetosis, and ataxia. *Spastic paralysis*, which is the most common form of cerebral palsy, forces the muscles into a state of permanent stiffness and contracture. When both legs are affected, the knees turn inward, causing the characteristic "scissor gait." *Athetosis* causes an involuntary writhing movement, usually affecting arms, feet, hands, and legs. If the patient's face is affected, the person may demonstrate drooling or grimacing. *Ataxic cerebral palsy* is the rarest form of the disease and causes problems with coordination of gait and balance.

In treating patients with cerebral palsy, keep this fact in mind: Many people with athetoid and diplegic cerebral palsy are highly intelligent. Do not automatically assume that a person with cerebral palsy cannot communicate with you. Also, as you might expect, many cerebral palsy patients rely on special devices to help them with their mobility. Diplegic patients, for example, may be dependent on wheelchairs.

When transporting patients with cerebral palsy, make accommodations to prevent further injury. If they experience severe contractions, the patients may not rest comfortably on a stretcher. Use pillows and extra blankets to pad extremities that are not in normal alignment. Have suction available if a patient drools. If a patient has difficulty communicating, make sure that the caregiver helps in your assessment. Be alert for patients with cerebral palsy who sign. If you do not know sign language, try to find someone who does and alert the emergency department.

Cystic Fibrosis (Mucoviscidosis)

Cystic fibrosis (CF or **mucoviscidosis**) is an inherited disorder that involves the exocrine (mucus-producing) glands, primarily in the lungs and the digestive system. Thick mucus forms in the lungs, causing bronchial obstruction and atelectasis, or collapse of the alveoli. In addition, the thick mucus causes blockages in the small ducts of the pancreas, leading to a decrease in the pancreatic enzymes needed for digestion. This results in malnutrition, even for patients on healthy diets.

Obtaining a complete medical history is important to the recognition of a patient with cystic fibrosis. A unique characteristic of CF is the high concentration of chloride in the sweat, leading to the use of a diagnostic test known as the "sweat test." A patient with CF may also suffer from frequent lung infections, clay-colored stools, or clubbing of the fingers or toes.

Recent medical advances have extended the lives of patients with CF so that some live well into their thirties. However, because of a poor prognosis, most of the patients with CF that you see will be children and adolescents. In treating these patients, remember that they have been chronically ill for their entire lives. The last thing they may want is another trip to the hospital. For this reason, transport can be difficult for both the patient and family members. To allay their fears, keep in mind the developmental stage of your patient. A child with CF is still a child, so recall everything you have learned about the treatment and comforting of pediatric patients.

Because of the high probability of respiratory distress in a patient with CF, some form of oxygen therapy may be necessary. You may need to have a family member or caregiver hold blow-by oxygen, rather than using a mask, if that is all the patient will tolerate. Suctioning may be necessary to help the patient clear the thick secretions from the airway. CF patients may be taking antibiotics to prevent infection and using inhalers or Mucomyst to thin their secretions. Make sure that you take along all medications so that the hospital staff can continue with the patient's regimen.

Multiple Sclerosis

Multiple sclerosis (MS) is a disorder of the central nervous system that usually strikes between the ages of 20 and 40, affecting women more often than men. The exact cause of MS is unknown, but it is considered to be an autoimmune disorder. Characteristically, repeated inflammation of the myelin sheath surrounding the nerves leads to scar tissue, which in turn blocks nerve impulses to the affected area.

The onset of MS is slow. It starts with a slight change in the strength of a muscle and numbness or tingling in the affected muscle. For example, a patient may start to drop things, blaming it on clumsiness. Doctors encourage patients with MS to lead as normal a life as possible, but the patients become increasingly tired. Their gait may become unsteady, and they may slur their speech. Patients with MS may also develop eye problems, such as double vision, owing to weakness of the eye muscles or eye pain due to neuritis of the optic nerve.

The initial signs of MS are usually temporary. However, they return and become more frequent and long lasting. As the symptoms progress, they become more permanent, leading to a weak extremity or paralysis. Over time, some patients may become bedridden and lose control of bladder function. Eventually an MS patient may develop a lung or urinary infection, which may lead to death. As with other chronically ill patients, people with MS may experience mood swings and seek medical attention for their feelings.

Transport of a patient with MS to the hospital may require supportive care, such as oxygen therapy. Make sure the patient is comfortable, by helping to position the person as necessary. Do not expect patients with MS to walk to the ambulance. Even if they normally are ambulatory, they may be in a more weakened

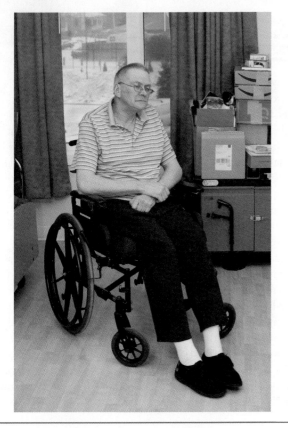

● **Figure 7-9** Patients with multiple sclerosis and muscular dystrophy may need to use wheelchairs.

state than usual. Again, be sure to bring assistive devices, such as a wheelchair or cane, so the patient can maintain as much independence as possible (Figure 7-9 ●).

Muscular Dystrophy

Muscular dystrophy (MD) is a group of hereditary disorders characterized by progressive weakness and wasting of muscle tissue. It is a genetic disorder, leading to gradual degeneration of muscle fibers. The most common form of MD is Duchenne muscular dystrophy, which typically affects boys between the ages of three and six. It leads to progressive muscle weakness in the legs and pelvis and to paralysis by age 12. Ultimately, the disease affects the respiratory muscles and heart, causing death at an early age. The other various MD disorders are classified by the age of the patient at onset of symptoms and by the muscles affected.

Because MD is a hereditary disease, you should obtain a complete family history. You should also note the particular muscle groups that the patient cannot move. Again, because patients with MD are primarily children, choose age-appropriate language. Respiratory support, such as oxygen, may be needed, especially in the later stages of the disease.

Poliomyelitis

Poliomyelitis, commonly called *polio*, is a communicable disease that affects the gray matter of the brain and the spinal cord. Although it is highly contagious, immunization has made outbreaks

of polio extremely rare in developed nations. However, it is important to know about polio because many people born before development of the polio vaccination in the 1950s have been affected by the disease.

Typically, the polio virus enters the body through the gastrointestinal tract. It circulates through the digestive tract and then enters the bloodstream. There, it is carried to the central nervous system where the virus enters and alters the nerve cells. In cases of paralytic poliomyelitis, patients experience asymmetrical muscle weakness that leads to permanent paralysis.

Although most patients recover from the disease itself, they are left with permanent paralysis of the affected muscles. You may recognize a polio victim by the use of assistive devices for ambulation or by the reduced size of the affected limb, which is a result of muscle atrophy. Some patients may have experienced paralysis of the respiratory muscles and require assisted ventilation. Patients on long-term ventilators will typically have tracheostomies.

A related disorder is called *post-polio syndrome*. Post-polio syndrome can develop in patients who suffered severely from polio more than 30 years ago. Although the cause of post-polio syndrome remains unknown, researchers think the condition results from the stress of long-term weakness in the affected nerves. Patients with this condition tire quickly, especially after exercise, and develop an intolerance for cold in their extremities. Unhappily, some persons who survived their original bout with polio die in later years from the effects of post-polio syndrome.

Many patients with polio or post-polio syndrome try to maintain their independence. They may insist on walking to the ambulance but should not be encouraged to do so. The idea of hospitalization will frustrate them, because many polio survivors have memories of spending months or even years in hospitals as children. Unlike other patients with chronic illnesses, most people who have had polio do not require frequent trips to the hospital. Therefore, this may be their first time in the back of an ambulance. Try to alleviate their anxiety as much as possible.

Previous Head Injuries

A patient with a previous head injury may not be recognized easily. You may not notice anything different about the patient until the person starts to speak. A patient who has had a head injury may display symptoms similar to those of a stroke, without the hemiparesis, or paralysis, to one side of the body. The presenting symptoms will be related to the area of the brain that has been injured. The patient may have aphasia, slurred speech, loss of vision or hearing, or a learning disability. Such patients may also exhibit short-term memory loss and may not have any recollection of their original injury.

Obtaining a medical history from these patients is very important, especially if you are responding to a traumatic event. Note any new symptoms the patient may be having or the recurrence of old ones. Conduct the physical assessment slowly. If the patient cannot speak, look for obvious physical signs of trauma or for facial expressions of pain. Transport considerations will depend on the condition for which you were called. However, information about the previous head injury, if you can obtain it, should be an important part of the patient's transfer.

Spina Bifida

Spina bifida is a congenital abnormality that falls under the category of neural tube defects. It presents when there is a defect in the closure of the backbone and the spinal canal. In *spina bifida occulta*, the patient exhibits few outward signs of the deformity. In *spina bifida cystica*, the failure of the closure allows the spinal cord and covering membranes to protrude from the back, causing an obvious deformity.

Symptoms depend on which part of the spinal cord is protruding through the back. The patient may have paralysis of both lower extremities and lack of bowel or bladder control. A large percentage of children born with spina bifida have hydrocephalus, which is the accumulation of fluid in the brain. If the patient has hydrocephalus, a shunt will need to be inserted to help drain off the excess fluid. Permanent disabilities cannot be assessed until the defect is surgically corrected.

When treating patients with spina bifida, keep several things in mind. Recent research has shown that between 18 and 73 percent of children and adolescents with spina bifida have latex allergies. For safety, assume that all patients with spina bifida have this problem. In transporting a patient with spina bifida, be sure to take along any devices that aid the patient. If you are called to treat an infant, safe transport to the hospital should be done in a car seat unless contraindicated.

Myasthenia Gravis

Myasthenia gravis is an autoimmune disease characterized by chronic weakness of voluntary muscles and progressive fatigue. The condition results from a problem with the neurotransmitters, which causes a blocking of nerve signals to the muscles. It occurs most frequently in women between the ages of 20 and 50.

A patient with myasthenia gravis may complain of a complete lack of energy, especially in the evening. The disease commonly involves muscles in the face. You may note eyelid drooping or difficulty in chewing or swallowing. The patient may also complain of double vision.

In severe cases of myasthenia gravis, a patient may experience paralysis of the respiratory muscles, leading to respiratory arrest. These patients will, of course, need assisted ventilations en route to the emergency facility. For patients with less severe cases, accommodations will vary based on presentation.

OTHER CHALLENGES

In addition to the challenges described in the preceding sections, you can expect to meet a whole range of special situations that will affect the quality of the patient service that you provide. The following are some of the special situations or conditions that you are likely to encounter, if you have not already done so.

Culturally Diverse Patients

As a health care provider, you are ethically required to take care of all patients in the same manner, regardless of their race, religion, gender, ethnic background, or living situation. What may make it difficult for you to treat culturally different patients may

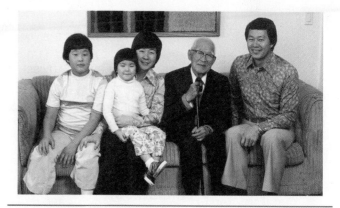

● **Figure 7-10**   The population of the United States is becoming increasingly diverse, with the largest number of immigrants coming from Asia and Latin America. (© *Michal Heron*)

not be the differences per se but your inability to understand them. Do not consider this a reason for refusing treatment. Rather, consider it a learning experience that will prepare you for a similar situation on another run. With American society becoming more diverse, instead of less diverse, the ability to tolerate cultural differences will become an important part of your professionalism as a paramedic (Figure 7-10 ●).

From time to time, you may encounter a patient who will make a decision about medical care with which you do not agree. For example, Christian Scientists do not believe in human intervention in sickness through the use of drugs or other therapies. You cannot force these patients to accept an IV or to take nitroglycerin if they are having chest pains. Remember, the patient who has decision-making capabilities has a right to self-determination. You should, however, obtain a signed document indicating informed refusal of consent (Figure 7-11 ●).

Accommodation of a culturally diverse population will require patience and, in some cases, ingenuity. If your patient does not speak English, and you do not speak the patient's language, communication may be a problem. You may need to rely on a family member to act as an interpreter or on a translator device, such as a telephone language line, for non-English-speaking people. In such cases, be sure to notify the receiving facility of the need for an interpreter.

Terminally Ill Patients

Caring for a terminally ill patient is an emotional challenge. Many times, the patient will choose to die at home, but at the last minute the family will compromise those wishes by calling for an ambulance. In other cases, the patient may call for an ambulance so that a newly developed condition can be treated or a medication adjusted. For more on caring for the terminally ill, either at home or in a hospice situation, see Chapter 8.

Patients with Communicable Diseases

When treating people with communicable diseases, you should withhold all personal judgment. Although you will have to take Standard Precautions just as you would with any patient,

REFUSAL OF TREATMENT AND TRANSPORTATION

I, THE UNDERSIGNED, HAVE BEEN ADVISED THAT MEDICAL ASSISTANCE ON MY BEHALF IS NECESSARY AND THAT REFUSAL OF SAID ASSISTANCE AND TRANSPORTATION MAY RESULT IN DEATH OR IMPERIL MY HEALTH. NEVERTHELESS, I REFUSE TO ACCEPT TREATMENT OR TRANSPORT AND ASSUME ALL RISKS AND CONSEQUENCES OF MY DECISION AND RELEASE GOLD CROSS AMBULANCE COMPANY AND ITS EMPLOYEES FROM ANY LIABILITY ARISING FROM MY REFUSAL.

_____
SIGNATURE OF PATIENT

_____
WITNESSED BY

_____
DATE SIGNED

● **Figure 7-11** If a patient refuses care because of cultural or religious beliefs, be sure to have the person sign a Refusal of Treatment and Transportation form.

keep in mind the heightened sensitivity of a person with a communicable disease. Most of these patients are familiar with the health care setting and understand why you must take certain protective measures. However, you should still explain that you take these measures with all patients who have similar diseases. Also, you do not need to take additional precautions that are not required by departmental policy. The patient will generally spot these extra measures and feel guilt, shame, or anger.

For more information on the etiologies and treatment of communicable diseases, see Volume 4, Chapter 10.

Patients with Financial Challenges

One of the exciting parts of a career in EMS is the opportunity to meet people of all backgrounds. You have the chance to get out into the street and see how people live, work, and play. This allows you to help and educate people who may not otherwise have access to health care. For example, you may get sent to a street corner where a homeless man has fallen and needs medical attention but cannot afford to pay the medical bills. It is your job to help the patient understand that he can receive health care regardless of his financial situation (Figure 7-12 ●).

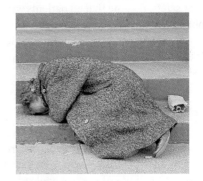

● **Figure 7-12** Homeless people sometimes refuse care, thinking they cannot afford to pay the medical bills. Become familiar with public hospitals and clinics that provide services to the needy. (© Michal Heron)

Become familiar with public hospitals and clinics that provide services to people without money or adequate insurance coverage. Calm a patient's fears by discussing this and providing as much helpful information as you can. In providing care, always keep this guideline in mind: Treat the patient, not the financial condition the patient is in.

◼ SUMMARY

As health care systems improve and make changes, more and more patients with impairments and challenges are beginning to live at home rather than in a medical facility such as a nursing home. EMS is now being summoned to residences for complications with chronic illnesses that were once handled in facilities. Because of this, it is important to be aware of the pathophysiology of diseases that you may encounter and the common complications and treatments seen with them. You will be called for a variety of situations ranging from critical emergencies to simple lifting assistance. In any event, the more you know about the specific situation, the better prepared you will be for the call.

Not all challenges you will face will include chronic illnesses or diseases. Some of these situations may be culturally driven or even financially driven. In any case, keep in mind the legal rights of the patient to accept or refuse treatment, no matter what the reasoning. Keeping patients' best interests in mind includes not only treating their physical being, but also treating their emotional, financial, and spiritual being as well. Remember that it is your responsibility to treat each of your patients with respect and dignity, even if you disagree philosophically with their decisions.

YOU MAKE THE CALL

You and your partner are called to the home of a 56-year-old female patient with a chief complaint of fever. You arrive on the scene to find the door unlocked and a woman calling to you to come to a back bedroom.

She stops you at the door of her bedroom and asks both you and your partner to put on a mask. She tells you that she is undergoing treatment for breast cancer (she has had a mastectomy, she tells you) and that the doctor told her that she shouldn't be around people who are sick because she has an increased risk of infection. She has a scarf around her head and you notice a wig on her bedside table.

She tells you that she has a fever of 102°F and her heart is beating very fast, and this is scaring her. She has had a decrease in appetite and some vomiting. The doctor told her that she should go to the hospital, but she lives alone and didn't have a ride so she called EMS.

Your partner has a cold, so he agrees to drive to the hospital while you ride with the patient. The short transport is uneventful. You arrive at the hospital and transfer patient care to the ED nurse.

1. Why did the patient's doctor tell her that she has an increased risk of infection from communicable diseases?

2. What signs indicate that this patient has cancer?

3. Is it necessary for all three of you to wear a mask? Explain.

4. Will you start a peripheral IV on this patient? Explain.

5. What information will you include in your patient report so the emergency department is prepared for this patient?

See Suggested Responses at the back of this book.

REVIEW QUESTIONS

1. Deafness caused by the inability of nerve impulses to reach the auditory center of the brain because of nerve damage either to the inner ear or to the brain is _____.
   a. otitis media
   b. transient deafness
   c. sensorineural deafness
   d. conductive deafness

2. _____ is a progressive sensorineural hearing loss that begins after age 20 but is significant only in people over age 65.
   a. Tinnitus   c. Labyrinthitis
   b. Presbycusis   d. Otitis media

3. _____, an opportunistic infection often seen in AIDS patients, can lead to blindness by causing retinitis.
   a. Glaucoma
   b. Enucleation
   c. Diabetic retinopathy
   d. Cytomegalovirus

4. _____ occurs when the patient cannot speak but can understand what is said.
   a. Visual aphasia   c. Global aphasia
   b. Motor aphasia   d. Sensory aphasia

5. A surgical diversion of the large intestine through an opening in the skin where the fecal matter is collected in a pouch is a _____.
   a. stoma   c. colectomy
   b. ileostomy   d. colostomy

6. Down syndrome presents with easily recognized physical features, including all of the following *except* _____.
   a. large face and features
   b. large and protruding tongue
   c. short and broad hands
   d. flattening of the back of the head

7. The most common form of cerebral palsy is _____.
   a. ataxia   c. athetosis
   b. aphasia   d. spastic paralysis

8. Myasthenia gravis results from a problem with the neurotransmitters and occurs most frequently in women between the ages of _____.
   a. 50 and 60   c. 10 and 20
   b. 40 and 50   d. 20 and 50

See Answers to Review Questions at the back of this book.

REFERENCES

1. Kom, J. "Servicing the Service Dogs." *Emerg Med Serv* 34 (2005): 56.

2. Haber, C. B. "Bariatric Transport Challenges: Part 1." *EMS Mag* 37(4) (2008): 67–71.

3. Haber, C. B. "Bariatric Transport Challenges: Part 2." *EMS Mag* 37(5) (2008): 73–75.

FURTHER READING

Barry, P. *Mental Health* and *Mental Illness.* 7th ed. Philadelphia: Lippincott, 2002.

Dresser, R. *When Science Offers Salvation: Patient Advocacy and Research Ethics.* Oxford, UK: Oxford University Press, 2001.

Early Identification of Hearing Impairment in Infants and Young Children, Program and Abstracts. Bethesda, MD: National Institutes of Health, 1993.

Phipps, W., et al. *Medical-Surgical Nursing: Health and Illness Perspective.* St. Louis: Mosby-Year Book, 2003.

8

Acute Interventions for the Chronic Care Patient

Bryan Bledsoe, DO, FACEP, FAAEM, EMT-P

STANDARD
Special Patient Populations (Patients with Special Needs)

COMPETENCY
Integrates assessment findings with principles of epidemiology and pathophysiology and knowledge of psychosocial needs to formulate a field impression and implement a comprehensive treatment/disposition plan for patients with special needs.

OBJECTIVES

Terminal Performance Objective
After reading this chapter, you should be able to effectively assess, manage, and take into consideration the psychosocial needs of chronically ill patients encountered in prehospital care.

Enabling Objectives
To accomplish the terminal performance objective, you should be able to:

1. Define key terms introduced in this chapter.

2. Describe factors that have contributed to the increase in home health care.

3. Relate the epidemiology of patients receiving home health care to paramedics' knowledge needs with respect to home health care.

4. Anticipate the psychosocial concerns of patients receiving home health care and of their family members.

5. Describe common reasons why paramedics are summoned to assist patients receiving home health care.

6. Anticipate common complications that occur with various types of home health care equipment.

7. Recognize home health care patients with signs and symptoms of infection and sepsis.

8. Describe the need to interact with other health care professionals when responding to patients receiving home health care.

9. Adapt techniques of scene size-up, patient assessment, and patient care interventions to the special situations of patients receiving home health care.

10. Consider the existence of a DNR/DNAR or other physician orders or instructions when caring for patients receiving home health care.

11. Address the special assessment and equipment troubleshooting needs for patients with each of the following situations:

    a. Respiratory problems
    b. Vascular access devices
    c. Cardiovascular problems

d. Gastrointestinal and genitourinary problems and devices

e. Maternal and newborn care

f. Hospice care

KEY TERMS

CASE STUDY

Desert Springs Paramedic 2 has just ordered a takeout dinner when dispatch reports an "elderly male, short of breath." With a shrug, the crew members cancel dinner and head to the address provided by the dispatcher. On arrival, they find the door slightly ajar and can see the patient sitting on the couch. As they pass through the vestibule, they notice several bottles of oxygen on the floor. They observe that their patient is on a nasal cannula. He is having obvious moderate dyspnea and is using some accessory muscles.

The patient speaks in four- to five-word sentences. He tells the crew that his name is Clarence Casey. Mr. Casey indicates that he is 74 years old. He complains that it has become increasingly difficult for him to breathe. He has used his "puffers" multiple times without relief. Although Mr. Casey says he has no chest pain, he feels as though his breathing has become "heavier."

While the EMT puts together a nebulizer, the paramedic auscultates lung sounds. She notes diminished breathing in all fields with inspiratory and expiratory wheezes. She also observes a prolonged expiratory phase with pursing of lips. The patient is not tripoding and has a respiratory rate of 30 breaths per minute. Use of a pulse oximeter indicates a reading of 86 percent on 4 liters oxygen. The patient's skin is warm, dry, and pale.

On questioning, Mr. Casey tells the crew that he has a history of emphysema, bronchitis, hypertension, glaucoma, and smoked a pack of cigarettes each day for 60 years. His medications include a Proventil inhaler, a Serevent inhaler, eye drops, and Cardura. He has no allergies. He usually uses oxygen only when walking around the house or doing light chores, such as washing dishes. He lives alone and has home care one day a week. Because of his end-stage COPD, Mr. Casey has authorized a valid prehospital do not resuscitate (DNR) order with his physician, which he shows to the EMS crew.

The paramedic administers nebulized albuterol (2.5 mg/mL) over 15 minutes. She also leaves the patient's nasal cannula at 4 liters per minute. She encourages the patient to take deep breaths. Vital signs indicate a blood pressure of 162/94 mmHg and a pulse rate of 110 beats per minute.

When Mr. Casey is moved to the cot, his dyspnea increases and he becomes more anxious. Reassessment in the ambulance shows that his respiratory rate has increased to 36 and there has been no subjective change in his wheezing. The patient now only speaks in one- to two-word sentences, even though his oxygen saturation has increased to 90 percent. Mr. Casey appears to be growing tired from the work of breathing. The EMT establishes an IV and draws blood. The paramedic contemplates intubating the patient, but the prehospital DNR precludes intubation, so the paramedic is forced to continue pharmacological interventions only.

En route to the hospital, the paramedic administers a second albuterol treatment and continues to encourage Mr. Casey to take deep breaths. Through gentle reassurances, she succeeds in calming him down. During the next 5 minutes, the patient's respiratory rate drops to 30, his wheezes become louder, and tidal volume increases. The patient appears less anxious and the SpO_2 rises slowly to 93 percent.

On arrival at the hospital, the crew administers a third albuterol treatment. The respiratory rate is now 28 breaths per minute, and the patient can again speak in four- to five-word sentences. In the emergency department, the admitting physician gives the patient 125 mg of Solu-Medrol and one more treatment of albuterol. The patient also receives blood tests, chest X-rays, arterial blood gas, and a 12-lead ECG. He is released 5 hours later with a diagnosis of exacerbation of COPD, the acute condition that Mr. Casey treats in a home care setting.

The crew, meanwhile, carefully documents the run and drops off their chart. Luckily, they get a chance to eat dinner before the next call arrives.

INTRODUCTION

One of the major trends in modern health care involves the shifting of patients out of the hospital and back into their homes as soon as possible. The result has been a huge increase in home health care needs and services. In 1963, approximately 1,100 health care agencies existed in the United States. Today, more than 20,000 agencies employ more than 665,000 caregivers: nurses, home health aides, physical therapists, occupational therapists, and other health care professionals. Experts predict that the trend toward home health care will increase in the future. As a result, more and more patients will receive treatment—even of terminal illnesses—in an out-of-hospital setting.[1]

EPIDEMIOLOGY OF HOME CARE

A number of factors have promoted the growth of home care in recent years:

● Enactment of Medicare in 1965

● The advent of health maintenance organizations (HMOs) and patient-centered medical homes (PCMHs)

● Improved medical technology

● Studies showing improved recovery rates and lower costs with home care

Supporters of home health care offer several arguments in its favor. First, they point out that patients often recover faster in the familiar environment of their homes than in the hospital. They also emphasize differences in the cost of home care versus hospital care. With total health expenditures on the rise, the savings promised by home health care continue to speed the dismissal of patients from hospitals and nursing homes.

The shift to home care has important implications for paramedics.[2] As patients and their families assume greater responsibility for their own treatment and recovery, the likelihood of ALS intervention for the chronic care patient increases. Calls may come from the patient, the patient's family, or a home health care provider.

In home care settings, you can expect to encounter a sometimes dizzying array of devices, machines, medications, and equipment designed to provide anything from supportive to life-sustaining care. As a paramedic, you should become familiar with the basic functions of the common home care devices and, just as important, recognize the underlying need for them. The failure or malfunction of this type of equipment has the potential to become a life-threatening or life-altering event. New technologies and machines are being developed constantly. It is your responsibility to stay informed of these changes and the assessment complications that may be involved with the use of each device.

Patients Receiving Home Care

In 1992, the National Center for Health Statistics conducted its first annual National Home and Hospice Care Survey (NHHCS). The survey grew out of the proliferation of home care agencies throughout the United States. The results gave health care professionals their first in-depth look at the home health care population. Key findings from the survey included the following two points:

● Almost 75 percent of home care patients were age 65 or older.

● Of the elderly home care patients, almost two-thirds were female.

Today some 8 million patients—receiving both acute and chronic care—receive formal health care treatment from paid providers. Millions of others receive unpaid assistance from family members or other volunteers. On average, these informal caregivers give up to 4 hours of assistance per day, 7 days a week. The Balanced Budget Act of 1997 called for a marked

CONTENT REVIEW

▶ Common Reasons for ALS
Intervention

• Equipment failure
• Unexpected complications
• Absence of a caregiver
• Need for transport
• Inability to operate a device

reduction in home health expenditures by Medicare. This resulted in a significant reduction in persons receiving Medicare-funded home health care, and thousands of home health agencies folded nationwide. This reduction in the home health care system has put a tremendous load on EMS and is partially responsible for overcrowding of hospital emergency departments. Many EMS systems are now developing innovative programs to deal with this segment of the population.

Patients require home care for a variety of reasons. Some simply do not need to recover from an injury or illness in a hospital or a rehabilitation facility. Their home care is transitory and their conditions usually improve. Other patients have chronic conditions that require varying degrees of home assistance so the patients can live relatively normal lives. These patients usually adjust to their illnesses or disabilities, but never completely recover. Still other patients have terminal illnesses that may or may not involve complicated supportive measures. Their conditions are expected to worsen, and these patients may in fact be waiting to die.

All these situations require sensitivity to the special needs of the patient and consideration of the people involved in the patient's care. Strong emotions may emerge during the call. A previously manageable condition may have suddenly become unmanageable or more complicated. Unlike in a hospital, the patient or home care provider cannot push a button and summon immediate help. Instead, that person often summons you, the ALS provider.

ALS Response to Home Care Patients

A number of situations may involve you in the treatment of a home care patient: equipment failure, unexpected complications, absence of a caregiver, need for transport, inability of the patient or caregiver to operate a device, and more. As already mentioned, you might also be called on to provide emotional support or intervention. Taking responsibility for an illness or an ill family member can be a stressful and overwhelming experience. Some people may be ill equipped to deal with complicated directions, mechanical problems, or the stress of long-term care. Do not minimize their frustrations or allow these frustrations to interfere with your care.

Your primary role as a paramedic is to identify and treat any life-threatening problems. An important source of information is the home care provider, whether that person is a nurse, nurse's aide, family member, or friend. Remember that this person usually knows the patient better than anyone else. The provider will often spot subtle changes in the patient's condition that may seem insignificant to the outsider. In assessing the patient, it is crucial that you listen carefully to what this person says (Figure 8-1 ●).

Home care providers are often health care professionals, but be sensitive in questioning their training or background.

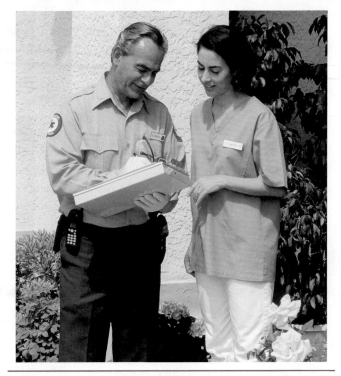

● **Figure 8-1** The home care provider usually knows the patient better than anyone else and will often spot subtle changes in the patient's condition.

LEGAL CONSIDERATIONS

Legal Considerations and the Home Care Patient

The line between home care and EMS is becoming increasingly fine. More and more people are cared for in a home setting, and the EMS system is the safety net when a home care patient deteriorates. Numerous legal considerations must be made when dealing with home care patients, especially those who are terminally ill. Various patient self-determination acts have made the terms living will, durable power of attorney for health care, do not resuscitate order, *and* Uniform Anatomical Gift Act *a part of our vocabulary. These documents often come into play when dealing with a home health care patient or hospice patient. Because of this, it is essential for EMS personnel to understand the intricacies of these documents and any applicable state and local regulations that may apply.*

You must obtain certain information to care for your patient, and the home care provider may be the only source you have for critical items such as the patient's baseline mental status. If you meet resistance, either from the home care provider's lack of training or from a misunderstanding of your needs, try rephrasing your question or using less technical language. You may also find evidence of neglect or improper patient care by the home care provider. Correct any immediate life threats that you find and document your findings in your patient report. You should also report the situation to your supervisors for corrective action. However, do not confront the home care worker yourself.

At all times, keep in mind the presence of the patient. Involve him in the questioning process. If the caregiver mentions a change or reaction, you might say: "Did you notice this change, too?" "How do you think you reacted?" Your role is to perform as complete and accurate an assessment as possible.

Typical Responses

Many of the medical problems that you will encounter in a home care setting are the same as the ones that you will encounter elsewhere in the field. However, you must always keep in mind that the home care patient is in a more fragile state to begin with. A member of the medical community has already decided that the person needs extra help. A home care patient is likely to decompensate and go into crisis more quickly than members of the general population. As a result, you need to monitor the home care patient carefully and be ready to intervene at all times. Some of the typical responses involve airway complications, respiratory failure, cardiac decompensation, alterations in peripheral circulation, altered mental status, GI/GU crises, infections and/or septic complications, and equipment malfunction. (For more specific information on examples of home care problems requiring acute intervention, see later sections of the chapter.)

Airway Complications   The airway is always your paramount concern, and the home care patient is no exception. In the absence of documentation proving the patient's request to withhold intubation and mechanical ventilation, you should protect the airway at all costs. However, even if the patient has a valid DNR order, remember that, in certain situations, you still can use basic airway techniques and suctioning to protect the airway.

Airway compromise can be the result of many different etiologies. Problems that you might encounter include inadequate pulmonary toilet, inadequate alveolar ventilation, and inadequate alveolar oxygenation. (For more on airway problems, see material later in the chapter.)

Respiratory Failure   As you will read later in the chapter, any number of respiratory problems can be treated in a home care setting. Some of the most common conditions that will lead to respiratory failure or acute crisis include:

- Emphysema
- Bronchitis
- Asthma
- Cystic fibrosis
- Congestive heart failure
- Pulmonary embolus
- Sleep apnea
- **Guillain-Barré syndrome**
- **Myasthenia gravis**

Cardiac Decompensation   Regardless of the setting, cardiac decompensation is a true medical emergency that can lead to life-threatening shock. This condition requires aggressive identification and treatment. Home care patients who have borderline cardiac output may be placed at risk if their cardiac

demand increases from stress or illness and their system cannot compensate. Some other common causes of cardiac decompensation include:

- Congestive heart failure
- Acute myocardial infarction (MI) (Home care patients are at higher risk.)
- Cardiac **hypertrophy**
- Calcification or degeneration of the heart's conductive system
- Heart transplant
- Sepsis

Alterations in Peripheral Circulation   You already know that the heart circulates blood throughout the body. However, in the case of home care patients, remember that bodily movement also aids in circulation. If a patient has limited mobility, expect the entire circulatory system to be less effective and weaker. As muscle tone declines, so does the flow of blood. When circulation slows, movement becomes more difficult, thus creating a vicious cycle that leads to poorer circulation overall.

Keep in mind that alterations in peripheral circulation can complicate or worsen the course of treatment for a home care patient. Slowed circulation may result in delayed healing, increased risk of infections, or even **gangrene**. Diabetes, a problem that affects some 16 million Americans, commonly results in poor circulation, especially to the extremities. These patients are at high risk of unhealed wounds or ulcers, particularly on the feet.

Altered Mental Status   A common ALS response to a home care patient involves some kind of subtle or obvious change in mental status. In the home care patient, always suspect an exacerbation of the condition as well as other causes. Never forget that these patients are at higher risk than the general population of developing new medical problems. Some common causes of altered mental status include:

- Hypoxia (from any number of respiratory or airway problems)
- Hypotension (from any number of cardiac problems or shock)
- Sepsis
- Altered electrolytes or blood chemistries (common in dialysis patients)
- Hypoglycemia (diabetes)
- Alzheimer's disease
- Cancerous tumor or brain lesions
- Overdose
- Stroke (brain attack)

GI/GU Crises   EMS personnel find themselves involved in a number of calls involving home care patients with gastrointestinal or genitourinary problems. The problem often revolves around a misplaced or removed catheter, such as a Foley catheter or a percutaneous endoscopic gastrostomy (PEG) tube. This may not seem like an emergency to you, but the inability to eat or urinate for a period of time can easily compromise an already weakened patient. In addition, home interventions such as peritoneal dialysis can alter fluid balances or electrolytes, creating a subtle but life-threatening problem.

Infections and Septic Complications You should always maintain a high index of suspicion for infection in a home care patient with a decreased immune response, either from poor general health or a specific disease. Be particularly alert to infections in patients with indwelling devices such as gastrostomy tubes, peripherally inserted central catheter (PICC) lines, Foley catheters, or colostomies. Also remember that patients with limited lung function or tracheotomies cannot clear their airways easily, putting them at a higher risk of lung infections.

Patients who have decreased **sensorium** from a variety of conditions may have wounds and ulcers that they are unaware of, especially if they have been bedridden or inactive for long periods of time. Surgically implanted drains or wound closures may become infected without the patient realizing it. A bedbound patient may also develop decubitus wounds, pressure sores, or bedsores (Figure 8-2 ●). If these problems are not identified or treated, they can progress from a generalized infection to gangrene and sepsis.

In identifying infections, look for the following general signs:

- Redness and/or swelling, especially at the insertion site of an indwelling device
- Purulent discharge at the insertion site
- Warm skin at the insertion site
- Fever

Infection at the cellular level is called **cellulitis** and is not life threatening. When an infection spreads systemically, however, it can lead to sepsis—a serious medical emergency. This may cause a patient's immune system to fail, resulting in septic shock. Signs and symptoms of sepsis include:

- Redness at an insertion site
- Fever
- Altered mental status
- Poor skin color or **turgor**
- Signs of shock
- Vomiting
- Diarrhea

Keep in mind that home care patients may already be receiving treatment for a generalized infection that has in fact

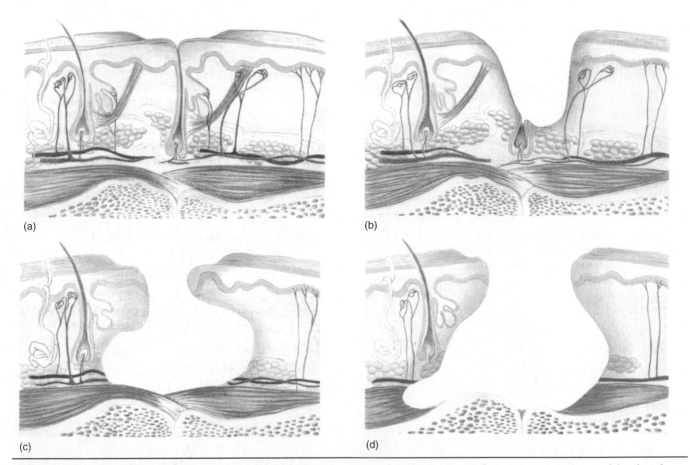

(a)

(b)

(c)

(d)

● **Figure 8-2** Pressure sores are classified by the depth of tissue destruction. (a) **Stage 1** Inflammation or redness of the skin that does not return to normal after 15 minutes of removal of pressure. Edema is present. It involves the epidermis. Skin may or may not be broken. (b) **Stage 2** Skin blister or shallow skin ulcer. Involves the epidermis. Looks like a shallow crater. Area is red, warm, and may or may not have drainage. (c) **Stage 3** Full-thickness skin loss exposing subcutaneous tissue, may extend into the next layer. Edema, inflammation, and necrosis present. Drainage is present, which may or may not have an odor. (d) **Stage 4** Full-thickness ulcer. Muscle and/or bone can be seen. Infection and necrosis are present. Drainage is present, which may or may not have an odor.

worsened or spread. Inquire whether a pattern of deterioration has been seen by the caregiver or home care provider. In cases of septic shock, ALS treatment is mainly supportive. Provide fluid for hypotension and necessary airway and oxygen support.

Equipment Malfunction   Home care equipment has the normal limitations of any machine. The power may go out and stop the machine from functioning. The machine may break and/or need maintenance. Some machines, if inoperative, can create a life threat to a patient. Common examples include home ventilators, oxygen delivery systems, apnea monitors, and home dialysis machines.

In cases of equipment malfunction, you may be called on to take the place of a device (such as a ventilator) or to treat problems that have arisen as a result of the malfunction. Even the malfunction of a glucometer can be a difficult situation for some diabetic patients to handle, especially if they suspect hypoglycemia. Your job is to assess the problem and take the appropriate actions.

Other Medical Disorders and Home Care Patients   As already mentioned, you can expect to find a wide variety of problems treated in the home care setting. They can range from an infant on an apnea monitor to progressive dementia in a family member to psychosocial support of the family of a home care patient. Some other conditions that may be treated at home include:

- Brain or spinal trauma
- Arthritis
- Psychological disorders
- Cancer
- Hepatitis
- AIDS
- Transplants (including patients awaiting transplants)

Commonly Found Medical Devices

As previously mentioned, home care patients use a vast number of devices (Figure 8-3 ●). They range from the simplicity of a nasal cannula to the complexity of a home ventilator. If you encounter an unfamiliar device, which may happen at some time in your career, don't panic. Find out what it is used for, and you will then have an idea on how to proceed. Don't be afraid to look foolish by asking questions. You won't. You will be foolish, and endanger the patient, if you pretend to understand a device, but actually do not. Some commonly used devices include:

- Glucometers
- IV infusions and indwelling IV sites
- Nebulized and aerosolized medication administrators
- Shunts, fistulas, and venous grafts

- Oxygen concentrators, oxygen tanks, and liquid oxygen systems
- Oxygen masks and nebulizers
- Tracheostomies and home ventilators
- G-tubes, colostomies, and urostomies
- Surgical drains
- Apnea monitors, cardiac monitors, and pulse oximeters
- Wheelchairs, canes, and walkers

Spend some time at the hospital talking with health care personnel about new devices being introduced for the home care setting. Study or make copies of the brochures that come with these devices. You might also talk with manufacturers or vendors, the people who commonly deliver equipment to home care patients.

Intervention by a Home Health Care Practitioner or Physician

Most calls involving home care patients will require acute intervention in problems such as inadequate respiratory support, acute respiratory events, acute cardiac events, acute sepsis, or GI/GU crises. Keep in mind, however, that you may not be the first person to provide intervention. If home care patients have a good relationship with their home health care practitioner or physician, they may contact this person first. In fact, they may be required to do so in order to receive reimbursement for medical services.

On any call involving a home care patient, be sure to ask whether a patient has called another health care professional. If so, find out what instructions or medications have been issued. Also inquire about written orders from the physician or the physician-approved health care plan. Health care agencies resubmit these plans to physicians at least every 62 days. So check the date to see when the plan was last revised.

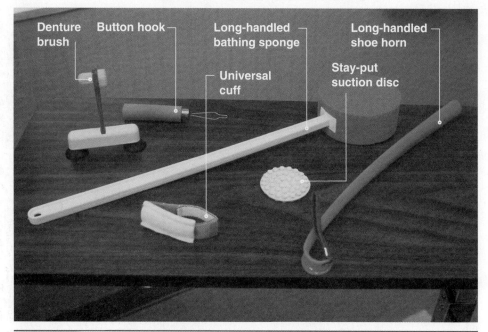

● **Figure 8-3**   EMS personnel must become familiar with the common medical devices that they may encounter when providing interventions for the chronic care patient.

In some cases, you may be called to a home care setting in which a home health practitioner or physician must intervene—that is, the scope of the treatment required is beyond your training. In such cases, your role will be mainly supportive. Examples of such conditions include:

- Chemotherapy
- Pain management
- **Hospice** care

Remain especially alert to home care patients receiving medications for pain management. They are at risk for pharmacological side effects and possible overdose. The patient may also be taking nonprescription drugs that could interact with prescribed medications. Substance abuse, especially in critically ill patients, is also a possibility.

Hospice patients have unique psychological needs due to the terminal nature of their illnesses. Although they and their families will have been counseled about the disease process, emotional support is still part of your job. If a call involves a hospice patient, the situation will almost always require intervention by specially trained health care professionals. Find out the names of these people as quickly as possible and determine the advisability of consultation versus rapid transport. (For more on hospice care, see the closing sections of this chapter.)

Injury Control and Prevention

As has been mentioned in Volume 5, the most effective intervention is prevention. Care of the patient begins even before he returns to the home. Some or all of the steps listed in Table 8–1 and Table 8–2 should be taken, depending on the patient's condition. You should also keep in mind a matrix, or strategy, for

TABLE 8–1 | Preparing the Home for Patient Care	
Room	**Strategies**
Bathroom	• Purchase a shower chair and/or tub seat. • Install grab bars. • Install a raised toilet seat. • Hang mirrors, shelves, and racks at wheelchair level. • Set water temperature at a safe level (no higher than 120°F/48.8°C).
Kitchen	• Install easy-to-reach stove dials, countertops, and storage areas. • Provide an easy-to-reach fire extinguisher. • Keep floors dry and nonslippery.
Living Room	• Arrange furniture for free access. • Provide sturdy seating at a suitable height.
Bedroom	• Install a telephone next to the bed. • Obtain a hospital-type bed. • Keep a nightlight or flashlight near the bed. • Keep a bedpan or commode chair within patient reach.
General	• Install smoke alarms. • Provide adequate heating and air conditioning. • Provide good lighting. • Remove all hazards to mobility—throw rugs, electrical wires, etc. • Install wheelchair ramps into house and over doorsills. • Secure all banisters and railings. • Provide a mobile phone.

TABLE 8–2 | Injury Control and Prevention	
Organize for Out-of-Hospital Care	• Find out about the patient's condition—length of time for recovery, possible impairments or limitations, prospects for recovery, prescribed treatment plan, frequency of checkups, and possible side effects of medications. • Determine available health care agencies, including home-to-hospital transportation services. • Prepare the home for patient care (Table 8–1). • Rent or purchase appropriate equipment and learn how it operates. • Arrange for help—Meals on Wheels, visiting nurses, adult day care, and so on.
Provide Proper Bed Care	• Apply restraints—safety vests, safety belts, limb holders, or mitts—as necessary. • Assist in elimination (and safe disposal of wastes). • Encourage exercise. • Look for bedsores or other infections.
Prepare for Emergencies	• Establish a patient baseline. • Learn the danger signs for the patient's particular condition. • Keep a list of emergency numbers at each phone (or program mobile or cell phones). • Notify fire and rescue squads of the patient's condition or special needs. • Obtain necessary Medic Alert identification. • Obtain a Vial of Life and post a decal on the refrigerator door.

injury prevention developed by William Haddon in 1972. His 10 steps to injury prevention are essential to all aspects of emergency medicine:

1. Prevent the creation of hazard to begin with.
2. Reduce the amount of the hazard brought into existence.
3. Prevent the release of the hazard that already exists.
4. Modify the rate of distribution of the hazard from the source.
5. Separate the hazard and that which is to be protected in both time and space.
6. Separate the hazard and that which is to be protected by a barrier.
7. Modify the basic qualities of the hazard.
8. Make that which is to be protected more resistant to the hazard.
9. Counter the damage already done by the hazard.
10. Stabilize, repair, and rehabilitate the object of the damage.

These 10 steps can be used to protect paramedics from the hazards they encounter in the workplace or to protect patients from injuries at home. The steps can be seen in such simple areas as Standard Precautions, the use of side rails to prevent falls, or the use of home rehabilitation to stabilize or repair a patient's injuries.

GENERAL SYSTEM PATHOPHYSIOLOGY, ASSESSMENT, AND MANAGEMENT

Assessment and management of home care patients can be challenging. You can gain confidence by becoming familiar with the pathophysiology of the diseases most commonly found in home care settings. You must also keep in mind the emotional needs of both the home care patient and the caregivers or family members affected by the patient's condition. Some caregivers love what they do and treat the patient's condition as part of their daily lives. Other households feel constant, unremitting stress, and possibly resentment toward the patient's condition.

Getting a feel for the emotional context of a patient's care should be a part of any call. However, in the case of home care patients, you must exhibit extra sensitivity. The way in which you interact with the patient and family can greatly affect the ease and efficiency with which you assess the patient and gather information. Developing a consistent, comprehensive approach to patient assessment and treatment can be your best strategy for dealing with these sometimes complicated responses. The one thing home care calls have in common is their diversity. Be prepared to draw on all your EMS skills and to think quickly as you figure out the most effective management plan.

Assessment

Assessment of the home care patient follows the same basic steps as any other patient: scene size-up, primary assessment, secondary assessment, reassessment, and continued management.

However, you will need to modify your mind-set for the home care patient—that is, observe for conditions that you might not ordinarily look for in the general population. This section highlights some of the points you should keep in mind or emphasize when assessing the home care patient. (For more on assessment, see Volume 3.)

Scene Size-Up

As with any call, your assessment of the scene begins before you get out of your vehicle. In the case of home care patients, note any special equipment you may observe on entering the home. This will alert you to any possible chronic problems that the patient might have. As you approach the scene, keep the following questions in mind:

- Is there a wheelchair ramp next to the front steps?
- Is oxygen equipment in view?
- Does a trail of oxygen tubing lead into the patient's bedroom?
- Are there infection control supplies on the counter?
- Is there a sharps container present? (This means there are sharps too!)
- Is the patient in a hospital bed?

Introduce yourself to any other medical personnel on the scene—nurse, aide, hospice worker, and so on. By making personal contact, you will help create a health care team that can pool resources and share information. It is a serious mistake to arrive on the scene with a "takeover" mentality that all but eliminates the home care provider from the assessment process.

Scene Safety After you have identified the scene as a home care situation, remain alert for special hazards that might be present. As mentioned earlier, emotions often run high in a home care situation. Evaluate whether any of the people present have a threatening attitude that could be directed toward you. If at any time you don't feel comfortable, withdraw and seek assistance, either from the police or additional personnel. Ask someone to put any pets in another room and have all sources of sound (TV, radio, and so on) turned off so you can work in a quiet, focused environment. As in any patient's home, look for weapons that the patient might use for self-defense, such as firearms, knives, or chemical sprays.

Other special hazards that you may face in a home care situation include infectious wastes, medical supplies such as needles, and potentially dangerous equipment. You would hope that all home care providers would be meticulous with the safe disposal of sharps. However, don't take it for granted. You cannot help any patients if you are on disability because you contracted hepatitis or AIDS from a needlestick. Look around carefully.

In responding to any home care situation, keep in mind the following guidelines:

- Any patient with limited movement may be contaminated with feces, urine, or **emesis**.
- Any bedbound patient may have weeping wounds, bleeding, or decubitus ulcers (bedsores).

- Sharps may be present.
- Collection bags for urine or feces sometimes leak.
- Tracheostomy patients clear mucus by coughing, which can spray.
- Any electrical machine has the potential for electric shock.
- A hospital bed, wheelchair, or walker could be contaminated with body fluid.
- Contaminated medical devices, such as a nebulizer, may be left around unprotected.
- Oxygen in the presence of flame has the potential for fire or explosion.
- Equipment may be in the way and cause you to fall, or it may be unstable and fall on you.
- Medical wastes may not be properly contained or discarded.

Do not minimize the impact of any of these hazards. You can always be contaminated by any patient, but treatment of the home care patient has the potential for a broader range of exposures. Be sure to remove any medical waste you generate so the patient does not return to an unsafe environment. If at all possible, you should also remove any medical waste that is already there for the same reason. Always use Standard Precautions and be careful!

Patient Milieu   Another important part of the scene size-up involves an evaluation of the patient's environment. Is the house clean or dirty? Is nutritious food available? Are the sanitary facilities clean? Is the house heated and/or air conditioned? Is there adequate electricity? Is there insect or vermin infestation? The answers to such questions obviously have an impact on the patient's health and ability to recover.

Also note the condition of the patient's specific medical devices. For example, is the nasal cannula clean? Is the wheelchair in good working order? Is the ventilator well situated for safety and effectiveness? Again, these observations provide important clues to the quality of the home care received by the patient and the ability or willingness of the patient to comply with a prescribed treatment regimen.

Remember that you not only have a responsibility to treat the patient, but to act as an advocate. If a patient is living in a hazardous or unhealthy environment, you have an obligation to notify the proper agency to ensure that the person receives the necessary help. Often hospital social services will be of assistance. The patient's home care agency or the police might also intervene, depending on the situation.

Remain alert to signs of abuse and/or neglect. In many states, you are required by law to report signs of child or elder abuse. (See Chapters 4, 5, and 6.) Know the laws that pertain to the practice of EMS in your state. Home care patients, whether old or young, may be helpless to improve their situations. It is the responsibility of all health care workers to look out for their safety and well-being.

Primary and Secondary Assessments

At this point in your assessment, you may already have a good base of information without actually having seen the patient! As you approach the patient, begin your primary assessment by observing the patient's general appearance, skin color and quality, quality of respiration, and level of distress. Also note any medical equipment that the patient may be currently using.

As you continue to assess the patient for the ABCs, try to ascertain from the primary care provider (if present) a baseline presentation for the patient. Were you called because an existing condition has gotten worse? Or are you here for a new problem? For some home care patients, respiratory distress may be a chronic condition. For example, a patient with chronic obstructive pulmonary disease (COPD) might always have difficulty breathing. Your first impulse may be to reach for your airway supplies only to find that this is the patient's norm and that you were called to treat an unrelated problem. You must be flexible in your judgments and listen carefully to the report provided by the caregiver or family member who summoned EMS.

As with any patient, treat it as you see it! Once you have established the patient's baseline, assess for changes from the norm. Airway and breathing are always your first concern, followed by circulation. If there are any serious threats to the ABCs, you must treat them. If you are unable to stabilize the patient, complete your rapid assessment and transport immediately. In such cases, your secondary assessment and reassessment will be performed en route to the hospital, if possible.

In noncritical patients, you might take the opportunity to compare vital signs with the bedside records, if they are kept. The focus of your exam should be on the chief complaint and how it might relate to the patient's chronic condition. Be meticulous in your exam, especially with the home care patient. As stated earlier, home care patients are more susceptible to complications than most other patients and can deteriorate rapidly—that is, a noncritical patient can quickly become a critical patient.

In examining a home care patient, be sure to inspect, palpate, and auscultate all potential problem areas. In bedbound patients, look for decubiti (pressure sores or bedsores) on parts of the body subjected to constant pressure or friction. As mentioned, decubiti pose a significant danger to the patient through infection or sepsis and may require surgical debridement.

Mental Status   If your patient has a preexisting altered mental status, such as dementia or Alzheimer's disease, you must have a good understanding of his normal mentation before transport. This information is vital to the physician evaluating and treating the patient at the receiving facility. As stressed in Chapter 5, depression can mimic senility and senility can mimic organic brain syndrome. Dementia can also be a sign or symptom of a number of other serious medical problems, such as hypoglycemia and AIDS.

In general, assessment of mental status follows the same general procedure as with other patients. However, you must tailor your questions to the home care setting (Figure 8-4 ●). For example, a person who does not work may be oriented but not know the date or even the day of the week. Also keep in mind the high level of stress in many home care situations and the effect this may have on patient confusion.

To avoid insulting the patient with what may appear to be childlike questions, preface your assessment by saying, "Since I don't know your condition very well, I need to ask you some very basic questions." If patients understand that you are

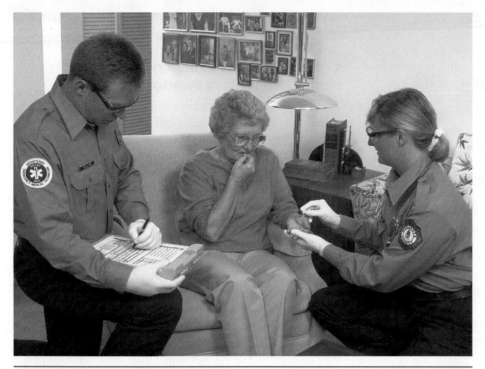

● **Figure 8-4** When assessing a chronic care patient, tailor your questions to the home care setting. Remember that the stress in many home care settings, or fear of removal from the home, can increase patient confusion.

following a systematic assessment, they usually cooperate in what, for them, is often a tedious process.

If a patient cannot or will not answer questions, rely on family members or health care providers to explain why the patient's current mental status is a departure from the norm. For example, belligerent behavior might be normal for a home care patient. If this is the case, find out what is different this time than other times. Perhaps, as pointed out earlier, nothing may be different—the family member or caregiver may have just reached the breaking point and is in need of outside assistance.

Remember that home care patients, especially older or terminal patients, are fearful of being removed from the home environment. This can trigger depression, which in turn worsens a preexisting altered mental status. The key in such cases is tactful questioning combined with your own powers of observation. Pay particular attention to body language and interactions between household members. Note any evidence that the altered mental condition may have been triggered or worsened by a treatable cause and present this information as part of your secondary assessment.

Other Considerations In preparing your history, take into account any long-term medical problems (i.e., the conditions that necessitated home care) and the specific events that led to the current crisis. Use the home health history and written orders from the physician, if available. The patient or family may have a discharge sheet with valuable information. As mentioned, talk to the health care provider and to the patient. What changes, if any, have taken place in the patient's life in the recent past? Has patient treatment and/or compliance changed? Are medical devices operating correctly?

Keep in mind that eating habits, fluid intake, and minor illnesses or injuries can have a dramatic effect on a seriously ill homebound patient. Have a high index of suspicion for any new conditions that the patient may be developing. For example, evidence of dementia in an AIDS patient is a serious sign. Correlate this with your physical exam and use this information in developing your treatment plan.

In the case of home care patients, you may more commonly encounter DNR orders, Do Not Attempt Resuscitation (DNAR) orders, living wills, and so on. Ascertain whether these documents are in place before beginning any lifesaving treatments. If that information is unavailable, act in the best interests of the patient. Also, keep in mind that a DNR or DNAR does not mean that you have to withhold *all* treatment. For example, if a congestive heart failure (CHF) patient with crackles and shortness of breath has a DNR, you may still be able to start a line, give nitroglycerin, administer an IV diuretic, and/or transport the patient to the hospital. However, you must read the specific instructions contained within the advance directives and consult with medical control.

Advance directives are designed to prevent unwanted treatment and invasion to the body when natural death or dying occurs. However, many people who have advance directives can be treated in crisis situations and recover. You must use your judgment on a case-by-case basis to determine what qualifies as a resuscitative or life-sustaining measure. (Additional material on advance directives appears later in the chapter.)

Transport and Management Treatment Plan

Transport and/or treatment of a home care patient often involves replacing home health treatment modalities with ALS modalities. Airway and ventilatory support should be straightforward, because EMS providers are usually equipped and trained in the use of most necessary supplies. Some home care interventions, such as Foley catheters, can simply be brought along with the patient. Other interventions, such as PEG tubes, must be flushed and capped, which you may not be trained or equipped to do. In this case, the home care provider should assist you.

In some instances, you may be forced to take the support mechanism on your ambulance if you cannot find a suitable replacement. Certain infusion pumps or other devices may be essential to the patient's well-being and you must bring them along. You should critically assess the risks of discontinuing the home care intervention versus transporting the mechanism. Seek advice from your base physician if you are unfamiliar with the intervention and if the home health provider is unable to help.

CONTENT REVIEW

► Common Acute Home Care
Situations

• Respiratory disorders
• Cardiac problems
• Use of VADs
• GI/GU disorders
• Acute infections

When taking a home care patient to a receiving facility, be sure to notify family members and caregivers, if they are not present. Before leaving the scene, secure the home, making sure that doors and windows are locked. In all likelihood, you will need to notify the patient's physician and/or the appropriate health care agency, if you have not already done so.

Document your findings and all care steps carefully. Your run report will become part of the home care patient's record and may, in fact, suggest modifications to the treatment plan. If the patient is not already using a home care agency, provide names of services in your community or refer the person to the proper social service agency. You might also mention nonmedical attendant care, such as housekeeping services and Meals on Wheels. As mentioned earlier, if you suspect the need for intervention in patient care, report your suspicions to the appropriate agency.

SPECIFIC ACUTE HOME HEALTH SITUATIONS

Although you will undoubtedly intervene in a wide variety of home care situations during your EMS career, you can expect to encounter certain conditions more commonly than others. The chronic care patients that will most likely require acute ALS intervention include those with respiratory disorders, cardiac problems, vascular access devices (VADs), GI/GU disorders, and acute infections. You may also be called on to intervene in the home care of mothers and their newborn infants and to provide assistance in hospice settings. A discussion of each of these situations will help you to prepare for your increasing involvement in the home health care system of the twenty-first century.

Respiratory Disorders

Respiratory disorders account for more than 630,000 of the hospital patients discharged for home care each year. Nearly 37 percent of patients with simple pneumonia and pleurisy and more than 50 percent of patients with COPD often receive home care within one day of their discharge from the hospital.

Some of the most common home care devices used to treat respiratory disorders include oxygen equipment, portable suctioning machines, aerosol equipment and nebulizers, incentive spirometers, various home ventilators, and tracheostomy tubes and collars. To provide intervention with these devices, you need to review pertinent respiratory anatomy and physiology as it relates to home oxygen and respiratory therapy. (See Volume 4, Chapter 1.) You also need to review the pathophysiology of the disorders that most frequently require home respiratory support.

Select respiratory disorders and the medical therapy used to treat them are discussed in the following sections. As you read this material, keep in mind earlier comments on the increased risk of airway infections and respiratory compromise in the home care patient.

Chronic Diseases Requiring Home Respiratory Support

Many home care patients have a lung capacity that is minimally able to meet their normal requirements. Sometimes even simple activities, such as climbing stairs, can severely stress their systems. Unlike patients with normal lung capacities, they simply do not have the ability for any increased workload. Even walking from one room to another may require use of oxygen equipment. The following is a review of some of the conditions you may find in the respiratory compromised patient.

COPD   As you know, COPD is a triad of diseases: emphysema, chronic bronchitis, and asthma. Some patients may have one, two, or all three disorders. All three are outflow obstructive diseases, impeding the exhalation of air from the lungs. This causes an increase in carbon dioxide and a decrease in oxygenation.

COPD patients work harder to breathe than healthy people, and they tire quickly. If home equipment fails for any reason, they often panic, thereby worsening their situation. As with any COPD patient, direct your treatment toward increasing oxygen flow. Be prepared to take over their breathing as soon as patients can no longer move enough oxygen to sustain themselves. In some cases, this may mean fixing or replacing home respiratory equipment and/or transport to the hospital (Figure 8-5 ●).

In treating the COPD patient, keep in mind the following disease-specific information.

Bronchitis and Emphysema These two diseases go hand in hand. Most often they result from smoking, but can have other causes as well. Bronchitis involves the chronic overproduction of mucus, which narrows bronchial passages and restricts air flow. Emphysema typically leads to a stiffening and enlargement of the alveoli. This loss of elasticity and compliance requires higher pressures in the lungs to facilitate gas exchanges at the alveolar level. Usually these patients are thin (because breathing takes up a large portion of their daily caloric intake) and barrel chested (due to the retention of air in the lungs as a result of outflow obstruction).

In cases of acute exacerbation, these patients have a difficult time compensating. They may exhibit wheezing with diminished lung sounds, use of accessory muscles, retractions, tripod positioning, and the inability to speak in full sentences. Home treatments that you may see include oxygen, nebulized or aerosol medications, and possibly a ventilator using positive end-expiratory pressure (PEEP), continuous positive airway pressure (CPAP), or bilevel positive airway pressure (BiPAP). PEEP is provided through an endotracheal tube, whereas CPAP and BiPAP are provided through a tightly fitted mask.

When providing intervention, do not forget that home care patients usually have a high dosing regimen, which may make them less responsive to their medications. Always provide these patients with high-concentration oxygen. Medications that may be helpful include:

● Nebulized beta$_2$-specific agonist bronchodilators, such as albuterol or metaproterenol

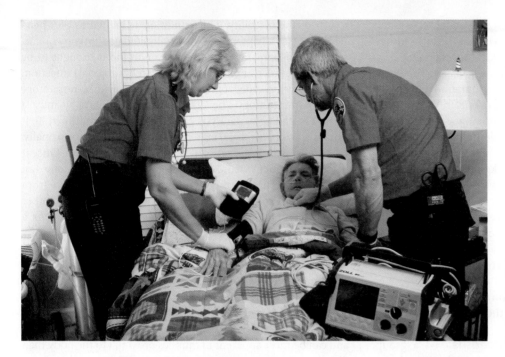

CONTENT REVIEW

► Common Home Respiratory Equipment

- Oxygen equipment
- Portable suctioning machines
- Aerosol equipment and nebulizers
- Incentive spirometers
- Home ventilators
- Tracheostomy tubes and collars

● **Figure 8-5**   If the home equipment for a COPD patient fails or is insufficient, you may have to replace it with equipment from the ALS unit.

- IV or oral corticosteroids, such as methylprednisolone (Solu-Medrol)

- Nebulized anticholinergics (ipratropium)

Asthma   Asthma, sometimes referred to as *reactive airway disease*, can be seen with patients of any age. A crisis often occurs when some reactant causes an acute constriction of the bronchial passages. Home care patients with asthma can usually handle these episodes on their own. If the episode becomes severe, however, you may be called by a caregiver or parent. (Asthma in children can be especially stressful for the family, so be sure to review its treatment in Chapter 4.)

With asthmatic patients, look for wheezing with diminished lung sounds, use of accessory muscles, and the inability to speak in full sentences. Head bobbing in children is an ominous sign of impending respiratory failure.

Home treatments you may see include oxygen, oral medications, and a variety of nebulizers and/or inhalers. In providing support, always administer high-concentration oxygen. Medications that may be helpful include the same ones used to treat bronchitis and emphysema. You may also consider epinephrine IV or SQ. However, use this medication with caution when treating the elderly or very weak patients.

Long-term care of asthma involves the avoidance or elimination of reactants that can trigger the problem. Try to gather as much information as possible about the cause of the attack so that the physician and patient can take action to avoid future episodes.

Congestive Heart Failure (CHF)   CHF often presents as a respiratory problem. For more information on this condition, see "Cardiac Problems" in Volume 4, Chapter 2.

Cystic Fibrosis (CF)   Cystic fibrosis is a genetic disorder usually identified during childhood, sometimes in the late teenage years. It is characterized by chronic and copious overproduction of mucus, inflammation of the small airways and hyperinflation of the alveoli, chronic infections, and erosion of the pulmonary blood vessels secondary to infection. CF is an **exocrine** disease that causes other systemic problems, such as GI disturbances, pancreatic disorders, and glucose intolerance.

Treatment of CF typically involves frequent postural drainage of mucus and chest percussion. Some patients may use mechanical vibrators to facilitate the percussions. They usually take medications aimed at mucus reduction and control of bacterial infection.

CF can be regarded as a terminal disease. Few patients live to the age of 40. Take this fact into account when treating the patient. At all times, remain sensitive to the emotional state of both the patient and any members of the family who may be present.

You may be summoned to help a patient with CF for a variety of reasons. The vigorous coughing associated with the disease can result in **hemoptysis** and pneumothorax. Severe or fatal pulmonary hemorrhage can occur at any time. Patients can also suffer **cor pulmonale**, or right ventricular hypertrophy secondary to pulmonary hypertension.

In treating a patient with CF, ascertain the stage of the disease and inquire about any standing medical orders. Also find out if the patient or family has initiated any advance directives. Your treatment will flow from this information and your own assessment. There is no specific in-field treatment for acute problems stemming from CF. As a general rule, you will provide respiratory support, ventilation, and intubation, if indicated. Be sure to counsel the family or summon the proper counselor to do so, especially if the patient is in the terminal stage of the disease.

Bronchopulmonary Dysplasia (BPD)   This disease affects primarily infants of low birth weight. It is characterized by an ongoing need for mechanical ventilation in newborns who have been treated for respiratory distress of any cause. These infants may simply fail to wean from mandatory ventilation or from O_2. They are also at increased risk of lower respiratory tract infections, especially viral infections, and may require immediate hospitalization if signs of respiratory infection or increased distress develop.

Home care providers will have been advised to wean infants to lower **intermittent mandatory ventilation (IMV)** settings. However, if the process occurs too quickly, the infant may be at risk of becoming hypoxemic. Arterial oxygenation should be maintained at or above 88 to 90 percent saturation and should be monitored continuously with a pulse oximeter.

Keep in mind that pulmonary congestion and edema may develop in infants with BPD if excessive fluids have been administered. Question caregivers about fluid intake, which may need to be restricted to about 120 mL/kg per day. Inquire, too, about the use of diuretic therapy, which is sometimes prescribed to these patients.

Even after an infant is weaned from a ventilator, supplemental oxygen may still be required for weeks or even months. In such cases, it is usually delivered by nasal cannula.

Remember that BPD is a serious condition in infants. Reduced lung compliance and increased airway resistance may persist for several years. The best treatment is adequate ventilatory support and prompt transport to the nearest neonatal unit.

Neuromuscular Degenerative Diseases As a group, these diseases affect respiratory action through degeneration of the muscles used for breathing. Patients who suffer from neuromuscular degeneration may at some point require respiratory support. Other problems, particularly an inability to ambulate, will have a huge impact on the patient's life.

Many patients with neuromuscular degenerative diseases will be cared for by family members. However, if the condition worsens, professional home care providers may be involved and ALS may be summoned. In cases of respiratory compromise, there is little that you can do other than provide airway and respiratory support and transport. Expect to see all manner of respiratory home care devices, including oxygen and ventilators.

In treating and transporting these patients, keep in mind the following information on the leading neuromuscular degenerative diseases.

Muscular Dystrophy This genetically inherited disorder causes a defect in the intracellular metabolism of muscle cells. (For more details, see Chapter 7.) The condition leads to degeneration and atrophy of muscles, which are eventually replaced by fatty and connective tissue. There is no cure as yet, and treatment is multidisciplinary because of the many muscle systems involved. These patients have difficulty moving and may need assistance with daily tasks. ALS involvement would almost certainly be for respiratory failure or accidental injuries, usually related to falls.

Poliomyelitis Poliomyelitis is an infectious disease rarely seen today because of effective vaccines. (For more details, see Chapter 7.) When it does occur, the disease causes destruction of motor neurons, leading to muscular atrophy, muscle weakness, and paralysis. Patients have difficulty ambulating. However, unless respiratory muscles are involved, there may be no systemic effects. Children who contract the disease may suffer permanent crippling or deformity. But once the disease is resolved, further degeneration will cease.

After polio patients recover normal functioning, they sometimes experience a **demyelination** of affected neurons and a

return of the disability. This condition is known as *post-polio syndrome* (see Chapter 7). Its pathophysiology is unknown.

Guillain-Barré Syndrome This syndrome is thought to be an autoimmune response to a viral (rarely bacterial) infection. It is usually preceded by a febrile episode with a respiratory and/or GI infection. The disease is characterized by muscle weakness leading to paralysis caused by nerve demyelination. It usually starts in the distal extremities and progresses proximally.

Progression of this disorder may take several days. Once it reaches the patient's trunk, respiratory involvement becomes an obvious concern. One way to differentiate Guillain-Barré from a spinal injury is the increased motor involvement. In other words, motor deficits are greater than sensory deficits. As a rule, there is no cognitive or CNS involvement with the disease. With supportive ventilatory care, the patient can be expected to recover.

Myasthenia Gravis Myasthenia gravis is a rare disease that affects the neuronal junction. (For more details, see Chapter 7.) Due to the breakdown in acetylcholine receptors, nerve impulses are dampened. This disease is characterized by muscle weakness and can be more apparent in muscles proximal to the body than distally.

There is no cure for this disorder, and treatment is aimed at relieving symptoms. If the disease progresses to the diaphragm or intercostal muscles, respiratory compromise can result. Sometimes patients may have an acute exacerbation of the disease brought on by infection or stress. In such cases, intubation or artificial ventilation may be required. These episodes are most commonly preceded by difficulty swallowing or breathing.

Sleep Apnea Sleep apnea is a complex condition not yet fully understood by experts. It is characterized by long pauses in the respiratory cycle that can be caused by a relaxation of the pharynx or lack of respiratory drive. It can result in hypertension, cardiac arrhythmias, and chronic fatigue.

As a general rule, the muscles of the airway become more relaxed as the mind falls deeper and deeper into sleep. This is what leads to snoring and, in some cases, blockage of the airway. With sleep apnea, decreased oxygen levels cause a partial awakening of the patient. Breathing then resumes and the patient returns to sleep, often with no memory of the incident. Repeated over and over, such interruptions destroy normal sleep patterns and the patient spends much of the sleeping period in a hypoxic state.

People with sleep apnea often suffer alterations in their blood pressure and stroke volume. They lose the normal effect of declining blood pressure as they sleep and their pulse oximetry may fall to 80 percent or less. In patients who have ingested alcohol, the reading can fall to 50 percent.

Treatment of sleep apnea may include surgical alteration of the airway, medications, prescribed loss of weight, avoidance of any CNS depressant or alcohol, or use of a CPAP ventilator.

Patients Awaiting Lung Transplants Patients receive lung transplants for a variety of cardiopulmonary diseases. Single-lung transplants are performed for pulmonary fibrosis, COPD, or reversible hypertension or cardiac disease. Double-lung transplants are performed for cystic fibrosis, COPD, or

bronchiectasis. Patients may also receive heart-lung transplants for primary pulmonary hypertension or various congenital diseases. Remember that patients awaiting organ transplants are in the end stages of their diseases and traditional therapies are unlikely to be effective.

Medical Therapy Found in the Home Setting

The treatment of chronic respiratory disorders in the home setting requires a wide range of devices. The following are some of the most common types of medical therapy that you can expect to encounter.

Home Oxygen Therapy   Oxygen therapy has many advantages for the home care patient. First, it is relatively simple to manage. Second, most patients tolerate it easily. Third, oxygen therapy can add much to the quality of a patient's life. Studies have shown that long-term oxygen use raises the life expectancy of COPD patients considerably. It also prevents hypoxic states that may result in permanent cognitive damage or degeneration.

A medical equipment supplier usually delivers, sets up, and educates patients on the home oxygen delivery systems that they will use. In most cases, the systems include:

- A source of oxygen (e.g., concentrator, cylinder, or liquid oxygen reservoir)
- Regulator–flow meter
- Nasal cannula, face mask, tracheostomy collar, oxygen tubing (large bore for face tents or tracheostomy collars)
- Humidifier
- Sterile water for respiratory therapy (Make sure it is sterile!)

Very few problems arise from the systems themselves. When problems do occur, patients or home care providers can usually correct the situation on their own (Table 8–3). However, you may be called on to provide oxygen while a home system is repaired or to transport the patient to the hospital until the system is replaced. You may also be summoned if a condition unexpectedly worsens and the home oxygen system proves insufficient.

When you arrive at the scene, review the physician's prescription for the type of therapy and the source of the oxygen supply. As already noted, the three sources are:

- *Oxygen concentrators.* These systems supply the lowest concentrations of home oxygen. They extract oxygen from room air and add to the flow received by the patient. Home concentrators usually provide no more than 6 liters of oxygen per minute.
- *Oxygen cylinders.* Cylinders or tanks are used by patients who may require more than 6 liters per minute or for some reason cannot have a concentrator. Cylinders involve the same technology as that used on EMS portable oxygen systems.
- *Liquid oxygen.* Patients who require constant oxygen may have a liquid oxygen system. This allows much more oxygen to be stored in the home. Patients will use this system as a reservoir to fill portable tanks that they may take outside the home.

Although these systems are relatively safe, any high-pressure tank or liquid system has the potential for explosion. In a polite manner, ensure that the patient and home care provider adhere to these safety tips:

- Alert the local fire department to the presence of oxygen in the home.
- Keep a fire extinguisher on hand.
- If a fire does start, turn the oxygen off immediately and leave the house.
- Don't smoke—and do not allow others to smoke—near the oxygen system. (No open flames or smoking within 10 feet of oxygen.)
- Do not use electrical equipment near oxygen administration.
- Store the oxygen tank in an approved, upright position.
- Keep oxygen tanks or reservoirs away from direct sunlight or heat.
- Ground all oxygen cylinders.

In terms of the oxygen therapy itself, keep these guidelines in mind:

- Ensure the ability of the patient/home care provider to administer oxygen and to check gauges for supply running low.
- Make sure the patient knows what to do in case of a power failure.

TABLE 8–3 | Common Technical Problems with Oxygen Systems

Problem	Possible Cause	Corrective Action
Oxygen not flowing freely	Faulty tubing	Check for obstruction or replace tubing.
	Dirty or plugged humidifier	Remove from oxygen supply, clean, and refill with sterile water or replace with prefilled bottle.
Buzzer goes off on oxygen concentrator	Unit unplugged	Check plug.
	Power failure	Check fuses, circuit breaker, or, in cases of power outages, use backup oxygen tank until power is restored. (Or call EMS, as necessary.)
Oxygen tank empties too quickly or hisses	Leak in tank	Open all windows, extinguish all flames, and summon help from the fire department, EMS, and/ or supplier.

- Evaluate sterile conditions, especially disinfection of reusable equipment.
- As with any patient with chronic respiratory problems, remain alert to signs and symptoms of hypoxemia.

Artificial Airways/Tracheostomies Patients who have long-term upper airway problems often have a tracheostomy. A **tracheostomy** is a small surgical opening that a surgeon makes from the anterior neck into the trachea. The tracheostomy may be temporary or permanent. The technique is used on any patient who requires artificial ventilation for a long period of time. (Endotracheal or nasal intubation can be used only on a short-term basis. Pressure on the tracheal tissues, from the inflated cuff, can cause necrosis.) Tracheostomies may also be used on patients who have had damage to their larynx, epiglottis, or upper airway structures from surgery or trauma. They may also be performed on patients who have cancer of the larynx or neck.

The tracheostomy consists of the surgical opening (stoma), an outer cannula, and an inner cannula. The outer cannula keeps the stoma open and is held in place by twill tape or Velcro around the neck. The inner cannula is similar to a mini ET tube and slides down into the trachea a few inches. Because of the small size of the airway, the inner cannula usually has a low-pressure cuff at the end to hold it in place and provide a good seal. In the case of infants, there is no inner cannula because of the small size of infant airways. In addition, the airways of infants are more pliable than those of older patients and more susceptible to blockage.

Tracheostomy patients who have had a laryngectomy may have some ability for speech, and some may have an air connection to the oropharynx or nasopharynx. Keep this in mind if you need to ventilate a person with a tracheostomy. It may be necessary to block off the nose and mouth to prevent air from escaping upwardly instead of being pushed into the lungs.

Patients who are unable to speak will use an artificial larynx. This device looks like a small flashlight. It creates an electronic vibration, which the patient manipulates by pressing the device up against the neck and by changing the shape of his mouth (much as you do when you speak). If the patient does not have an artificial larynx, you will need to resort to writing or signing for communication. Remember that an inability to communicate can create a great deal of stress and frustration for the patient. Try to be part of the solution, not part of the problem.

Routine care of the tracheostomy includes:

- Keeping the stoma clean and dry
- Periodically changing the outer cannula
- Changing and cleaning the inner cannula from every few weeks to every few months, depending on the patient
- For ventilator patients, routine changing of the ventilator hose connections
- Frequent suctioning, because of increased secretions

Remember that a tracheostomy eliminates a large part of the normal air-filtering process. The trapping of bacteria in the nasopharynx and oropharynx no longer occurs; neither does the humidification and heating of air by the nasal passages. This means that bacteria have a more direct route to the lungs, and the air received in the lungs is drier and cooler than normal. Therefore, people with a tracheostomy have a higher incidence of lung infections, mucus production, and irritation. Because they have less control over their airway, it is also more difficult for them to clear blocked airways.

If a patient is not currently using a tracheostomy, it may be closed with a Trach-Button. This device simply plugs up the opening until it is needed again.

Common Complications The most common problems faced by tracheostomy patients include blockage of the airway by mucus and a dislodged cannula. The patient can usually clear the obstructing mucus by coughing. (Be careful—the mucus can fly out of the stoma for quite a distance.) Sometimes suctioning, either by the patient or by the caregiver, will suffice. Cannulas can become dislodged by patient movement, or, in the case of children, by their growth. In assessing a child with a cannula problem, find out when it was last changed. Maybe the child is ready for the next size. Children can also have their stoma blocked by foreign objects that enter by accident or are put there by a sibling. Other complications include infection of the stoma, drying of the tracheal mucus leading to crusting or bleeding, and tracheal erosion from an overinflated cuff (causing necrosis).

Management If EMS has been called, it means that neither the patient nor the caregiver has been able to solve the problem. If the tracheostomy patient is on a ventilator, you must rapidly determine if the problem is with the ventilator or with the airway itself. If the problem is simply a loose fitting or disconnected tube, fix it. If the problem is not immediately apparent, do not waste time trying to troubleshoot the machine, unless you are qualified and authorized by local protocols to do so. Your bag-valve device will connect directly to where the ventilator tubing connects. Remove the tubing, connect the bag-valve device to the trach connector, and ventilate (Figure 8-6 ●).

If the problem is with the patient's airway, you will need to clear it. If the patient is hypoxic, always hyperventilate before suctioning. Be sure to evaluate any postural or positional considerations. If the patient is slumped over, straighten him up. Remember to ensure that ventilations are directed downward into the lungs, not upward into the mouth. (Ask the home care provider if there is a connection from the trachea to the upper airway.)

If you are unable to ventilate, clearing the airway is your first priority. Visualize as much of the airway as possible and check for obstructions. If none are visible, introduce a suction catheter and suction while withdrawing—no more than 10 to 15 seconds for an adult, 5 seconds for a child. Again, always hyperventilate before and after suctioning.

If it appears that the inner cannula is blocked or dislodged, you may remove it. If cuffed, you must first deflate the cuff. Connect a 10-mL syringe to the cuff valve and withdraw the air. If a syringe is unavailable, you can cut off the valve and the air will escape. You can then remove the inner cannula, hyperventilate, and continue to suction as needed.

If necessary, you may intubate the stoma. The inner cannula must always be removed first. Use an appropriately sized tube to pass through the outer cannula, and advance so the ET cuff

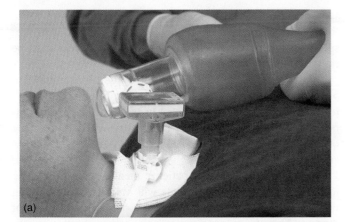

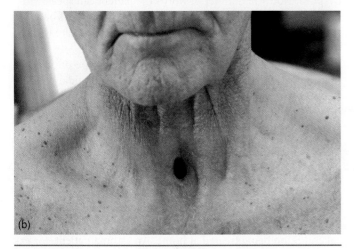

● **Figure 8-6** (a) Artificial ventilation can be accomplished in the patient with a tracheostomy tube by attaching the bag-valve device directly to the tube. (b) Photo shows the site of the stoma.

(if a cuffed tube is used) is 1 to 2 cm inside the trachea. Inflate the cuff and verify placement by auscultating the epigastrium and both lungs. Add an end-tidal CO_2 device to the end of the tube. Pulse oximetry should also be used to monitor patient oxygenation.

Once the airway is secure, you may proceed with the rest of your assessment. It is inappropriate to proceed until you have protected the airway.

Home Ventilation

Although you will see positive-pressure ventilators with most home care patients, you may also encounter negative-pressure ventilators. Both devices are used to ventilate patients for a wide variety of diseases and conditions.

Some of the most common reasons patients may be on a ventilator include:

- Decreased respiratory drive
  - Spinal cord injury
- Ventilatory muscle weakness
  - Muscular dystrophy
  - Poliomyelitis
  - Myasthenia gravis
  - Guillain-Barré syndrome

- Obstructive pulmonary disorders
  - COPD
  - Sleep apnea
  - Cystic fibrosis
  - Bronchopulmonary dysplasia
- Other disorders
  - Pediatric sleep apnea
  - Chest wall deformities

Ventilators provide ventilation in several different ways. They also have a number of operating controls and options, depending on the manufacturer. Volume-cycled ventilation, for example, has long been the standard type of ventilatory support for all forms of severe respiratory failure. All modern ventilators can provide this feature as well as several other modes that vary in ventilatory waveform, method of terminating the machine-aided cycle, and so on.

Positive-Pressure Ventilators According to current practice, positive-pressure ventilation (PPV) is the recommended form of support for acute respiratory disorders. A positive-pressure ventilator pushes air into the lungs, through either a face mask, nasal mask, or tracheostomy. Features of this type of ventilator include variations in tidal volume, respiratory rate, flow rate, and pressure. Optional connectors will be available for oxygen and a humidifier.

There are too many types of positive-pressure ventilators to list here. However, any home care provider should be familiar with a patient's particular machine, including the small ventilators that attach to a mobile patient's wheelchair.

Negative-Pressure Ventilators Ventilators that apply negative pressure to the chest—tank, cuirass, or poncho-wrap—require a rigid structure to support the vacuum compartment. When they expand, they pull on the chest, causing it to expand and allowing air to flow into the lungs. This mimics the normal breathing process.

The iron lung is one of the best known examples of negative-pressure ventilators. However, some home care patients may also be fitted with a poncho-wrap, which is a suit that is sealed at all openings. Patients most commonly use this device at night.

PEEP, CPAP, and BiPAP

These three ventilator options add pressure at various times in the respiratory cycle. They may be used by full-time or part-time ventilator patients. Keep in mind that the danger of pneumothorax exists because of the increased pulmonary pressure. Take this into account during your assessment of PEEP.

PEEP Positive end-expiratory pressure (PEEP) is used to keep alveoli from collapsing. It works by providing a little back pressure at the end of expiration. This option can be used for newborns—usually premature ones—who have insufficient surfactant to keep the alveoli inflated or in adults who have surfactant washout from acute pulmonary edema, **ARDS**, or drowning.

PEEP also has a use in treating COPD. However, because of stiffening and degeneration of the alveoli in emphysema, patients require higher diffusion pressures for gas exchange. If you ever see COPD patients pursing their lips as they exhale, they are providing their own PEEP. By blowing against a slight resistance, they will keep their alveoli open. A COPD patient who is getting worse may deteriorate to the point at which he needs occasional assistance from a ventilator with PEEP.

CPAP Continuous positive airway pressure (CPAP) is used to keep pharyngeal structures from collapsing at the end of a breath. This option is often prescribed for sleep apnea patients who need help in keeping their airways open. Most of these patients will use nasal CPAP, which is a mask that encompasses the nose (Figure 8-7 ●). In these cases, patients must learn to keep their mouths closed for the mask to work correctly. Otherwise, the pressure will be lost. The idea behind mask CPAP or nasal CPAP is the same as PEEP, except that CPAP is provided via a mask, whereas PEEP is provided via an endotracheal tube.

BiPAP Bilevel positive airway pressure (BiPAP) provides two levels of pressure, one on inspiration and one on exhalation. This option is used for patients who require more or higher levels of pressure than CPAP. Although the settings on the patient's home ventilator may be useful to the ED or to follow-up patient care, they are not essential to your assessment. Try to gather this information at the scene, but don't let it delay your management of any serious airway or breathing problems.

As you may already have inferred, a home care patient with a chronic respiratory problem might eventually progress from home oxygen to occasional ventilator support (PEEP, CPAP, BiPAP) to full ventilator dependency. Knowing each stage of the illness and how it relates to the various ventilatory options will give you a more complete understanding of the patient's clinical progress.

General Assessment Considerations Assessment of the respiratory patient should focus on the patient's entire respiratory apparatus. Any deficit found in the system must be rapidly identified and managed.

As you approach the patient, look at the effort required to breathe. Observe for head bobbing, retractions, respiratory rate, tripod posturing, pursed lips, quality and effort of speech, cyanosis, and depth of respiration. Listen for sounds of wheezing or crackles. Note any devices or medications that the patient is currently using.

Immediately assess the patient's mental status by talking to him as you approach. Patients will indicate understanding with their eyes even if they are unable to speak as a result of dyspnea. Note the number of words the patient can speak without stopping for a breath. Rapidly confirm the patient's baseline respiratory effort and mental status from the home care worker, if present.

Next, auscultate the lungs to identify the type of problem that the patient may be having and to determine tidal volume. Look at the patient's chest to spot any irregularities, retractions, or abdominal breathing. You can use pulse oximetry as an adjunct to your assessment, but do not rely on it alone. If the patient has poor peripheral circulation, pulse oximetry may not give an accurate reading.

Finally, complete your assessment by considering the full range of problems that might have caused the patient's current complaint. Whenever assessing a home care patient, you must remain vigilant for complications other than the chronic medical condition being treated at home. An asthma patient, for example, might be having a myocardial infarction (MI).

General Management Considerations As always, your first considerations when intervening in the care of a chronically ill patient center on the ABCs. In the absence of documentation or a valid prehospital DNR, you must maintain a patent airway or improve on the airway that is already in place. This may be as simple as suctioning secretions from an airway device, such as a tracheostomy tube. You should also assess the placement of airway devices that you did not insert. It is easy for a device to become dislodged, obstructing the airway or failing to ensure patency. You may be forced to remove home airway devices and replace them with your own interventions, such as endotracheal tubes.

Ventilatory problems are traditionally easy to fix in the prehospital environment. If a home ventilator fails, you should begin manual PPV immediately. The failure may be easy to remedy, such as in the case of unplugged power cords or a temporary loss of electricity. If you are trained to work with the ventilator, you can adjust the settings to restore or improve ventilations. However, if you are unfamiliar with the ventilator, play it safe and support ventilations with your own equipment.

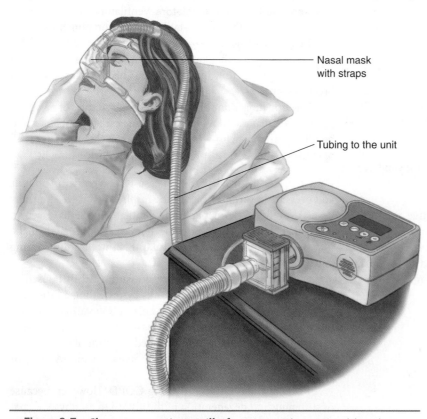

Nasal mask with straps

Tubing to the unit

● **Figure 8-7**   Sleep apnea patients will often use continuous positive airway pressure (CPAP) to keep their airways open.

As with ventilation, oxygenation problems are also generally easy for EMS providers to fix. First, assess the patency of the patient's home oxygen delivery system. The power may be off, the tubing damaged, or the oxygen supply depleted. You can adjust the flow rate of an intact home oxygen delivery system or replace it with your own system.

Whatever interventions you choose, you will have to make arrangements for the devices to be transported with you to the hospital. Flexibility is the key to transporting home care patients. You should reassure patients that you will properly care for their needs, because they will be physically as well as psychologically dependent on their home care systems.

Vascular Access Devices

Vascular access devices (VADs) are used to provide any parenteral treatment on a long-term basis. The type of device and treatment depend on the disease process involved. Patients may have chemotherapy, hemodialysis, peritoneal dialysis, total parenteral nutrition (TPN) feedings, or antibiotic therapy provided through a VAD.

Types of VADs

Approximately 500,000 long-term therapy catheters are inserted each year. Some of the most common VADs that you can expect to find in the home are described in the following sections. Consult your local protocols and procedures for accessing VADs.

Hickman, Broviac, and Groshong Catheters These catheters may have single, double, or triple lumens and can be inserted into any central vein in the trunk of the body. The subclavian vein is the most common anatomic insertion site, because it is usually easy to locate and secure.

Although these catheters have slight differences, each has an external port that looks like a typical intravenous port. The external hub of the catheter is sutured to the skin and has a cuff that promotes fibrous ingrowth. This growth helps anchor the catheter to the body and prevents infection from traveling down the catheter. The highest risk of infection or accidental removal of the catheter is during the first two weeks after insertion. Care of these devices consists of keeping the site clean and dry and the administration of anticoagulant therapy to prevent clot formations.

Peripherally Inserted Central Catheters Peripherally inserted central catheters, or PICC lines, are inserted into a peripheral vein, such as the median cubital vein in the antecubital fossa. These veins are easily accessible and allow a physician to thread a catheter from the insertion site into central venous circulation. PICC lines are inserted under fluoroscopy by radiology rather than in an operating room. As a result, the procedure has a relatively low complication rate (Figure 8-8 ●).

Surgically Implanted Medication Delivery Systems Surgically implanted devices, such as the Port-A-Cath or Medi-Port, are similar to Hickman-style catheters. However, the infusion port is implanted completely below the skin. These devices are disk-shaped and have a diaphragm that requires a specially

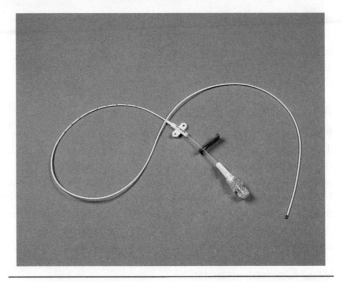

● **Figure 8-8** A peripherally inserted central catheter (PICC). These are usually inserted through an antecubital vein and advanced into the central circulation.

shaped needle, such as the Huber needle, to access. They are typically found in the upper chest and can be felt through the skin.

Never access a surgically implanted port unless local protocols allow you to do so. If such protocols exist, only properly trained personnel with proper equipment should complete the procedure. A regular intravenous catheter or needle will permanently damage an implanted port. Surgically implanted medication delivery devices should only be accessed using sterile technique.

Dialysis Shunts Dialysis shunts are used for patients undergoing hemodialysis to filter their blood. An A-V shunt is a loop connecting an artery and a vein, usually in the distal arm, where the dialysis apparatus draws out and returns blood (Figure 8-9 ●). A fistula connects an artery and a vein, creating an artificially large blood vessel for access. It is also usually found in the upper extremity.

Both shunts and fistulas are created surgically and are very delicate. As a result, you should avoid vascular access and application of blood pressure cuffs in the extremity where they are located. Some jurisdictions allow shunt access by paramedics

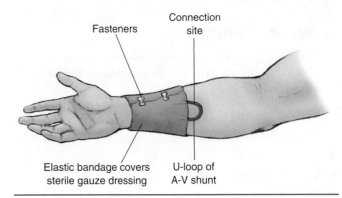

● **Figure 8-9** An A-V shunt is a loop connecting an artery and a vein, usually in the distal arm, where the hemodialysis apparatus draws and returns blood. It is used in home care patients requiring hemodialysis.

during life-threatening emergencies. You will be able to see the shunt in the extremity, and you should be able to auscultate a bruit over the area. Failure to auscultate a bruit over the shunt area may indicate an obstruction, either a thrombus that has formed or an embolus that has lodged there.

Anticoagulant Therapy

Patients with VADs will be on some type of anticoagulant therapy. The most commonly found anticoagulants are those used to flush the device to prevent clot formation. Some patients may be on systemic anticoagulants as well. Because VADs are artificial, the body's natural clotting mechanism must be suppressed to ensure that the devices function properly. As a result, these patients will be much more prone to bleeding disorders. The most common sites for hemorrhage are GI bleeding, strokes, and extremity bruising.

VAD Complications

In treating patients with VADs, keep in mind possible complications. The most common complications result from various types of obstructions. A thrombus may form at the catheter site, or an embolus may lodge there after formation elsewhere in the body. Inactivity increases the risk for clot formation. Other obstructive problems include catheter kinking or catheter tip embolus.

With central venous access devices, you should always be aware of the potential for an air embolus. The devices provide a clear pathway for air to enter central circulation. Signs and symptoms of an air embolus include:

- Headache
- Shortness of breath with clear lungs
- Hypoxia
- Chest pain
- Other indications of myocardial ischemia
- Altered mental status

Of course, any device implanted in the body has a risk of infection or hemorrhage. Look for redness, swelling, tenderness, localized heat, or discharge at a potentially infected catheter site. Because these catheters provide a channel into the central circulation, patients may quickly become septic, especially if they are weakened or immunosuppressed.

Cardiac Conditions

Many chronic care patients receive treatment for a wide variety of cardiac conditions. You may be called to intervene in the following situations:

- Post-MI recovery
- Postcardiac surgery
- Heart transplant
- Congestive heart failure (CHF)
- Hypertension
- Implanted pacemaker
- Atherosclerosis
- Congenital malformation (pediatric)

Home care for the cardiac patient can consist of oxygen, monitoring devices, and regular visits by a home health care provider. You can expect to find a variety of medications associated with the specific cardiac problem: bedside cardiac monitors (for adults and children), diagnostic devices such as a halter monitor, and possibly a defibrillator. For a review of the assessment, treatment, and management of cardiac problems, see Volume 4, Chapter 2.

GI/GU Crisis

Patients with various long-term devices to support gastrointestinal or genitourinary functions may need ALS intervention. Your response may be directly related to a problem with the GI or GU device, or you may simply need to be aware of the device and support during transport.

Urinary Tract Devices

Various medical devices have been designed to support patients with urinary tract dysfunction. External devices, such as Texas catheters (also called condom catheters), attach to the male external genitalia to collect urine (Figure 8-10 ●). Because these devices are not inserted into the urethra, they reduce the risk of infection. However, they do not collect urine in a sterile manner, nor are they adequate for long-term use.

Internal catheters, such as Foley or indwelling catheters, are the most commonly used devices for urinary tract dysfunction. They are long catheters with a balloon tip that is inserted through the urethra into the urinary bladder. The balloon is then inflated with saline to keep the device in place (Figure 8-11 ●). Internal catheters are well tolerated for long-term use and are frequently found in hospitals, skilled nursing facilities, or home care situations.

Suprapubic catheters are similar in purpose to internal catheters. However, they are inserted directly through the abdominal wall into the urinary bladder. Suprapubic catheters may be used instead of indwelling catheters in the event of surgery or other problems with the genitalia or bladder.

Urostomies are a surgical diversion of the urinary tract to a stoma, or hole, in the abdominal wall. A collection device will be attached to the stoma outside the body to collect urine.

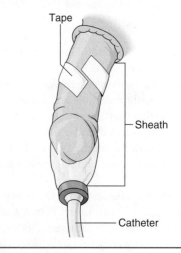

● **Figure 8-10** A condom catheter.

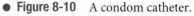

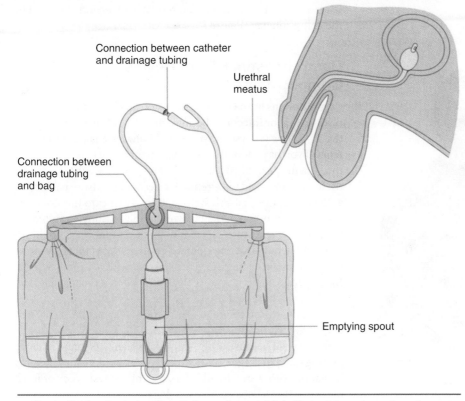

Connection between catheter and drainage tubing

Urethral meatus

Connection between drainage tubing and bag

Emptying spout

● **Figure 8-11** An indwelling Foley catheter with balloon. Note sites where bacteria can enter.

Urostomies are used when the bladder is unable to collect urine effectively.

Urinary Device Complications

Most complications related to urinary tract support devices result from infection or device malfunctions. Infection is a very common problem with urinary tract devices because the area is rich with pathogens and because the catheter provides a pathway directly into the body. Remain alert to foul-smelling urine or altered urine color, such as tea-colored, cloudy, or blood-tinged urine. Also look for signs and symptoms of systemic infection, or urosepsis, because urinary infections can quickly spread in the immunocompromised patient. Suprapubic catheters or urostomies may also have infections at the abdominal wall site. You should note redness, swelling, heat, discharge, or loss of skin integrity.

Device malfunctions typically include accidental displacement of the device, obstruction, balloon ruptures in devices that use a balloon as an anchor, or leaking collection devices. Changes in the patient's anatomy, such as a shortened urinary tract or tissue necrosis, can also cause malfunctions. Ensure that the collection device is empty and record the amount of urine output. Look for kinks or other obstructions in the device, and make sure that the collection bag is placed below the patient.

Gastrointestinal Tract Devices

You can expect to encounter a wide variety of devices to support the gastrointestinal tract. Nasogastric (NG) tubes are commonly seen by EMS personnel because they are often used to decompress gastric contents in the prehospital environment (Figure 8-12 ●). NG tubes may also be used to lavage the GI system in various situations, such as GI bleeding or substance ingestion. NG tubes are not usually long-term devices, because they cause discomfort and may lead to tissue necrosis in the nasal passages if left intact for an extended period.

Feeding tubes are more substantial than NG tubes and come to rest in either the duodenum or jejunum. Often they are weighted to help them pass through the pyloric sphincter and have a steel filament to facilitate insertion. Feeding tubes are used for supplemental nutrition when a person cannot swallow because of dysphagia, paralysis, or unconsciousness.

For longer-term supplemental nutrition, a gastric tube may be inserted through the abdominal wall into the small intestine (Figure 8-13 ●). Indications for a gastrostomy tube include Alzheimer's disease, neurologic deficits from strokes or head trauma, or mental retardation. Gastrostomy tubes come in many forms, such as percutaneous endoscopic gastrostomy tubes, surgical gastrostomy tubes, and jejunal tubes, to name a few. These tubes have different means of insertion (surgical vs. endoscopic), location (stomach vs. duodenum), and function (feeding vs. aspiration prevention).

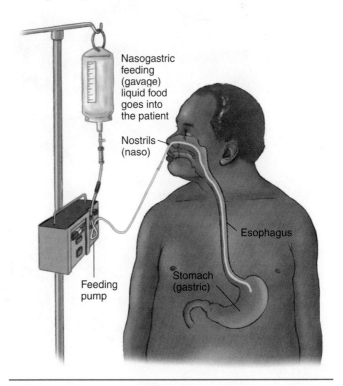

Nasogastric feeding (gavage) liquid food goes into the patient

Nostrils (naso)

Esophagus

Stomach (gastric)

Feeding pump

● **Figure 8-12** A nasogastric feeding tube.

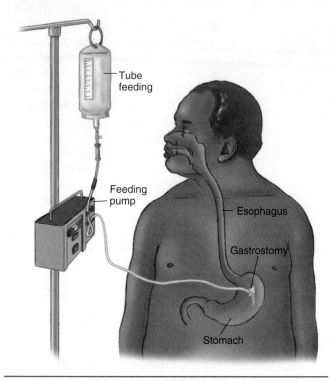

Tube feeding

Feeding pump

Esophagus

Gastrostomy

Stomach

● **Figure 8-13**   A gastrostomy feeding tube.

A **colostomy** is used to bypass part of the large intestine and allow feces to be collected outside the body in a collection bag, either on a temporary or permanent basis. Indications for a colostomy include cancer of the bowel or rectum, diverticulitis, Crohn's disease, or trauma. A surgical connection of the bowel to an ostomy created in the skin results in diversion of feces into the collection bag (Figure 8-14 ●).

Gastrointestinal Tract Device Complications

Complications from GI tract devices include tube misplacement, obstruction, or infection. Because misplaced tubes can obstruct the airway or GI system, you should always ensure device patency if you have doubts about placement of the tube. First, have the patient speak to you. If he cannot speak, the tube may be in the airway and need to be removed. Second, to ensure patency of an NG tube, use a 60-mL syringe to insert air into the stomach. Use your stethoscope to listen over the epigastrium for air movement within the stomach. A low-pitched rumbling should be heard. You may also note stomach contents spontaneously moving up the tube or they may be aspirated with a 60-mL syringe. In such cases, patients may be repositioned to return patency, or the device may be reinserted.

Tubes are also prone to obstructions. Colostomies may become clogged or otherwise obstructed. Feeding tubes can become clogged because of the thick consistency of supplemental feedings or pill fragments. As a result, the tubes may require irrigation with water. In addition, the thick consistency of food may cause bowel obstructions or constipation.

As might be expected, ostomies can become infected (or lose skin integrity from pressure). Look for signs and symptoms of skin or systemic infection. In addition, remember that digestive enzymes may leak from various ostomies and begin to digest the skin and abdominal contents.

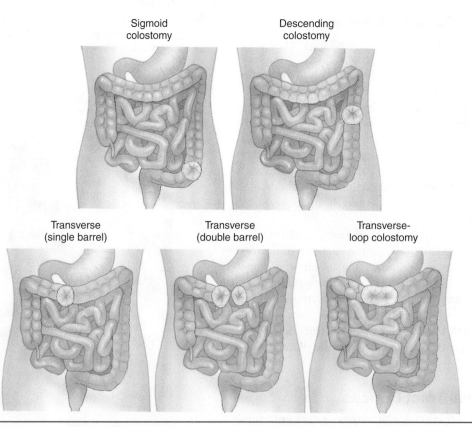

Sigmoid colostomy

Descending colostomy

Transverse (single barrel)

Transverse (double barrel)

Transverse-loop colostomy

● **Figure 8-14**   Examples of colostomy stoma locations.

Psychosocial Implications

Many patients with GI or GU support devices lead active and otherwise normal lives. These patients may be understandably self-conscious about their conditions and many experience embarrassment, avoidance, anger, or discomfort when questioned. You should be sensitive to the patient's emotions during your patient assessment and treatment.

Acute Infections

After physicians or hospital personnel treat open wounds, they typically release patients to home care. These wounds may be surgical wounds or loss of skin integrity for other reasons. In such instances, you may see dressings covering wounds to protect against infection, absorb drainage, or immobilize the wound area. Gauze packing may also be inserted in infected spaces to absorb drainage.

Drains may sometimes be inserted in a wound site to remove blood, serum bile, or pus from the area. Drains are typically soft rubber tubes that have one end in the wound and the other end attached to a bag or suction device. Common drains include the Penrose drain, which is a simple rubber tube, and the Jackson-Pratt drain, which includes a suction bulb.

Wounds are typically closed with sutures, wires, staples, or cyanoacrylate adhesives. The type of closure used depends on the wound and the preferences of the physician closing it. Sutures are the most common device used to secure a wound, but staples and adhesives are becoming more widespread because of their ease of use. Wires are typically used to secure musculoskeletal structures, such as ribs or the sternum after a sternotomy.

In assessing wounds, always be aware of the potential for improper wound healing. As already mentioned, home care patients are at increased risk of infection. The immunologic response and rate of wound healing expected in the general population are compromised in the home care patient by poor peripheral perfusion, a sedentary existence, the presence of percutaneous and implanted medical devices, the existence of chronic diseases, and more.

An infected superficial wound may quickly lead to major infections or sepsis in the immunocompromised or weakened patient. Keep in mind that chronically ill or homebound patients, particularly the elderly, often have a decreased ability to perceive pain or to perform self-care. Pay particular attention to signs of infection in wounds found in home care patients. If you inspect a wound, be sure to use sterile technique and redress the wound.

Maternal and Newborn Care

Today, many women who deliver their babies in a hospital will be discharged in 24 hours or less. This trend, fueled by rising health care costs, greatly shortens the transition time from hospital to home. Some parents, especially first-time parents, may not yet be emotionally prepared to care for a new baby. Rapid discharge may also leave a mother or newborn with an unrecognized problem or complication stemming from delivery. As a result, you, the ALS provider, might be summoned to the home

and called on to use the neonatology and pediatrics skills that you learned in Chapters 3 and 4 of this volume.

Common Maternal Complications

For the mother, postpartum bleeding and embolus (especially after a cesarean section) are the most common complications. Management of an embolus would be the same as with any patient with a similar complaint. Postpartum bleeding can be a serious condition. Management steps include:

- Massage of uterus, if not already contracted
- Administration of fluids to correct hypotension
- Administration of certain medications, such as Pitocin (if ordered)
- Rapid transport to the hospital, if necessary

Mothers may also experience **postpartum depression**. In such cases, women may have difficulty caring for both themselves and their newborns. In extreme cases, babies have been neglected or even harmed.

When entering the home, be sensitive to the needs of the parents. First-time mothers and/or fathers may be inexperienced in child rearing and may call EMS for what a more experienced parent might regard as normal. It is important that you always take any parent's concerns seriously, and if no medical support is needed, provide emotional reassurance. If you suspect neglect or abuse of the newborn, take the actions recommended in Chapters 1, 2, and 4.

Common Infant/Child Complications

As pointed out in Chapter 3, newborns must rapidly adapt to a new environment and may well not have reached a state at which they can thrive on their own. Newborns must be positioned properly to breathe, their noses must be clear (newborns are nose breathers), and they must be kept warm because of immature thermoregulation. Newborns also have immature immune systems and can develop rapid, life-threatening infections or septicemia.

Infants with recognized problems may already be receiving home care. They may have cardiac or respiratory abnormalities or other congenital defects. Premature or low-birth-weight babies, as well as babies with any number of respiratory disorders, are at risk for sleep apnea. Such babies may wear apnea monitors around their chests so that an alarm sounds at any pause in their breathing pattern. Some infants may also be on pulse oximetry. If you are summoned because of an alarm and find a normal breathing pattern, still encourage the parents or caregivers to have the baby examined as soon as possible.

As noted, newborns may also be discharged from the hospital with an undetected cardiac or respiratory condition. Signs and symptoms of cardiac or respiratory insufficiency include:

- Cyanosis
- Bradycardia (<100 beats per minute)
- Crackles
- Respiratory distress

In such cases, resuscitation should be initiated immediately. Management should be toward respiratory support with a bag-valve-mask (BVM) unit or intubation, as necessary. If any newborn has a heart rate <80 beats per minute despite 30 seconds or more of oxygenation, start CPR. Preserve warmth and obtain a record from the parents of feeding intake since birth. If the infant has not been feeding or has been vomiting with diarrhea, the infant may be dehydrated. In this case, a fluid bolus of 20 mL/kg is indicated. If a peripheral IV cannot be obtained in two attempts or 2 minutes, obtain access via the intraosseous route. If blood sugar is below 80 mg/dL administer $D_{10}W$ at a dosage of 0.5 mg/kg.

For a newborn with infection or septicemia, look for fever, tachycardia, and irritability. If septicemia progresses to septic shock, you should initiate resuscitation as previously described.

Children who have serious, long-term health problems are usually cared for by their parents at home, with or without the help of a home care professional. Commonly found medical therapies for children who are home care patients include:

- Mechanical ventilators
- IV medications or nutrition
- Oxygen therapy
- Tracheostomies
- Feeding tubes
- Pulse oximeters
- Apnea monitors

Education of the parents or caregivers by doctors and nurses forms a critical component in their ability to deal with a crisis. Some people adapt well to the task and can deal with their child's chronic problems in a professional manner. Others, however, may become panicked or, either through misunderstanding or denial, have little comprehension of the situation. As with any difficult call, maintain a professional demeanor at all times.

When dealing with children, remember to keep the parents or caregivers informed of your assessment and treatment plans. Children quickly pick up on a person's emotions. As a result, it is part of your job to act in a supportive and controlled manner. Calming a child could make a huge difference in the long-term effects of the current episode.

Hospice and Comfort Care

Today more than 5,000 hospice providers—and hundreds of volunteer agencies—provide support for the terminally ill and their families. Initially philanthropic, these programs are now covered by Medicare. Most states also include them under Medicaid. Most programs are home based, with Medicare and Medicaid stipulating that at least 80 percent of an agency's care be provided to patients in their homes.[3]

Up to 450,000 patients per year receive services from hospices funded by Medicare or Medicaid. (Thousands more receive help from private or volunteer agencies.) Although the majority of Medicare patients are age 70 and older (Table 8–4), children receive benefits, too. Reimbursement is extended to patients with a life expectancy of six months or less.

TABLE 8–4 | Percentage of Hospice Patients by Age

Age	Percent
Less than 45 years	8.1
45–54 years	7.9
55–64 years	14.8
65–69 years	8.7
70–74 years	15.6
75–79 years	14.5
80–84 years	12.3
85 years and older	16.4

Source: *National Center for Health Statistics.*

The goal of hospices is to provide palliative or comfort care, rather than curative care. This is a very different role from that of most other branches of the health care profession, including EMS. For an ALS team, care is usually geared toward aggressive and lifesaving treatment. A hospice team, on the other hand, seeks to relieve symptoms, manage pain, and give patients control over the end of their lives. It is important to remember that these patients have, for the most part, exhausted or declined curative resources.

ALS Intervention

Involvement in a hospice situation can be a difficult and stressful call. In most cases, family members, caregivers, and health care workers have been instructed to call a hospice rather than EMS. However, you may be summoned for intervention, particularly in situations involving transport. You should always keep in mind that the hospice patient is in the end stages of his disease and has already expressed wishes to withhold resuscitation. However, even a valid DNR order should not prevent you from performing palliative and/or comfort care.

Common diseases that you can expect to see in hospice include:

- CHF
- Cystic fibrosis
- COPD
- AIDS
- Alzheimer's disease
- Cancer

In some instances, particularly with cancer, you may also be confronted with patients on high dosages of pain medications. In cases of cancer, for example, morphine is the drug of choice. It is important for you to know that patients using morphine (often taking doses of up to 3,000 mg a day) will have few side effects other than constipation. They will have grown used to the drug and normal side effects will not be seen. Other drugs that may be administered include hydromorphone (Dilaudid), oxycodone (Percocet, Oxycontin), or a fentanyl (Duragesic) patch. Some patients may also have a portable pump that provides a continuous infusion of medication through a PICC line. The pumps can be small and hidden by clothing.

In a hospice, you need to establish communication with the home health care worker as quickly as possible. Your inclination may be to intubate, start a line, or administer medications. However, as noted, palliative care supersedes curative care. A hospice worker, when faced with the end stage of a disease, may do nothing, in accordance with the patient's wishes. Therefore, it is vital that you gain a clear understanding of these wishes, whether through a family member or a written document. If you are called to the house, it is your responsibility to respect the wishes of the patient and the ideals of hospice care.

In a hospice situation, family members might panic at a patient's imminent death and appropriate care might involve support for the family rather than resuscitation of the patient. Local protocols may also vary with respect to DNRs, DNARs, living wills, and durable power of attorney documents. Be sure that you are familiar with these legal statements and their implications for care of the terminally ill. (See Volume 1, Chapter 7.)

Terminally ill patients who are not involved in a hospice present a potentially gray area. Remember that although hospice prepares families for the impending death of their loved ones, families without hospice may be ill prepared for the end stages of life. Don't assume that all terminal patients are under hospice care. A simple question to determine the presence of hospice may alter your course of treatment and approach to the family.

Regardless of whether a patient is in hospice or not, keep in mind the stages of the grief process: denial, anger, depression, bargaining, and acceptance. Remember that both the patient and the family will go through these stages, and, in the case of the terminally ill, the patient may have reached acceptance well ahead of those who remain behind.

CONTENT REVIEW

▶ Stages of Response to Death and Grief

- Denial
- Anger
- Depression
- Bargaining
- Acceptance

SUMMARY

The shift toward home health care is one of the most important trends of the early twenty-first century and will have a great impact on the ALS profession. You can expect in your career to provide acute intervention for a growing number of chronic care patients of all ages and in all stages of the disease process. These calls will challenge you to use all of your assessment skills in developing an effective management plan, which in many cases will be based on input from an extended team of home health care workers.

YOU MAKE THE CALL

Pridemark Paramedic 4 receives a call to assist a patient who has fallen out of a wheelchair. En route to the scene, dispatch informs the crew that the patient is a 32-year-old female with possible head injuries. A home health care worker is with the patient.

On arrival, the crew finds the patient supine on the floor, A/O × 3, with a relatively minor amount of blood caked into her hair over the left temple. The health care worker introduces herself as the nursing assistant who regularly visits the patient. When she arrived for her normal visit about 20 minutes earlier, she knocked on the door and heard the patient call out for help. She then opened the door with a key and found the patient on the floor.

While the EMT assesses the patient, the paramedic interviews the home care worker for a complete history and baseline presentation. During this time, the fire department arrives with three firefighters to assist per local protocol. The Pridemark crew notes that the patient's apartment is messy and dirty.

The home care worker explains that the patient has a left-sided neurologic deficit from a right-sided head injury caused by a motor vehicle crash when the patient was 18 years old. The patient does have sensation on her left side, but movement is limited. Her left arm is normally contracted, and she has a left-sided facial droop. The home care worker shows the paramedic where the patient keeps her medications, but does not know what they are. Examination of the bottles reveals that the patient takes Tegretol, Glucophage, and Zoloft.

Firefighters offer further history because they know the patient from past runs. They explain that the patient smokes heavily, uses marijuana, and can be hostile at times.

Members of the Pridemark crew meet to share what they have learned. The EMT reports that the patient fell out of her wheelchair last night, approximately 14 hours before the crew's arrival. She apparently lost her balance and was not dizzy, weak, or sick. She complains of being cold and demands a cigarette. There is blood on the left side of her temple, but the wound cannot be visualized due to matted hair. The patient denies loss of consciousness and does not want to go to the hospital. Blood pressure is 110/84 mmHg; pulse is 72, normal and regular; and respirations are normal and unlabored. Skin is cool, dry, and normal in color. The patient's eyes are equal and reactive. The abdomen is soft and nontender. No other injuries are noted.

The EMT reports that the patient is lying in a pool of urine. The home care worker states that the patient is normally incontinent. However, she seems quieter than usual.

Although the patient has no neck or back pain, C-spine stabilization is taken. The paramedic talks to the patient and attempts to get her consent for treatment and transport. After explaining that she could have a possible C-spine injury, the patient changes her mind and gives her approval. Although C-spine clearance is allowed in the local protocol, the paramedic feels that, due to the patient's baseline neurologic deficits, more caution is required.

The crew applies a rigid cervical collar. They then log-roll the patient onto a long spine board and secure her in place. En route to the hospital, the crew conducts a secondary assessment with no new findings. On further questioning, the patient vehemently denies a history of diabetes or seizures, despite medications to the contrary. She repeatedly states, "I am normal!" She also denies allergies. A blood glucose test is not done because of the patient's strong emotional response to the procedure.

At the emergency department, the crew gives a full report and transfers care of the patient to the hospital staff. The patient is later released from the hospital with a butterfly bandage for a 1-inch head laceration and returned home by wheelchair van.

1. What does the condition of the apartment tell you?

2. Why is it important to immediately interview the home care worker?

3. What are some of the causes of urinary incontinence?

4. How can you rule out spinal injury to this patient?

5. Why do you think the patient denies a history of diabetes and seizures if she takes Tegretol and Glucophage?

6. Why is it acceptable to defer the glucose test when patient medications indicate a possible blood sugar problem?

7. Was there any need for an IV?

8. Should the patient have been placed on oxygen?

See Suggested Responses at the back of this book.

REVIEW QUESTIONS

1. Diabetes commonly results in poor circulation, especially to the _____.
   a. head
   b. neck
   c. trunk
   d. extremities

2. Infection at the cellular level is called _____ and is often not life threatening.
   a. sepsis
   b. necrosis
   c. cellulitis
   d. gangrene

3. Pressure sores are classified by _____.
   a. the degree of necrosis present
   b. the depth of tissue destruction
   c. the amount of drainage present
   d. the number of blisters around the area

4. Some of the most common home care devices used to treat respiratory disorders include _____.
   a. oxygen equipment
   b. incentive spirometers
   c. various home ventilators
   d. all of the above

5. _____ in children is an ominous sign of impending respiratory failure.
   a. Retraction
   b. Head bobbing
   c. Use of accessory muscles
   d. Abdominal breathing

6. Which genetically inherited disorder causes a defect in the intracellular metabolism of muscle cells and leads to degeneration and atrophy of muscles?
   a. poliomyelitis
   b. myasthenia gravis
   c. muscular dystrophy
   d. Guillain-Barré syndrome

7. According to current practice, _____ is the recommended form of support for acute respiratory disorders.
   a. PPV
   b. BVM
   c. CPAP or BiPAP
   d. PEEP

8. Which option is often prescribed for sleep apnea patients who need help in keeping their airways open?
   a. PPV
   b. CPAP
   c. BiPAP
   d. PEEP

9. The _____ vein is the most common anatomic insertion site for a central catheter—such as a Hickman, Broviac, or Groshong catheter—because it is usually easy to locate and secure.
   a. cephalic
   b. subclavian
   c. saphenous
   d. external jugular

See Answers to Review Questions at the back of this book.

REFERENCES

1. Centers for Disease Control and Prevention. *Home Health Care*. [Available at http://www.cdc.gov/nchs/fastats/homehealthcare.htm]
2. Arendts, G., M. Sim, S. Johnston, and R. Brightwell. "ParaMED Home: A Protocol for a Randomized Controlled Trial of Paramedic Assessment and Referral to Access Medical Care at Home." *BMC Emerg Med* 8 (2011): 7.
3. National Hospice and Palliative Care Organization. *Advancing Care at the End of Life*. [Available at http://www.nhpco.org]

FURTHER READING

Neal, L. J., and S. E. Guillet. *Care of the Adult with a Chronic Illness or Disability: A Team Approach.* St. Louis, MO: Mosby-Year Book, 2004.

Redman, B. K. *Patient Self-Management of Chronic Disease: The Health Care Provider's Challenge.* Sudbury, MA: Jones and Bartlett Publishers, 2003.

Spratt, S. J., et al., eds. *Home Health Care: Principles and Practices.* Delray Beach, FL: GR/St. Lucie Press, 1997.

PRECAUTIONS ON BLOODBORNE PATHOGENS AND INFECTIOUS DISEASES

Prehospital emergency personnel, like all health care workers, are at risk for exposure to blood-borne pathogens and infectious diseases. In emergency situations it is often difficult to take or enforce proper infection control measures. However, as a paramedic, you must recognize your high-risk status. Study the following information on infection control carefully.

Infection control is designed to protect emergency personnel, their families, and their patients from unnecessary exposure to communicable diseases. Laws, regulations, and standards regarding infection control include:

- *Centers for Disease Control and Prevention (CDC) Guidelines.* The CDC has published extensive guidelines on infection control. Proper equipment and techniques that should be used by emergency response personnel to prevent or minimize risk of exposure are defined.
- *The Ryan White Act.* The Ryan White Act of 1990 allows emergency personnel to find out if they were exposed to an infectious disease while rendering patient care. Employers are required to name a "designated officer" to coordinate communications with the treating hospital.
- *Americans with Disabilities Act.* This act prohibits discrimination against individuals with disabilities, including those with contagious diseases. It guarantees equal employment opportunities and job protection if the infected individual can perform essential job functions and does not pose a threat to the safety and health of patients and coworkers.
- *Occupational Safety and Health Administration (OSHA) Regulations.* OSHA has enacted a regulation entitled Occupational Exposure to Bloodborne Pathogens that classifies emergency response personnel as being at the greatest risk of occupational exposure to communicable diseases. This regulation requires employers to provide hepatitis B (HBV) vaccinations free of charge, maintain a written exposure control plan, and provide personal protective equipment. These requirements primarily apply to private employers. Applicability to local and state governmental employees varies by locality. Many states have developed their own OSHA plans.
- *National Fire Protection Association (NFPA) Guidelines.* This is a national organization that has established specific guidelines and requirements regarding infection control for emergency response agencies, particularly fire departments and EMS services.

STANDARD PRECAUTIONS AND PERSONAL PROTECTIVE EQUIPMENT

Emergency response personnel should practice Standard Precautions by which ALL body substances are considered to be potentially infectious. To practice Standard Precautions, all emergency personnel should utilize personal protective equipment (PPE). Appropriate PPE should be available on every emergency vehicle. The minimum recommended PPE includes the following:

- *Gloves.* Disposable gloves should be donned by all emergency response personnel BEFORE initiating any emergency care. When an emergency incident involves more than one patient, you should attempt to change gloves between patients. When gloves have been contaminated, they should be removed as soon as possible. To properly remove contaminated gloves, grasp one glove approximately 1 inch from the wrist. Without touching the inside of the glove, pull the glove halfway off and stop. With that half-gloved hand, pull the glove on the opposite hand completely off. Place the removed glove in the palm of the other glove, with the inside of the removed glove exposed. Pull the second glove completely off with the ungloved hand, only touching the inside of the glove. Always wash hands after gloves are removed, even when the gloves appear intact.
- *Masks and Protective Eyewear.* Masks and protective eyewear should be present on all emergency vehicles and used in accordance with the level of exposure encountered. Masks and protective eyewear should be worn together whenever blood spatter is likely to occur, such as during arterial bleeding, childbirth, endotracheal intubation, invasive procedures, oral

suctioning, and cleanup of equipment that requires heavy scrubbing or brushing. Both you and the patient should wear masks whenever the potential for airborne transmission of disease exists.

- *HEPA and N-95 Respirators.* Due to the resurgence of tuberculosis (TB), prehospital personnel should protect themselves from TB infection through use of an N-95 or a high-efficiency particulate air (HEPA) respirator, as approved by the National Institute of Occupational Safety and Health (NIOSH). It should fit snugly and be capable of filtering out the tuberculosis bacillus. An N-95 or HEPA respirator should be worn when caring for patients with confirmed or suspected TB. This is especially true when performing "high-hazard" procedures such as administration of nebulized medications, endotracheal intubation, or suctioning on such a patient.
- *Gowns.* Gowns protect clothing from blood splashes. If large splashes of blood are expected, such as with childbirth, wear impervious gowns.
- *Resuscitation Equipment.* Disposable resuscitation equipment should be the primary means of artificial ventilation in emergency care. Such items should be used once, then disposed of.

Remember, the proper use of personal protective equipment ensures effective infection control and minimizes risk. Use ALL protective equipment recommended for any particular situation to ensure maximum protection.

Consider ALL body substances potentially infectious and ALWAYS practice Standard Precautions.

The following are suggested responses to the "You Make the Call" scenarios presented in each chapter of Volume 6, Special Patients. Each represents an acceptable response to the scenario but should not be interpreted as the only correct response.

Chapter 1—Gynecology

1. What is your first priority?

Your first priority is to assess the patient, obtain intravenous access, and prepare the patient for transport to the local emergency department by placing her on your stretcher in the position of comfort.

2. What else should you do?

You should try to obtain information regarding who performed the abortion so you can relay the information to the receiving facility. The receiving facility will most likely want to consult with the person who performed the abortion and even have him or her come in to see the patient right away.

3. What do you suspect is the likely cause of her signs and symptoms?

The fever is most likely secondary to an infection that is related to the recent abortion. The foul-smelling discharge, as well, is most likely necrotic tissue left over from the abortion.

In your assessment, you should determine whether the patient's "abortion" was an actual procedure or the result of her ingesting an "abortion pill." With an abortion pill, at some point the patient will be expected to bleed and slough off the results of pregnancy. Most procedure-based abortions will include removing the tissue and fetus. In any event, it is imperative to treat and transport the patient.

4. Because your patient is a minor, do you have any legal requirements to notify her parents or obtain their consent before treating her?

No. In this case, the patient is a minor who is in need of medical attention and treatment. It is implied that the parents would give consent (implied consent) for you to treat and transport the patient.

Chapter 2—Obstetrics

1. What is your first priority?

Your first priority is to apply oxygen and package the patient, being prepared for aggressive airway maneuvers if necessary.

2. What do you suspect is the likely cause of the patient's signs and symptoms?

This patient is clearly suffering from preeclampsia (hypertensive disorders of pregnancy) and could be subject to eclampsia and seizures if not treated quickly.

3. Your patient's husband is very concerned about the well-being of his wife and baby. What should you tell him?

Tell him the truth. Explain what you have found and that it is serious, but it is also a common situation that typically has normal births and outcomes if treated appropriately.

4. How should this patient be transported to the hospital?

She should be placed on the stretcher in a left lateral recumbent position with padding under her abdomen. The lights in the back of the unit should be kept down to a minimum, if not turned off completely. Consider magnesium sulfate administration if indicated. The transport should be made routine, without sirens or anything else that could aggravate or agitate the patient any more than she already is.

Chapter 3—Neonatology

1. Should you stimulate this baby to breathe as soon as it is delivered? Why or why not?

No. When thick meconium is present, and the infant is nonvigorous, consider intubation and suctioning prior to stimulation of the first breath.

2. What is the major danger associated with this type of problem?

Meconium can cause airway obstruction. In addition, the infant could inhale the meconium, potentially setting up an infection that could be life threatening.

3. Once you have stabilized this infant, where should he be transported?

This infant should be transported to a facility with a NICU.

Chapter 4—Pediatrics

1. What are your assessment priorities for this patient?

Initial assessment priorities are to determine the patient's level of consciousness, apply pressure to the bleeding scalp wound, and stabilize the cervical spine before doing a more thorough assessment.

2. What interventions would you perform on scene and en route to the receiving hospital?

On-scene interventions would be kept to a minimum, only handling the bleeding scalp wound, spinal precautions, and any other significant findings; otherwise, the majority of the treatment would be performed en route to the hospital.

3. Describe possible transport considerations, including a potential refusal of transport by the angry parents.

Clearly, in this case the patient should be transported for further evaluation and to give the proper authorities time to assess the situation for possible abuse. There is a possibility that the parents will refuse treatment and transport for the patient. In this case, the only option you will have is to contact the proper authorities and notify them of what you have found, making sure to thoroughly document your objective findings.

4. What are the important factors in reporting this incident and documenting the call?

It is very important that you do not accuse or confront the parents while on scene. Make sure you pay attention to the surroundings and scene. Document only the things you see, hear, touch, or smell. Do not document any feelings or assumptions.

Chapter 5—Geriatrics

1. What general impression do you have of this patient?

Your first impression should be of a possible stroke. It would be prudent, if possible, to determine when the symptoms began in order to determine whether the patient is within an interventional treatment window.

2. Do you suspect that this is an acute or chronic problem? Explain.

This is probably an acute problem because the patient's wife says that he normally takes care of her. Additionally, the house is in immaculate condition. Even if they have a housekeeper or housecleaner, there would be a few things out of place if he was normally like this, considering that the wife is very arthritic and can barely ambulate around the home.

3. Aside from the patient's presentation and response to your interventions, what other information should be included in your hospital report?

It would be important to record the inability of Mrs. Jones to navigate the home, the location of the patient, and, most important, to record the last known time the patient was "normal."

4. What support do you provide for Mrs. Jones?

If there is no one immediately available to come help take care of Mrs. Jones, you should allow her to ride with you to the hospital, where she would be able to receive assistance. Additionally, check with your local resources to see if an elder assistance program may exist that you or the hospital could contact to help. It would not be out of line to ask her whether she has someone she would like for you to contact, such as family members or a religious group.

Chapter 6—Abuse, Neglect, and Assault

1. What do you suspect is taking place?

This situation is highly indicative of child abuse.

2. What physical evidence do you have to support this suspicion?

Bruises on the child's arms and back in various stages of healing.

3. *What emotional evidence do you have to support this suspicion?*

The fact that the boy has a flat affect and does not look toward his parents.

4. *What other clues lead you to believe that abuse might be taking place?*

Additional clues that may not individually be representative of abuse but can be confirming evidence would include law officers being on scene for "domestic disturbance," and the fact that the boy is dressed only in underwear in the winter.

5. *What are your priorities in this case?*

In this case, the priorities are the child's welfare and making sure that he is not suffering from any medical emergency. Carefully document your findings in the patient care report.

Chapter 7—The Challenged Patient

1. *Why did the patient's doctor tell her that she has an increased risk of infection from communicable diseases?*

The medical treatments she is receiving (e.g., chemotherapy)—including the recent mastectomy, which includes a removal of lymph nodes responsible for helping with infections—all put her at high risk for obtaining an infection.

2. *What signs indicate that this patient has cancer?*

You would notice that she has a recent mastectomy and is wearing a scarf around her head with a wig at her bedside, indicating that she most likely has lost her hair from the cancer treatment.

3. *Is it necessary for all three of you to wear a mask? Explain.*

It is safer for the patient if all three of you wear masks. This will provide additional filtration for the patient and protection from communicable disease. Once in the ambulance, the patient compartment can be secluded by closing doors separating it from the cab and turning on the ventilation system. Once this has been accomplished, it would then be acceptable for the driver to remove his or her mask.

4. *Will you start a peripheral IV on this patient? Explain.*

Most likely, this patient will not require a peripheral IV. If she does, it would be important to avoid the side from which she has had her mastectomy. Mastectomies involve the removal of lymph nodes, which, in turn, makes the patient very susceptible to lymphedema secondary to any trauma or pressure on the arm.

5. *What information will you include in your patient report so the emergency department is prepared for this patient?*

You should include information about the additional respiratory precautions that you are taking.

Chapter 8—Acute Interventions for the Chronic Care Patient

1. *What does the condition of the apartment tell you?*

A messy, dirty apartment may indicate that the patient is on her own and has little support from family or friends. It may also show that she is receiving inadequate home care. These social factors may help you understand the patient's state of mind and interact with greater compassion.

2. *Why is it important to immediately interview the home care worker?*

The home care worker usually knows the patient well and can tell you exactly what is different, if anything, about the patient. If you don't fully understand the patient's baseline mental status and disability, you cannot adequately assess and compare your own findings.

3. *What are some of the causes of urinary incontinence?*

Causes include seizures, spinal injury, abdominal trauma, and overdose, among others.

4. *How can you rule out spinal injury to this patient?*

You can't. The possibility of spinal injury in a patient with a preexisting neurologic deficit cannot be ruled out without knowing the exact nature of his or her baseline deficit. That decision is best left to the patient's own physician or the ED staff.

5. *Why do you think the patient denies a history of diabetes and seizures if she takes Tegretol and Glucophage?*

Imagine how you would feel if confined to a wheelchair at age 18 for the rest of your life. Such patients can become unhappy, lonely, resentful, and bitter. They may also deny certain aspects of their disability in an attempt to feel better or to gain acceptance. In this case, because the patient exhibited no complicating factors related to diabetes or seizures, the crew decided not to argue with her. However, they had a responsibility to report all medications—and suspicions—as a part of their transfer of care.

6. *Why is it acceptable to defer the glucose test when patient medications indicate a possible blood sugar problem?*

The patient seems to be sensitive to her condition. Because she shows no signs of hypoglycemia, it is probably better to keep the patient calm than to argue with her about the test. If the crew had any doubts about their actions, they should, of course, consult with medical direction.

7. *Was there any need for an IV?*

No. The patient was showing no signs of shock, nor did she need to have any medications given.

8. *Should the patient have been placed on oxygen?*

Oxygen would not have hurt the patient in any way, but there was no indication for its use. The patient exhibited no shortness of breath, was in no distress, and had good skin color. (She was getting enough oxygen from room air.)

ANSWERS TO REVIEW QUESTIONS

Below are the answers to the Review Questions presented in each chapter of Volume 6.

**CHAPTER 1—
GYNECOLOGY**
1. b
2. c
3. c
4. b
5. c
6. c
7. c
8. d

**CHAPTER 2—
OBSTETRICS**
1. b
2. d
3. b
4. c
5. d
6. c
7. a
8. a
9. c
10. d

**CHAPTER 3—
NEONATOLOGY**
1. a
2. b

3. c
4. d
5. d
6. d
7. b
8. b
9. c
10. d

**CHAPTER 4—
PEDIATRICS**
1. b
2. c
3. b
4. b
5. b
6. b
7. a
8. b
9. a
10. d
11. d
12. d
13. b
14. c
15. c
16. c
17. c

18. d
19. b
20. c

**CHAPTER 5—
GERIATRICS**
1. a
2. a
3. b
4. b
5. d
6. d
7. b
8. c
9. b
10. b

**CHAPTER 6—
ABUSE, NEGLECT,
AND ASSAULT**
1. c
2. b
3. b
4. c
5. a
6. b
7. d
8. d

**CHAPTER 7—THE
CHALLENGED
PATIENT**
1. c
2. b
3. d
4. b
5. d
6. a
7. d
8. d

**CHAPTER 8—
ACUTE
INTERVENTIONS
FOR THE
CHRONIC CARE
PATIENT**
1. d
2. c
3. b
4. d
5. b
6. c
7. a
8. b
9. b

GLOSSARY

abortion   termination of pregnancy before the 20th week of gestation. The term refers to both miscarriage and induced abortion. Commonly, abortion is used for elective termination of pregnancy and miscarriage for the loss of a fetus by natural means. A miscarriage is sometimes called a "spontaneous abortion."

acrocyanosis   cyanosis of the extremities.

acute respiratory distress syndrome (ARDS)   respiratory insufficiency marked by progressive hypoxemia, due to severe inflammatory damage.

advance directive   legal document prepared when a person is alive, competent, and able to make informed decisions about health care. The document provides guidelines on treatment if the person is no longer capable of making decisions.

afterbirth   the placenta and accompanying membranes that are expelled from the uterus after the birth of a child.

ageism   discrimination against aged or elderly people.

Alzheimer's disease   a progressive, degenerative disease that attacks the brain and results in impaired memory, thinking, and behavior. It affects 4 million American adults.

amniotic fluid   clear, watery fluid that surrounds and protects the developing fetus.

amniotic sac   the membranes that surround and protect the developing fetus throughout the period of intrauterine development.

aneurysm   abnormal dilation of a blood vessel, usually an artery, due to a congenital defect or a weakness in the wall of the vessel.

ankylosing spondylitis   a form of inflammatory arthritis that primarily affects the spine.

anorexia nervosa   eating disorder marked by excessive fasting.

anoxic hypoxemia   an oxygen deficiency due to disordered pulmonary mechanisms of oxygenation.

antepartum   before the onset of labor.

aortic dissection   a degeneration of the wall of the aorta.

APGAR score   a numerical system of rating the condition of a newborn. It evaluates the newborn's heart rate, respiratory rate, muscle tone, reflex irritability, and color.

aphasia   absence or impairment of the ability to communicate through speaking, writing, or signing as a result of brain dysfunction; occurs when the individual suffers a brain injury due to stroke or head injury and no longer has the ability to speak or read. In *sensory aphasia*, the patient cannot understand the spoken word. In *motor aphasia*, the patient can understand what is said but cannot speak. A patient with *global aphasia* has both sensory and motor aphasia.

ARDS   acute respiratory distress syndrome.

assisted living   housing for the elderly or disabled that provides nursing care, housekeeping, and prepared meals as needed.

asthma   a condition marked by recurrent attacks of dyspnea with wheezing due to spasmodic constriction of the bronchi, often as a response to allergens or to mucus plugs in the arterial walls.

autonomic dysfunction   an abnormality of the involuntary aspect of the nervous system.

bacterial tracheitis   bacterial infection of the airway, subglottic region; in children, most likely to appear after episodes of croup.

bend fractures   fractures characterized by angulation and deformity in the bone without an obvious break.

bias-motivated crime   a hate crime based on bias.

BiPAP   bilevel positive airway pressure.

birth injury   avoidable and unavoidable mechanical and anoxic trauma incurred by the newborn during labor and delivery.

brain ischemia   injury to brain tissues caused by an inadequate supply of oxygen and nutrients.

bronchiectasis   chronic dilation of a bronchus or bronchi, with a secondary infection typically involving the lower portion of the lung.

bronchiolitis   viral infection of the medium-sized airways, occurring most frequently during the first year of life.

buckle fractures   fractures characterized by a raised or bulging projection at the fracture site.

cardiogenic shock   the inability of the heart to meet the metabolic needs of the body, resulting in inadequate tissue perfusion.

cataracts   medical condition in which the lens of the eye loses its clearness.

cellulitis   inflammation of cellular or connective tissue.

central IV line   intravenous line placed into the superior vena cava for the administration of long-term fluid therapy.

chain of evidence   legally retaining items of evidence and accounting for their whereabouts at all times to prevent loss or tampering.

child abuse   physical or emotional violence or neglect toward a person from infancy to 18 years of age.

choanal atresia   congenital closure of the passage between the nose and pharynx by a bony or membranous structure.

cleft lip   congenital vertical fissure in the upper lip.

cleft palate   congenital fissure in the roof of the mouth, forming a passageway between oral and nasal cavities.

colostomy   a surgical diversion of the large intestine through an opening in the skin where the fecal matter is collected in a pouch; may be temporary or permanent.

comorbidity   having more than one disease at a time.

conductive deafness   deafness caused when there is a blocking of the transmission of the sound waves through the external ear canal to the middle or inner ear.

congenital   present at birth.

congregate care   living arrangement in which the elderly live in, but do not own, individual apartments or rooms and receive select services.

cor pulmonale   congestive heart failure secondary to pulmonary hypertension.

CPAP   continuous positive airway pressure.

croup laryngotracheobronchitis; a common viral infection of young children, resulting in edema of the subglottic tissues; characterized by barking cough and inspiratory stridor.

crowning the bulging of the fetal head past the opening of the vagina during a contraction; it is an indication of impending delivery.

cystitis infection of the urinary bladder.

deafness the inability to hear.

DeLee suction trap a suction device that contains a suction trap connected to a suction catheter. The negative pressure that powers it can come either from the mouth of the operator or, preferably, from an external vacuum source.

delirium an acute alteration in mental functioning that is often reversible.

dementia a deterioration of mental status that is usually associated with structural neurologic disease. It is often progressive and irreversible.

demyelination destruction or removal of the myelin sheath of nerve tissue; found in Guillain-Barré syndrome.

diabetic ketoacidosis complication of diabetes due to decreased insulin secretion or intake; characterized by high levels of blood glucose, metabolic acidosis, and, in advanced stages, coma; often referred to as diabetic coma.

diabetic retinopathy slow loss of vision as a result of damage done by diabetes.

diaphragmatic hernia protrusion of abdominal contents into the thoracic cavity through an opening in the diaphragm.

distributive shock marked decrease in peripheral vascular resistance with resultant hypotension; examples include septic shock, neurogenic shock, and anaphylactic shock.

domestic elder abuse physical or emotional violence or neglect when an elder is being cared for in a home-based setting.

ductus arteriosus channel between the main pulmonary artery and the aorta of the fetus.

dysmenorrhea painful menstruation.

dyspareunia painful sexual intercourse.

dysphagia inability to swallow or difficulty swallowing.

dysphoria an exaggerated feeling of depression or unrest, characterized by a mood of general dissatisfaction, restlessness, discomfort, and unhappiness.

dysuria painful urination often associated with cystitis.

ectopic pregnancy the implantation of a developing fetus outside the uterus, often in a fallopian tube.

effacement the thinning and shortening of the cervix during labor.

elderly a person age 65 or older.

Emergency Medical Services for Children (EMSC) federally funded program aimed at improving the health of pediatric patients who suffer from life-threatening illnesses and injuries.

emesis vomitus.

endometriosis condition in which endometrial tissue grows outside the uterus.

endometritis infection of the endometrium.

endometrium the inner layer of the uterine wall where the fertilized egg implants.

enucleation removal of the eyeball after trauma or illness.

epiglottitis bacterial infection of the epiglottis, usually occurring in children older than age four; a serious medical emergency.

epistaxis nosebleed.

estimated date of confinement (EDC) the approximate day the infant will be born. This date is usually set at 40 weeks after the date of the mother's last menstrual period (LMP).

exocrine disorder involving external secretions.

extrauterine outside the uterus.

febrile seizures seizures that occur as a result of a sudden increase in body temperature; occur most commonly between the ages of six months and six years.

fibrosis the formation of fiber-like connective tissue, also called scar tissue, in an organ.

foreign body airway obstruction (FBAO) blockage or obstruction of the airway by an object that impairs respiration; in the case of pediatric patients, tongues, abundant secretions, and deciduous (baby) teeth are likely to block airways.

functional impairment decreased ability to meet daily needs on an independent basis.

gangrene death of tissue or bone, usually from an insufficient blood supply.

geriatric abuse a syndrome in which an elderly person is physically or psychologically injured by another person.

geriatrics the study and treatment of diseases of the aged.

gerontology scientific study of the effects of aging and of age-related diseases on humans.

glaucoma group of eye diseases that results in increased intraocular pressure on the optic nerve; if left untreated, it can lead to blindness.

glomerulonephritis a form of nephritis, or inflammation of the kidneys; primarily involves the glomeruli, one of the capillary networks that are part of the renal corpuscles in the nephrons.

glottic function opening and closing of the glottic space.

greenstick fractures fractures characterized by an incomplete break in the bone.

growth plate the area just below the head of a long bone in which growth in bone length occurs; the epiphyseal plate.

Guillain-Barré syndrome acute viral infection that triggers the production of autoantibodies, which damage the myelin sheath covering the peripheral nerves; causes rapid, progressive loss of motor function, ranging from muscle weakness to full-body paralysis.

gynecology the branch of medicine that deals with the health maintenance and the diseases of women, primarily of the reproductive organs.

hate crime a crime of hatred or prejudice in which the perpetrator targets a particular victim or victims because of the victim's perceived membership in a certain social group.

heatstroke life-threatening condition caused by a disturbance in temperature regulation; in the elderly, characterized by extreme fever and, in extreme cases, delirium or coma.

hemoptysis expectoration of blood arising from the oral cavity, larynx, trachea, bronchi, or lungs; characterized by sudden coughing with production of salty sputum with frothy bright-red blood.

hepatomegaly   enlarged liver.

herniation   protrusion or projection of an organ or part of an organ through the wall of the cavity that normally contains it.

herpes zoster   an acute eruption caused by a reactivation of latent varicella virus (chickenpox) in the dorsal root ganglia; also known as shingles.

hiatal hernia   protrusion of the stomach upward into the mediastinal cavity through the esophageal hiatus of the diaphragm.

hospice   program of palliative care and support services that addresses the physical, social, economic, and spiritual needs of terminally ill patients and their families.

hyperbilirubinemia   an excessive amount of bilirubin—the orange-colored pigment associated with bile—in the blood. In newborns, the condition appears as jaundice. Precipitating factors include maternal Rh or ABO incompatibility, neonatal sepsis, anoxia, hypoglycemia, and congenital liver or gastrointestinal defects.

hyperglycemia   abnormally high concentration of glucose in the blood.

hypertrophy   an increase in the size or bulk of an organ or structure; caused by growth rather than by a tumor.

hypochondriasis   an abnormal concern with one's health, with the false belief of suffering from some disease, despite medical assurances to the contrary; commonly known as hypochondria.

hypoglycemia   abnormally low concentration of glucose in the blood.

hypovolemic shock   decreased amount of intravascular fluid in the body; often due to trauma that causes blood loss into a body cavity or frank external hemorrhage; in children, can be the result of vomiting and diarrhea.

immune senescence   diminished vigor of the immune response to the challenge and rechallenge by pathogens.

incontinence   inability to retain urine or feces because of loss of sphincter control or cerebral or spinal lesions.

institutional elder abuse   physical or emotional violence or neglect when an elder is being cared for by a person paid to provide care.

intermittent mandatory ventilation (IMV)   respirator setting in which a patient-triggered breath does not result in assistance by the machine.

intracerebral hemorrhage   bleeding directly into the brain.

intractable   resistant to cure, relief, or control.

intrapartum   occurring during childbirth.

isolette   also known as an incubator; a clear plastic enclosed bassinet used to keep prematurely born infants warm. The temperature of an isolette can be adjusted regardless of the room temperature. Some isolettes also provide humidity control.

kyphosis   exaggeration of the normal posterior curvature of the spine.

labor   the time and processes that occur during childbirth; the physiologic and mechanical process in which the baby, placenta, and amniotic sac are expelled through the birth canal.

labyrinthitis   inner ear infection that causes vertigo, nausea, and an unsteady gait.

life-care community   communities that provide apartments/homes for independent living and a range of services, including nursing care. Usually the elderly own their own homes.

lochia   vaginal discharge following birth that contains blood, mucus, and placental tissue.

maceration   process of softening a solid by soaking it in a liquid.

Marfan syndrome   hereditary condition of connective tissue, bones, muscles, ligaments, and skeletal structures characterized by irregular and unsteady gait, tall lean body type with long extremities, flat feet, and stooped shoulders. The aorta is usually dilated and may become weakened enough to allow an aneurysm to develop.

meconium   dark green material found in the intestine of the full-term newborn. It can be expelled from the intestine into the amniotic fluid during periods of fetal distress.

melena   a dark, tarry stool caused by the presence of "digested" free blood.

menarche   the onset of menses, usually occurring between ages 10 and 14.

Ménière's disease   a disease of the inner ear characterized by vertigo, nerve deafness, and a roar or buzzing in the ear.

meningomyelocele   herniation of the spinal cord and membranes through a defect in the spinal column.

menopause   the cessation of menses and ovarian function due to decreased secretion of estrogen.

menorrhagia   excessive menstrual flow.

menstruation   sloughing of the uterine lining (endometrium) if a fertilized egg is not implanted. It is controlled by the cyclical release of hormones. Menstruation is also called a period.

mesenteric ischemia or infarct   death of tissue in the peritoneal fold (mesentery) that encircles the small intestine; a life-threatening condition.

miscarriage   commonly used term to describe a pregnancy that ends before 20 weeks' gestation; may also be called spontaneous abortion.

mittelschmerz   abdominal pain associated with ovulation.

mucoviscidosis   cystic fibrosis, so called because of the abnormally viscous mucoid secretions associated with the disease.

myasthenia gravis   disease characterized by episodic muscle weakness triggered by an autoimmune attack of the acetylcholine receptors.

myometrium   the thick middle layer of the uterine wall made up of smooth muscle fibers.

nasogastric tube/orogastric tube   a tube that runs through the nose or mouth and esophagus into the stomach; used for administering liquid nutrients or medications or for removing air or liquids from the stomach.

neonatal abstinence syndrome (NAS)   a generalized disorder presenting a clinical picture of central nervous system (CNS) hyperirritability, gastrointestinal dysfunction, respiratory distress, and vague autonomic symptoms. It may be due to intrauterine exposure to heroin, methadone, or other less potent opiates. Nonopiate CNS depressants may also cause NAS.

neonate   an infant from the time of birth to one month of age.

nephrons   the functional units of the kidneys.

neutropenia   a condition that results from an abnormally low neutrophil count in the blood (less than 2,000/mm^3).

newborn   a baby in the first few hours of its life; also called a newly born infant.

nocturia   excessive urination during the night.

noncardiogenic shock   types of shock that result from causes other than inadequate cardiac output.

obstetrics   the branch of medicine that deals with the care of women throughout pregnancy.

old-old   an elderly person age 80 or older.

omphalocele   congenital hernia of the umbilicus.

osteoarthritis   a degenerative joint disease, characterized by a loss of articular cartilage and hypertrophy of bone.

osteoporosis   softening of bone tissue due to the loss of essential minerals, principally calcium.

otitis media   middle ear infection.

ovulation   the release of an egg from the ovary.

Parkinson's disease   chronic, degenerative nervous disease characterized by tremors, muscular weakness and rigidity, and a loss of postural reflexes.

partner abuse   physical or emotional violence from a man or woman toward a domestic partner.

PEEP   positive end-expiratory pressure.

pelvic inflammatory disease (PID)   an acute infection of the reproductive organs that can be caused by a bacterium, virus, or fungus.

perimetrium   the serosal peritoneal membrane which forms the outermost layer of the uterine wall.

persistent fetal circulation   condition in which blood continues to bypass the fetal respiratory system, resulting in ongoing hypoxia.

personal-care home   living arrangement that includes room, board, and some supervision.

phototherapy   exposure to sunlight or artificial light for therapeutic purposes. In newborns, light is used to treat hyperbilirubinemia or jaundice.

Pierre Robin syndrome   unusually small jaw, combined with a cleft palate, downward displacement of the tongue, and an absent gag reflex.

pill-rolling motion   an involuntary tremor, usually in one hand or sometimes in both, in which fingers move as if they were rolling a pill back and forth.

placenta   the organ that serves as a lifeline for the developing fetus. The placenta is attached to the wall of the uterus and the umbilical cord.

polycythemia   an excess of red blood cells. In a newborn, the condition may reflect hypovolemia or prolonged intrauterine hypoxia.

polypharmacy   multiple drug therapy in which there is a concurrent use of a number of drugs.

postpartum depression   the "let down" feeling experienced during the period following birth, occurring in 70 to 80 percent of mothers.

premenstrual dysphoric disorder   condition in which a woman has severe depression symptoms, irritability, and tension before menstruation.

premenstrual syndrome (PMS)   a variety of signs and symptoms, such as weight gain, irritability, or specific food cravings, associated with the changing hormonal levels that precede menstruation.

presbycusis   progressive hearing loss that occurs with aging.

pressure ulcer   ischemic damage and subsequent necrosis affecting the skin, subcutaneous tissue, and often the muscle; result of intense pressure over a short time or low pressure over a long time; also known as pressure sore or bedsore.

pruritus   itching; often occurs as a symptom of some systemic change or illness.

puerperium   the time period surrounding the birth of the fetus.

rape   penile penetration of the genitalia or rectum without the consent of the victim.

retinopathy   any disorder of the retina.

senile dementia   general term used to describe an abnormal decline in mental functioning seen in the elderly; also called "organic brain syndrome" or "multi-infarct dementia."

sensorineural deafness   deafness caused by the inability of nerve impulses to reach the auditory center of the brain because of nerve damage either to the inner ear or to the brain.

sensorium   sensory apparatus of the body as a whole; also the portion of the brain that functions as a center of sensations.

sexual assault   unwanted oral, genital, rectal, or manual sexual contact.

shunt   surgical connection that runs from the brain to the abdomen for the purpose of draining excess cerebrospinal fluid, thus preventing increased intracranial pressure.

Shy-Drager syndrome   chronic orthostatic hypotension caused by a primary autonomic nervous system deficiency.

sick sinus syndrome   a group of disorders characterized by dysfunction of the sinoatrial node in the heart.

silent myocardial infarction   a myocardial infarction that occurs without exhibiting obvious signs and symptoms.

spondylosis   a degeneration of the vertebral body.

status epilepticus   prolonged seizure or multiple seizures with no regaining of consciousness between them.

Stokes-Adams syndrome   a series of symptoms resulting from heart block, most commonly syncope. The symptoms result from decreased blood flow to the brain caused by the sudden decrease in cardiac output.

stoma   a permanent surgical opening in the neck through which the patient breathes.

stroke   injury to or death of brain tissue resulting from interruption of cerebral blood flow and oxygenation.

subarachnoid hemorrhage   bleeding that occurs between the arachnoid and dura mater of the brain.

substance abuse   misuse of chemically active agents such as alcohol, psychoactive chemicals, and therapeutic agents; typically results in clinically significant impairment or distress.

sudden infant death syndrome (SIDS)   illness of unknown etiology that occurs during the first year of life, with the peak at ages two to four months.

thyrotoxicosis   toxic condition characterized by tachycardia, nervous symptoms, and rapid metabolism due to hyperactivity of the thyroid gland.

tinnitus   ringing or tingling sound in the ear.

tocolysis   the process of stopping labor.

tracheostomy   small surgical opening that a surgeon makes from the anterior neck into the trachea, held open by a metal or plastic tube.

transient ischemic attack (TIA)   reversible interruption of blood flow to the brain; often seen as a precursor to a stroke.

turgor   ability of the skin to return to normal appearance after being subjected to pressure.

two-pillow orthopnea   the number of pillows—in this case, two—needed to ease the difficulty of breathing while lying down; a significant factor in assessing the level of respiratory distress.

umbilical cord   structure containing two arteries and one vein that connects the placenta and the fetus.

urosepsis   septicemia originating from the urinary tract.

urostomy   surgical diversion of the urinary tract to a stoma, or hole, in the abdominal wall.

vagal stimulation   stimulation of the vagus nerve causing a parasympathetic response.

Valsalva maneuver   forced exhalation against a closed glottis, such as with coughing. This maneuver stimulates the parasympathetic nervous system via the vagus nerve, which in turn slows the heart rate.

varicosities   an abnormal dilation of a vein or group of veins.

vertigo   the sensation of faintness or dizziness; may cause a loss of balance.

INDEX

Hydrocortisone (Hydrocortone), side effects in elderly, 174
Hydromorphone (Dilaudid)
    for hospice patients, 235
    side effects in elderly, 174
Hymen, 4
Hyperbilirubinemia, 55
Hyperglycemia, 119, 120
Hyperoxia, 89
Hypertension
    elderly, 161–162
    management, 31
    obstetric patient, 24, 25, 30–31
Hyperthermia (heatstroke), 171
Hyperthyroidism, 166
Hypochondriasis, 175
Hypoglycemia, 32, 66, 118–119
Hypoperfusion. *See* Shock
Hypoplastic left heart syndrome, 52
Hypotension, pediatric patient, 88
Hypothermia
    elderly, 170–171, 177
    newborn, 65–66
Hypothyroidism, 166
Hypovolemia, newborn, 64–65
Hypovolemic shock, 101, 113

Imipramine (Tofranil), 173
Immobilization
    C-spine, 103, 104, 105
    child, 123
    elderly, 178
Immune senescence, 157
Immune system, age-related changes, 154, 157
Impairments, patients living with. *See* Challenged patients
Incomplete abortion, 28
Incontinence, 147–148
Indwelling catheters, 230
Inevitable abortion, 28
Infants. *See also* Neonates; Newborn
    anatomic and physiologic characteristics, 77, 78
    bronchopulmonary dysplasia (BPD), 223–224
    deafness, 197
    of diabetic mothers, 25
    growth and development, 74–75
    with special needs, 129–132
    sudden infant death syndrome, 127
Infarct, 167
Infections
    children, 106
    home care patient, 216
    newborn, 233
Inferior vena cava, uterus compression of, 26
Infusions, preparation, 103
Injury prevention, pediatrics, 72–73
Institutional elder abuse, 186
Integumentary system, age-related changes, 154, 156
Intermittent mandatory ventilation (IMV), 224
Internal genitalia, 4–6
Intracerebral hemorrage, 163
Intracranial pressure, signs of increased, 125
Intraosseous infusion, for child, 99, 101

Intrapartum, 49
Intrauterine device (IUD), 9
Introitus, 4
Ipratropium, 223
Irreversible shock, 113
Ischemia, 163, 167
Ischemic colitis, 167
Ischemic phase of menstrual cycle, 6
Isocarboxazie (Marplan), 173
Isolette, 61
Itching, 167

Jaw-thrust method, 83
JumpSTART system for pediatric triage, 132–133
Juvenile rheumatoid arthritis (JRA), 203

Kendrick extrication device (KED), 103
Ketamine, 191
Kidneys. *See* Renal system
King LT-D, 99
Kyphosis, 156

Labetalol, 171
Labia, 4
Labor, 33–34
    active, 25
    false, 32
    maternal complications, 43–44
    patient management, 35
    preterm, 32–33
    stopping, 33
Labyrinthitis, 197
Language disorders, 199
Lanoxin, side effects in elderly, 172–173
Laryngeal mask airway (LMA), 99
Laryngoscope, placement of, 97
Laryngotracheobronchitis, 107–108
Larynx
    artificial, 226
    cancer, 199
    pediatric patient, 79
Lasix (furosemide), 197
Legal issues
    abuse and assault, 191
    child *vs.* adult, 81
    for gynecologic physical exam, 10
    home care patient, 191
Leiomyomas, 12
Librium (chlordiazepoxide), 173
Life support skills, advanced, in pediatrics, 73
Ligamentum arteriosum, 49
Ligamentum teres, 49
Ligamentum venosum, 49
Limb presentation, 41
Liquid Ecstasy, 191
Liquid X, 191
Lisinopril, 172
Lithium carbonate, 173
Liver
    age-related changes, 156
    pediatric patient, 79, 126
Living environments, 140–142
Living will, 221, 235
Local government, hospital and clinic funding, 142

Lochia, 34
Loneliness, elderly, 140–141
Lorazepam (Ativan), 173
Los Angeles Prehospital Stroke Screen, 163
Lower airway distress, children, 110–112
Lung cancer, 160
Lung transplants, patients awaiting, 224–225
Lungs. *See also* Respiratory system
    pediatric patient, 79
    tracheostomy and infection, 226
Luteinizing hormone (LH), 6, 19

M, 191
Magnesium sulfate
    for inhibiting uterine contractions, 33
    for pediatric advanced life support, 102
    for seizures, 31
Male victims, of sexual assault, 13
Mallory-Weiss tear, 166
Marfan syndrome, 161
Marplan (isocarboxazie), 173
Maternal drug abuse, 189
Maternal narcotic use, and newborn distress, 60
Maternal-fetal circulation, 23
McRobert's maneuver, 42, 43
MD (muscular dystrophy), 206
MDMA (3,4-Methylenedioxymethamphet-amine), 191
Mechanism of injury (MOI), 80
Meconium, presence at birth, 42–43, 54, 55–56, 62
Medi-Port, 229
Mediastinum, of pediatric patient, 79
Medicaid, 142–143, 234
Medicare, 142, 234
Medications
    antiseizure, 163
    date rape, 190–191
    for elderly, 146
    for home care patient, 218
    for pediatric resuscitation, 101–102
    and skin disorder, 167
    toxicity in elderly, 156
Melena, 167
Mellaril (thioridazine), 173
Menarche, 6
Ménière's disease, elderly, 150
Meningitis, 65, 117
Meningomyelocele, 53
Menopause, 8
Menorrhagia, 12
Menstrual cramps, 6
Menstrual cycle, 6–8, 19
Menstrual period (menses), 5, 8
Menstruation, 6–7
Mental status, 202, 220
Meperidine (Demerol), side effects in elderly, 174
Mesenteric ischemia, 167
Metabolic system
    disorders in elderly, 165–166
    pediatric patient, 80, 118–119
Metaproterenol, 222
Methylprednisolone, 223
Metoprolol, 171
Midazolam (Versed), 98